1986

My

Cardiovascular Problems in Pediatric Critical Care

CLINICS IN CRITICAL CARE MEDICINE

Series Editors: *Dr. Ake Grenvik*
Dr. Iain McA. Ledingham

Volumes Already Published

Chapman: Acute Renal Failure
Grenvik & Safar: Brain Failure and Resuscitation
Gregory: Respiratory Failure in the Child
Spence: Respiratory Monitoring in Intensive Care
Geelhoed & Chernow: Endocrine Aspects of Acute Illness
Meakins: Surgical Infections
Sprung & Grenvik: Invasive Procedures in Critical Care
Cousins & Phillips: Acute Pain Management
Williams: Liver Failure

Forthcoming Volumes in the Series

Imrie & Moosa: Gastrointestinal Emergencies
Farber: Infection Control in Intensive Care
Shires: Fluids and Electrolytes
Guthrie: Neonatal Intensive Care
Kaye & Bircher: Cardiopulmonary Resuscitation

Cardiovascular Problems in Pediatric Critical Care

EDITED BY

David B. Swedlow, M.D.

Assistant Professor of Anesthesia and Pediatrics
The University of Pennsylvania School of Medicine
Senior Anesthesiologist
Department of Anesthesia and Critical Care
The Children's Hospital of Philadelphia
Philadelphia, Pennsylvania

Russell C. Raphaely, M.D.

Associate Professor of Anesthesia and Pediatrics
The University of Pennsylvania School of Medicine
Senior Anesthesiologist and Director
Pediatric Intensive Care Complex
Department of Anesthesia and Critical Care
The Children's Hospital of Philadelphia
Philadelphia, Pennsylvania

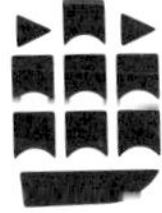

CHURCHILL LIVINGSTONE
NEW YORK, EDINBURGH, LONDON, MELBOURNE 1986

Library of Congress Cataloging in Publication Data

Cardiovascular problems in pediatric critical care.

(Clinics in critical care medicine ; 10)
Includes bibliographies and index.
1. Cardiovascular system—Diseases—Treatment.
2. Pediatric intensive care. I. Swedlow, David B.
II. Raphaely, Russell C. III. Series. [DNLM:
1. Cardiovascular System—physiology. 2. Critical Care
—in infancy & childhood. 3. Heart Diseases—in
infancy & childhood. 4. Heart Diseases—therapy.
W1 CL831AI v.10 / WS 290 C2675]
RJ421.C27 1986 618.92′1 86-17146
ISBN 0-443-08321-5

Distributed in the United Kingdom by Churchill Livingstone, Robert Stevenson House, 1–3 Baxter's Place, Leith Walk, Edinburgh EH1 3AF, and by associated companies, branches, and representatives throughout the world.

Accurate indications, adverse reactions, and dosage schedules for drugs are provided in this book, but it is possible that they may change. The reader is urged to review the package information data of the manufacturers of the medications mentioned.

Acquisitions Editor: *Kim Loretucci*
Copy Editor: *Leslie Burgess*
Production Designer: *Michiko Davis*
Production Supervisor: *Jane Grochowski*

Printed in the United States of America

First published in 1986

Preface

This monograph was written with the belief that a solid understanding of the principles behind cardiovascular physiology, pharmacology and monitoring technology is necessary to deliver optimal care to the child with existing or impending failure of the circulation. The contributors to this monograph were chosen for their ability to present the material with that focus.

The first chapter describes in detail the current knowledge of normal cardiovascular physiology, with special attention to cardiac muscle physiology and pharmacology.

Next, a description of noninvasive evaluation of the failing circulation takes the reader through the normal physical examination of the pediatric heart with special attention to the interpretation of abnormal findings suggesting congestive heart failure. As this is not a monograph on congenital heart disease per se, description and interpretation of murmurs is kept to a minimum. The author then reviews interpretation of technology for the noninvasive assessment of the circulation, including such techniques as M-mode and 2-D echocardiography. Wherever possible, noninvasive methodologies are compared to available "gold standards."

The third chapter deals with invasive assessment of the failing circulation. The technologies of pressure monitoring, cardiac output measurements, and oxygen transport are covered in detail, along with a discussion of pitfalls in interpretation of the invasive monitoring and a discussion of risks and contraindications.

Chapter 4 covers an important area that should be of great interest to those who care for critically ill infants and children—anesthetic considerations for the child undergoing surgery for congenital heart disease. The child suffering from congenital heart disease is often scheduled for surgery, either elective or urgent, without a complete understanding of the preanesthetic issues or the intraoperative considerations facing the anesthesiologist. This chapter describes in detail the issues surrounding the anesthetic care of the child.

Chapters 5 through 8 deal with the manipulation of the four determinants of cardiac output, namely, preload augmentation, afterload reduction, contractility augmentation, and correction of heart rate and rhythm abnormalities. The authors review their respective subjects and describe the means available to the clinician to manipulate and improve these parameters.

The last chapter describes the current knowledge in the field of pediatric CPR, and offers recommendations based on that knowledge combined with clinical experience.

Our objective in this monograph is to present current information in a format that is both useful and convenient. We hope that you will find this volume a useful and often-referenced addition to your library.

David B. Swedlow, M.D.
Russell C. Raphaely, M.D.

Contributors

Nick G. Anas, M.D.

Assistant Professor of Pediatrics, University of California, Irvine, California College of Medicine, Irvine; Associate Director, Pediatric Intensive Care, Children's Hospital of Orange County, Orange, California

Richard A. Browning, M.D.

Clinical Assistant Professor of Anesthesia, Division of Surgery, Brown University Program in Medicine; Staff Anesthesiologist, Department of Anesthesia, Rhode Island Hospital, Providence, Rhode Island

David E. Cohen, M.D.

Assistant Professor of Anesthesia, The University of Pennsylvania School of Medicine; Assistant Anesthesiologist, Department of Anesthesia and Critical Care, The Children's Hospital of Philadelphia, Philadelphia, Pennsylvania

Robert G. Kettrick, M.D.

Associate Professor of Anesthesiology, The University of Pennsylvania School of Medicine; Senior Anesthesiologist, Department of Anesthesia and Critical Care, The Children's Hospital of Philadelphia, Philadelphia, Pennsylvania

Stephen Ludwig, M.D.

Associate Professor of Pediatrics, The University of Pennsylvania School of Medicine; Director, Emergency Medicine, The Children's Hospital of Philadelphia, Philadelphia, Pennsylvania

Roger A. Moore, M.D.

Assistant Professor of Anesthesiology, The University of Pennsylvania School of Medicine, Philadelphia, Pennsylvania; Co-Chairman, Department of Anesthesiology, Director of Pediatric Anesthesiology, Deborah Heart and Lung Center, Browns Mills, New Jersey

Ronald M. Perkin, M.D.

Assistant Professor of Pediatrics, University of California, Irvine, California College of Medicine, Irvine; Director, Pediatric Intensive Care, Children's Hospital of Orange County, Orange, California

William H. Perloff, M.D., Ph.D.

Associate Professor of Pediatrics and Anesthesiology, Director of Pediatric Critical Care Medicine, University of Wisconsin Medical School; Director, Pediatric Critical Care Unit, University of Wisconsin Hospital and Clinics, Madison, Wisconsin

Russell C. Raphaely, M.D.

Associate Professor of Anesthesia and Pediatrics, The University of Pennsylvania School of Medicine; Senior Anesthesiologist and Director, Pediatric Intensive Care Complex, Department of Anesthesia and Critical Care, The Children's Hospital of Philadelphia, Philadelphia, Pennsylvania

Mark C. Rogers, M.D.

Professor and Chairman, Department of Anesthesiology and Critical Care Medicine; Professor of Pediatrics and Director of Pediatric Intensive Care Unit, The Johns Hopkins Medical Institutions, Baltimore, Maryland

Richard A. Schieber, M.D.

Associate Professor of Pediatrics and Anesthesiology, Director, Pediatric Critical Care Medicine, Emory University School of Medicine; Medical Director, Pediatric Intensive Care Unit, Henrietta Egleston Hospital for Children, Atlanta, Georgia

Mark S. Schreiner, M.D.

Assistant Professor of Anesthesiology, The University of Pennsylvania School of Medicine; Assistant Anesthesiologist, Department of Anesthesia and Critical Care, The Children's Hospital of Philadelphia, Philadelphia, Pennsylvania

David J. Steward, M.B., F.R.C.P. (C)

Professor, University of British Columbia Faculty of Medicine; Chief, Department of Anesthesia, Children's Hospital, Vancouver, British Columbia

Judith L. Stiff, M.D.

Associate Professor, Department of Anesthesiology and Critical Care Medicine, Chief, Anesthesia Services, The Johns Hopkins Medical Institutions at the Francis Scott Key Medical Center, Baltimore, Maryland

David B. Swedlow, M.D.

Assistant Professor of Anesthesia and Pediatrics, The University of Pennsylvania School of Medicine; Senior Anesthesiologist, Department of Anesthesia and Critical Care, The Children's Hospital of Philadelphia, Philadelphia, Pennsylvania

Randall C. Wetzel, M.D.

Assistant Professor, Department of Anesthesiology and Critical Care Medicine; Chief, Pediatric Anesthesia, The Johns Hopkins Medical Institutions, Baltimore, Maryland

Contents

Cardiovascular Problems in Pediatric Critical Care

1
Physiology of the Heart and Circulation

William H. Perloff

Since William Harvey's observation that the heart pumped blood in a continuous circuit, the function of the cardiovascular system has been the subject of intensive study. Many landmark developments leading to the present advanced, but still incomplete understanding of the circulation have been reviewed by Leake[225] and Neil.[292] This chapter summarizes selected aspects of normal cardiovascular physiology which are likely to have diagnostic or therapeutic implications in the intensive care unit. As the available range of therapeutic modalities has broadened, an appreciation of the physiologic basis for their application has become increasingly important. The pediatric population with cardiovascular dysfunction comprises a heterogeneous group, from both developmental and etiologic perspectives. Consequently, emphasis has also been given to postnatal developmental aspects of circulatory function, where possible.

The broad scope of this subject insures that its treatment is incomplete. Among the important omissions is consideration of electrophysiology and its development, which are discussed in Chapter 8. Where appropriate, economy of space has been effected by reference to reviews of specific areas.

POSTNATAL PHYSICAL DEVELOPMENT OF THE HEART

Anatomic Development

Determination and development of the cardiac anatomy during fetal life are described elsewhere.[429] The only normal anatomic change in the heart following birth is the eventual permanent closure of the foramen ovale. At autopsy, approximately 50 percent of five-year-olds and 25 percent of adults possess a probe-patent foramen ovale (PFO).[361] This has little clinical significance in normal individuals. However, in circumstances where pulmonary artery hypertension induces elevated right atrial pressure, right-to-left interatrial shunting of blood may result in hypoxemia.[186,282] Such shunting can be induced by the Valsalva maneuver in healthy subjects with a PFO.[246]

Morphologic Development

General description

The mature myocardium consists of a complex interwoven meshwork of elongate myocytes connected end-to-end by "intercalated discs."[381] These collections of cells are grouped into fibers forming a three-dimensional continuum in a nested

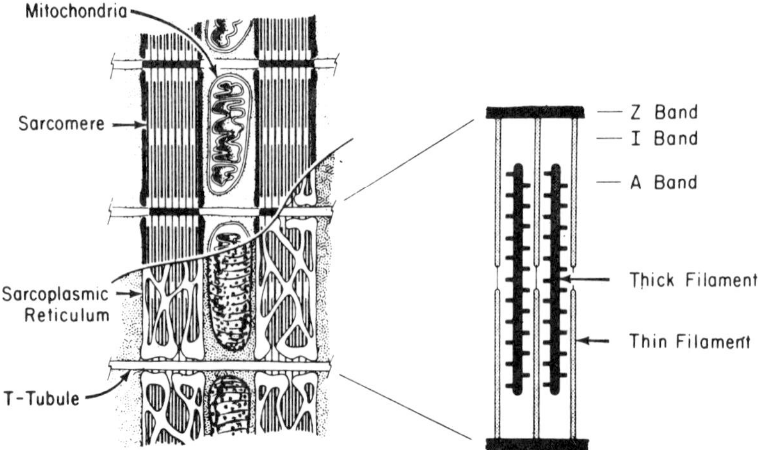

Fig. 1.1. Anatomy of the cardiac muscle cell. (Morkin E, LaRaia, PJ 1974 Biochemical studies on the regulation of myocardial contractility. New England Journal of Medicine 290: 445.

figure-eight pattern involving both ventricles.[403] Thus the septum consists of fibers from both ventricles, a thin right ventricular (RV) segment and a much thicker left ventricular (LV) segment.[110,17] Most LV myocardial fibers are circumferentially oriented, consistent with the direction of the forces to be resisted. This promotes uniformity of changes in fiber length across the thickness of the wall.[444] The papillary muscles are invaginations of the continuous fiber chains[403] with a relatively linear organization of fibers.[44]

Capillaries parallel the myocytes with nearly a 1 : 1 ratio.[41,444] A collagen network in the extracellular space interlaces to bind the myocytes into bundles, maintaining their alignment relative to each other and their capillaries.[84]

The myocyte itself, shown schematically in Figure 1.1, contains myofibrils which are linear organelles consisting of the basic contractile elements, the sarcomeres, arranged in series. As shown in the right panel of the figure, the sarcomere consists of interdigitating structures which on electron microscopy appear to be thick and thin filaments.[381] The thick filaments are constructed of myosin molecules tail-to-tail, arranged so that their globular heads project out of the filament.[454] The thin filaments are composed of actin as well as troponin and tropomyosin. Contraction is caused by interaction of the projecting myosin heads and actin, leading to sliding of the thin and thick filaments relative to each other.[280] Some important biochemical features of this process are discussed in the section *Contractility*.

Fetal morphologic development is reviewed elsewhere.[249] Postnatal development is due largely to the response of the cardiac tissues to changing hemodynamic demands occasioned by birth and body growth.[14,116,146,313,461] Most significant is the increased work required of the left ventricle and the decrease in that of the right ventricle at birth. The disparity increases during the early neonatal period as pulmonary vascular resistance diminishes, as described in the section *Components of the pulmonary circulation*. The nature of the response is modified by the time-limited capacity for myocyte replication.[14,64,65,461]

Development at the cellular level

The newborn myocyte is smaller, more rounded, and more primitive in appearance than its mature counterpart. Mitoses occur frequently along with active synthesis of intracellular components.[14,65,229,372,392] Development during early infancy in the rat, dog, and sheep differs between the right and left ventricles. After birth a rapid proliferation of LV myocytes occurs, doubling in number in the first 11 days of life in the rat.[14] Additional hyperplasia of the LV can be stimulated by experimentally increased pressure loading in the neonatal period.[86,460]

Myocyte replication ceases in early infancy in other mammalian species,[14,229,461] and is complete by 3 to 6 months of age in humans.[460] Nutrition studies suggest that a genetically programmed number of mitoses does not exist; rather the process is a response to hemodynamic and other stimuli.[461] The biochemical basis for this is not known, but the abrupt increase in tissue PO_2 at birth has been suggested.[129] Whatever the reason, essential enzymes for cell replication, including deoxyribonucleic acid (DNA) polymerase, disappear from the myocyte in infancy.[64,65] Once lost, the capacity for mitosis has never been shown to return.[461]

Early postnatal left ventricular growth then consists of combined cell proliferation and growth. Subsequent ventricular development is associated only with increased myocyte size and maturation,[313] though hyperplasia of supporting elements continues.[229,230] Myocyte growth involves both greater number and length of myofibrils which lead to increased width and length of the cell. In the rat, myocyte volume nearly triples in the first 11 days of life with the length/width ratio approximately doubling to the adult value of five.[14] The major proportion

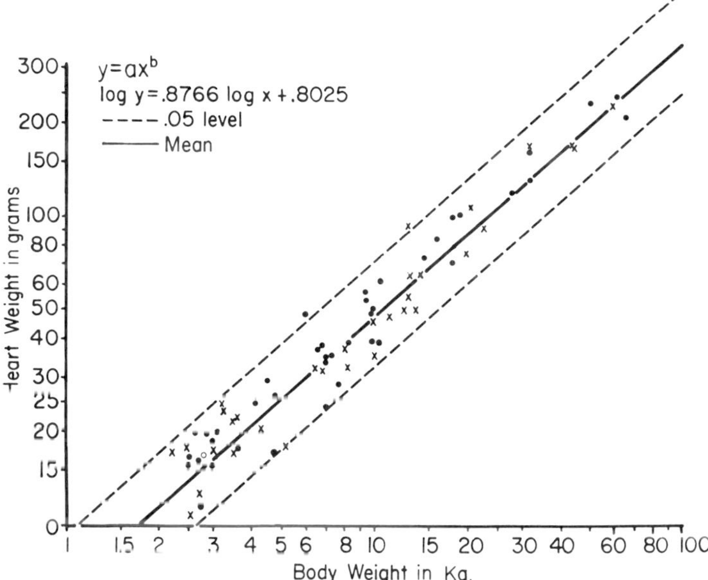

Fig. 1.2. Relationship between heart weight and body weight. Autopsy specimens for children from newborn to 15 years old. Key: ●, males; ○, females; ×, unknown. (Rowlatt UF, Rimoldi HJA, Lev M 1963 The quantitative anatomy of the normal child's heart. Pediatric Clinics of North America 10, 499.)

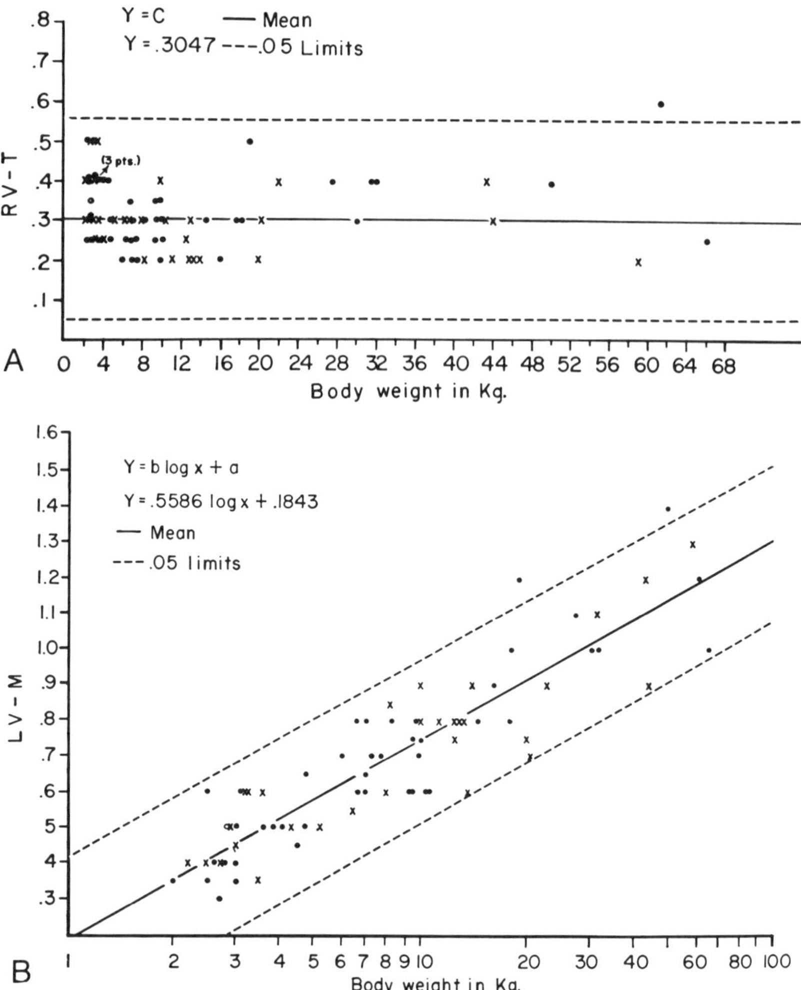

Fig. 1.3. Effect of growth on the thickness of normal cardiac ventricles. Autopsy specimens for children from newborn to 15 years old. (A) Right ventricular thickness, in centimeters, near the tricuspid valve. (B) Maximum thickness of left ventricle, in centimeters. Key: ●, males, ○, females, ×, unknown. (Rowlatt UF, Rimoldi HJA, Lev M 1963 The quantitative anatomy of the normal child's heart. Pediatric Clinics of North America 10: 499.)

of the twentyfold increase in heart weight from birth to adulthood is due to growth of a constant number of myocytes.[146]

The biochemical mediator for this physiologic hypertrophy is undefined,[146,370] but norepinephrine has been suggested.[222] This is discussed further in the section *Afterload*.

Right ventricular myocytes are the same or larger in diameter at birth than those of the LV, but grow more slowly throughout early development.[14,229,230] Cell proliferation is minimal,[14] even in response to congenital pressure loading such as in tetralogy of Fallot.[416]

The proportion of the cross-sectional area of cardiac tissue occupied by myocytes

Table 1.1. Selected Cardiovascular Data for Normal Infants and Children

	Infants ≤1–2 yr	Children ≥2 yr
Cardiac index (L/min/M^2)	4.53 ± 0.94 (all ages)	
Right heart:		
RVEDV (ml/M^2)	39.8 ± 8	70 ± 13
RVEF	0.66 ± 0.07	0.64 ± 0.09
Left heart:		
LVEDV (ml/M^2)	42 ± 10	73 ± 11
LVEF	0.68 ± 0.05	0.63 ± 0.05
LA_{max} (ml/M^2)	26 ± 5	38 ± 8

Abbreviations: RVEDV and LVEDV, right and left ventricular end-diastolic volumes, respectively; RVEF and LVEF, right and left ventricular ejection fraction, respectively; LA_{max}, maximum left atrial size.

Data shown are ± one standard deviation.

Data from Graham and Jamarkani[139] and Graham et al.[140] Similar but not identical results have been presented by others (see text).

is remarkably constant in both ventricles throughout development at 80 percent, despite the major changes in myocyte size and contents.[229]

Cardiac growth

Developmental changes in mass and thickness of the human myocardium have been studied in recent years at autopsy,[21,78,95,202,341,396] by angiography[106,138,140,203,257,269,422] and by echocardiography.[97,159,165,296,297,331,395,394] Despite different techniques and variability in the way the septum is attributed to the two ventricles, the concusions are relatively consistent.

Total heart weight is shown as a function of body weight in Figure 1.2 for infants and children with presumably normal hearts. The ratio of heart to body weight varies from about 0.05 at birth to 0.04 in adolescence. Males' hearts tend to be slightly heavier than females' at the same body weight.

The profound difference in growth of the two ventricles during infancy and childhood is illustrated in Figure 1.3. Figure 1.3A shows the RV thickness at the tricuspid valve is essentially unchanged at 0.3 cm for children from birth to 15 years old. During the same time period the maximum LV posterior wall thickness more than doubles to approximately 1.1 cm. The LV growth is most rapid early, with the increase in thickness exceeding 50 percent the first 6 months.[97,297,341] Chamber weights reflect the overall cardiac growth. The RV/LV weight ratio diminishes from approximately 1.0 to 1.2 at birth to the adult value of 0.5 to 0.6 by 2 months of age.[95,341]

Ventricular cavity volumes have been historically difficult to determine due to the complex shape changes during the cardiac cycle.[106,322,355] The use of biplane[140,141,142] and radionuclide angiography[66] have improved the accuracy of such estimates. Interpretation of the significance of ventricular volumes requires an appreciation of the myocardial contractile state and its history. This is illustrated by the differences in end-diastolic volume between infants and children shown in Table 1.1 and discussed further in the section *Preload*. Of note is the fact that LV shape, as reflected by the ratio of LV posterior wall thickness to end-diastolic diameter, is unchanged from birth to adult life. By echocardiography, this ratio is constant at about 0.18.[97,159,296,395] The significance of this fact to myocardial mechanics is considered in the section *Afterload.*

CARDIAC PHYSIOLOGY

The Heart as a Pump

The pumping action of the heart delivers oxygen, nutrients, and other essential materials via the blood to the tissues, including the heart itself, and removes CO_2 and wastes produced there. This occurs via a complex system which normally satisfies the metabolic needs of tissues throughout the body, despite wide variations in these local requirements. Major elements of this part of the circulatory system are depicted in Figure 1.4. The figure indicates that the outcome of the heart's contractile activity is blood flow, the cardiac output (CO), which is distributed to the tissues. This output is the product of the volume of blood pumped each beat, the stroke volume (SV), and the frequency of contraction, the heart rate (HR). These are discussed in the following sections. Features of the peripheral circulation are considered in the section *Integrated systemic circulatory function.*

Factors Affecting Stroke Volume

Introductory concepts

The SV results from the integration of the active shortening of ventricular myocardial fibers, the LV ejecting into the systemic circulation, the RV into the pulmonary circuit. The magnitude of the fiber shortening and consequent stroke

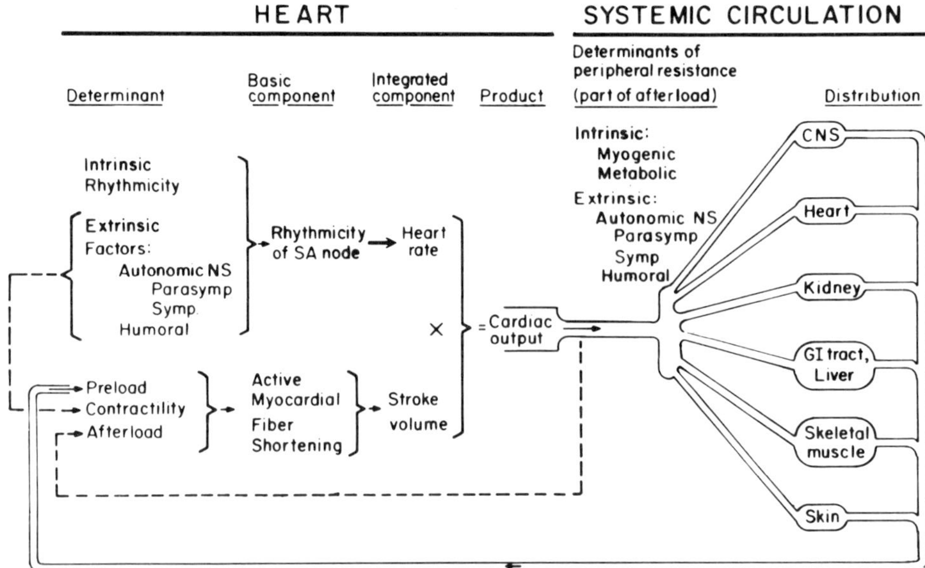

Fig. 1.4. Simplified diagram of the major components of the normal postnatal systemic circulation. The neural control loop is not shown. A full discussion is given in the text. (Adapted from Braunwald, E 1974 Regulation of the circulation. New England Journal of Medicine 290: 1124.)

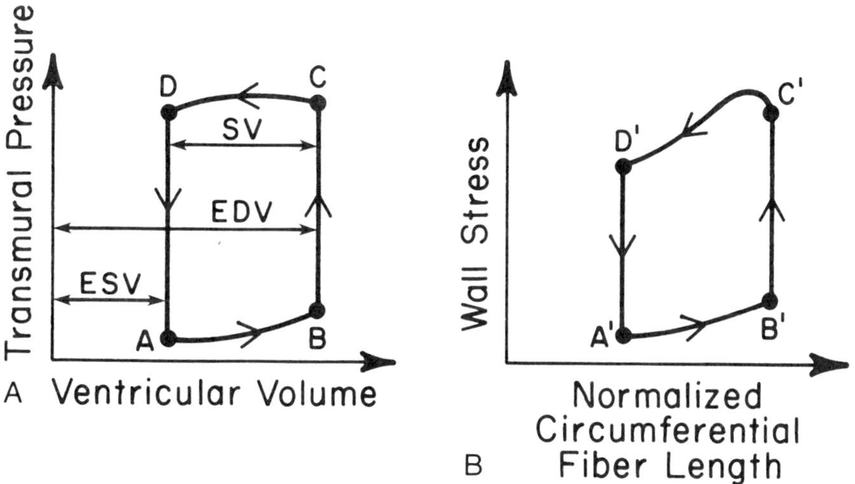

Fig. 1.5. Representations of the cardiac cycle. (A) Ventricular pressure-volume diagram for the cardiac cycle. (B) Ventricular wall stress-circumferential fiber length diagram for the same cardiac cycle in (A). Details are discussed in the text.

volume is determined by the interaction of three key elements: the end-diastolic volume (preload), the impedance to ventricular outflow (afterload) and the inherent contractile state of the myocardium (contractility). Their effects can be visualized by considering the instantaneous ventricular pressure and volume throughout the cardiac cycle[188,304] depicted schematically in Figure 1.5A. Each point on the closed loop describes a combination of intraventricular pressure and ventricular volume. The loop shown is traced by all such states during a single cardiac cycle. The concepts embodied apply equally to both ventricles, but for simplicity the discussion will focus on the LV.

At point A, when LV pressure drops below that in the left atrium (LA) the mitral valve opens and diastolic filling of the ventricle occurs along the path A–B. The volume at point B is the end-diastolic volume (LVEDV) as shown. At point B, ventricular contraction is initiated, accompanied by closure of the mitral valve as the LV pressure exceeds that of the LA. Contraction is isovolumic as shown by the vertical path B–C. When intracavitary pressure exceeds that in the aorta, the aortic valve opens, point C, and systolic ejection occurs along path C–D. At point D the intraventricular pressure falls below aortic pressure, the aortic valve closes and isovolumic relaxation takes place, path D–A. The SV is shown in the figure as the width of the loop; the end-systolic volume (LVESV) is indicated as the ventricular volume at points D and A. The external stroke work is the area within the loop. Note that the diagram does not convey information about the rates at which the parts of the cardiac cycle occur. Also, the figure is idealized and assumes no valve incompetence. The pressure-volume loop for a normal child is illustrated in Figure 1.6, in which volume has been normalized by body surface area. The other parts of this figure are discussed below.

The pump function described by the pressure-volume loop derives from the mechanical behavior of the myocardium itself. Thus it is useful to establish that

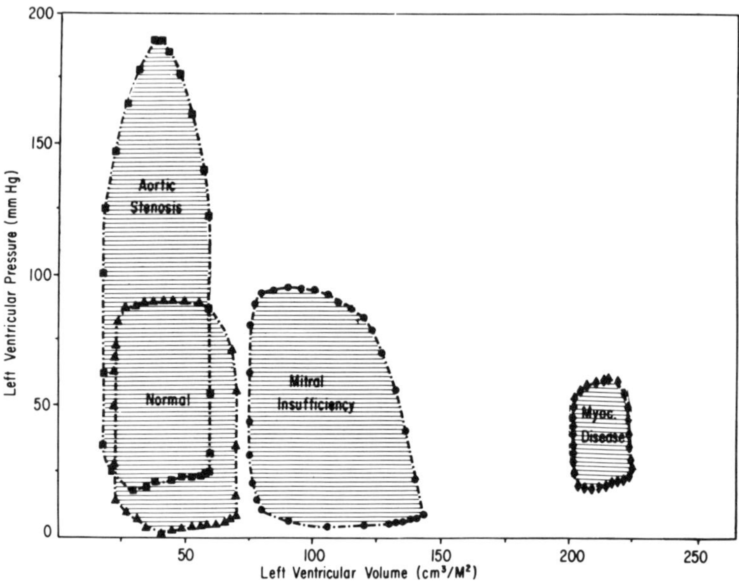

Fig. 1.6. Pressure-volume diagrams for the cardiac cycle in normal and asymptomatic children with pressure loading, volume loading, and myocardial disease. (Graham TP Jr, Jarmakani JM 1971 Evaluation of ventricular function in infants and children. Pediatric Clinics of North America 18: 1109.)

the pressure-volume diagram is analogous to that resulting from an analysis of the behavior of the muscle fibers during a contraction-relaxation cycle. This is illustrated in Figure 1.5B, in which the fiber-related equivalent of the volume is the circumferential fiber length relative to the unloaded length. The analogue of the pressure is the wall stress, i.e., the circumferential force applied to a unit cross-sectional area of muscle. The points A′, B′, C′, D′ correspond respectively to A, B, C, D in the pressure-volume diagram. The shape of the systolic ejection curve is somewhat different because the maximum wall stress occurs near the beginning of ejection.[84,148,356] This is considered further in the section describing *Afterload*.

The roles played by the three major determinants of stroke volume are indicated in Figure 1.7. These sketches are hypothetical but the concepts have been confirmed under carefully controlled experimental conditions[389,412,413,442,443] and in patients.[84,254,262]

The effect of preload is shown in Figure 1.7A in which three pressure-volume loops for the same ventricle with unchanged contractility are depicted. The preload is different in each case (points B, B′, B″) but the ventricle is ejecting against the same end-systolic pressure (afterload). Consequently, in each case the end-systolic volume is also the same (point D). The increased preload results in augmented stroke volume by an amount *equal* to the increase in end-diastolic volume (preload). Note that the ejection fraction (LVEF), the proportion of end-diastolic volume ejected, increased with preload in this example despite unchanged contractility.

Illustrated in Figure 1.7B is the effect of afterload when preload (point B) and contractility are unchanged. Three pressure-volume loops are shown. Loop A–B–

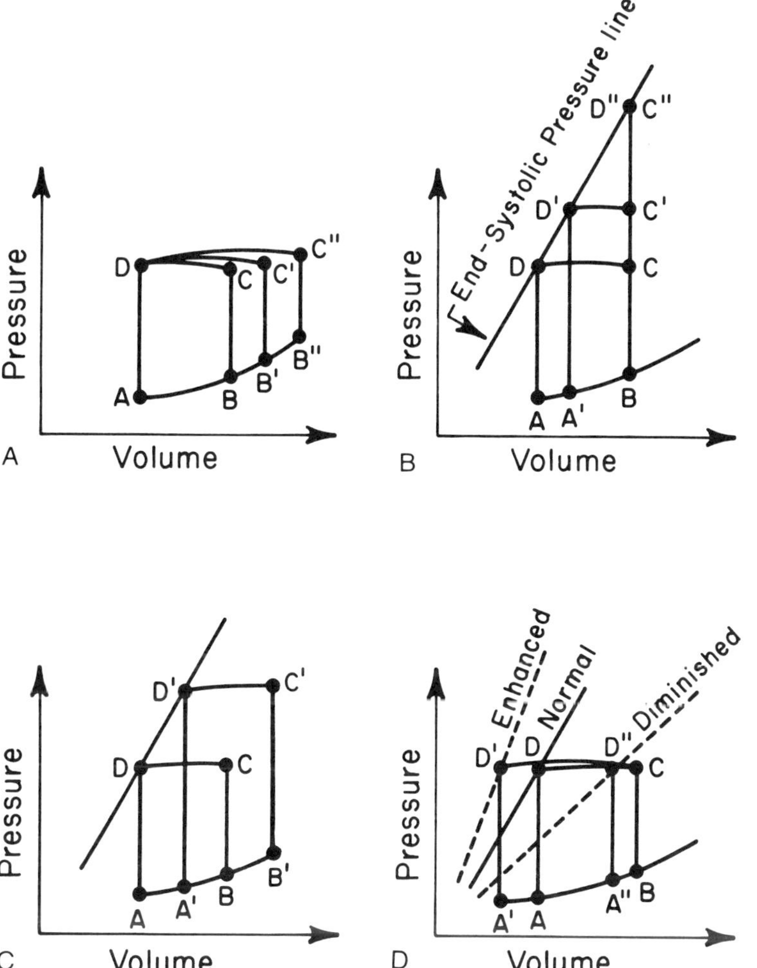

Fig. 1.7. Factors affecting the pressure-volume loop and the end-systolic pressure line. (A) Effect of preload with constant end-systolic pressure. (B) Effect of afterload with constant preload. (C) Maintenance of stroke volume by increased preload in response to increased afterload. (D) Effect of contractility with constant preload and end-systolic pressure.

C–D represents a cycle in which the end-systolic volume is indicated by point D and the SV is the change in abscissa from C to D. For loop A′–B–C′–D′ the preload at point B is the same, but the ventricle is forced to eject against higher aortic pressure (afterload), as depicted by the curve C′–D′. Consequently, SV is reduced as shown. The third pressure-volume loop illustrated is the special case of an isovolumic contraction B–C″–D″–B which corresponds to the classical isometric contraction of isolated muscle preparations.[388] With outflow from the ventricle prevented, the systolic points C″ and D″ coincide at a pressure higher than for either of the other two loops, the maximum value of the developed pressure for the preload selected. Indeed, each end-systolic point (D, D′, D″) is at the maximum developed pressure corresponding to the end-systolic volume. The locus of all such points forms a straight line for the intact ventricle.[262,350,412,443] Termed the end-systolic pressure-volume (P-V_{es}) line or the isovolumic pressure-volume line, it is the limiting envelope of pressure corresponding to any instantaneous volume so long as contractility is unchanged.

In the normal heart, an increase in end ejection pressure can be compensated by the development of increased preload as shown in Figure 1.7C. The initial conditions are indicated by loop A–B–C–D, with SV equal to the difference in the abcissas of points C and B. In the face of an end-systolic pressure corresponding to point D′, a gradual increase in preload to that for point B′ produces the loop A′–B′–C′–D′ with preservation of the stroke volume. The effects described above are manifestations of the *Frank-Starling law of the heart.*[117,399]

Figure 1.7D illustrates the effect of changes in myocardial contractility on the pressure-volume loop with preload and end-systolic pressure held constant. Loop A–B–C–D represents a normal contractile state, with the end-systolic pressure point D lying on the P-V_{es} line shown. Because preload is constant, point B is unchanged. With constant end-ejection pressure, point C is approximately the same for all loops too. Increased contractility augments ejection leading to an increased SV as seen for loop A′–B–C–D′. Point D′ lies on a P-V_{es} line with increased slope as shown. The slope of the corresponding line for a state of diminished contractility is less, as defined by the pressure-volume loop A″–B–C–D″. The slope of this limiting curve has been suggested as a measure of contractile state.[350,412]

In the following sections, specific features of the determinants of stroke volume and their developmental changes are discussed.

Preload

The historical development of the key concepts of cardiac muscle function by Bowditch and Frank[117] in the late 19th century and by Wiggers, Straub, Starling and colleagues[398,399] in the early 20th century has recently been reviewed.[364] It is now apparent that the *Frank-Starling law of the heart* as described above can be related usefully to ultrastructural features of the myocardial cell.

Ultrastructural basis of Starling's law It has been shown that preload is in fact a measure of the extent of overlap of the active portions of the actin and myosin molecules at the onset of contraction, and that the strength of contraction is directly related to the extent of overlap.[387] Using cat papillary muscles, Sonnenblick et al[388] found that a sarcomere length of 2.2 μm led to maximal isometric force development; increasing initial length to 2.3 μm or decreasing it to 1.8 μm produced a reduction in force exceeding 25 percent. The effect of fiber stretch thus appears to influence primarily the number of actin-myosin interactive (force-generating) sites, not the magnitude of force generated at each site.[364]

Passive diastolic behavior of the ventricle The passive pressure-volume relationship for the normal ventricle is shown schematically in Figure 1.8A. Note that the shape differs somewhat at low volumes from the normal filling curve in Figure 1.6. The discrepancy is due to the fact that diastolic relaxation is continuing during the early phase of ventricular filling in the cardiac cycle and pressure actually declines, known as "diastolic suction."[155]

The normal LV passive pressure-volume curve in Figure 1.8A is taken from

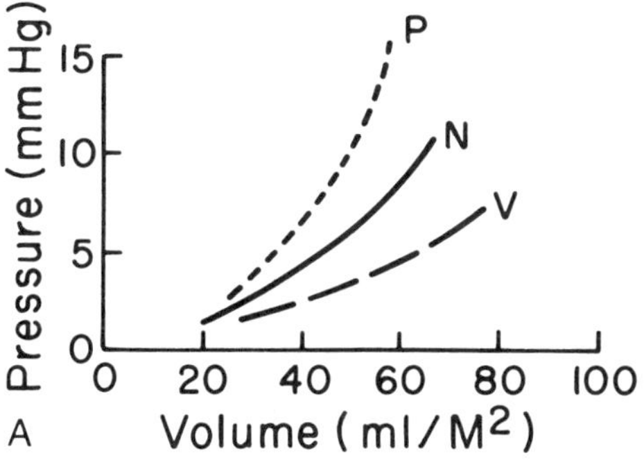

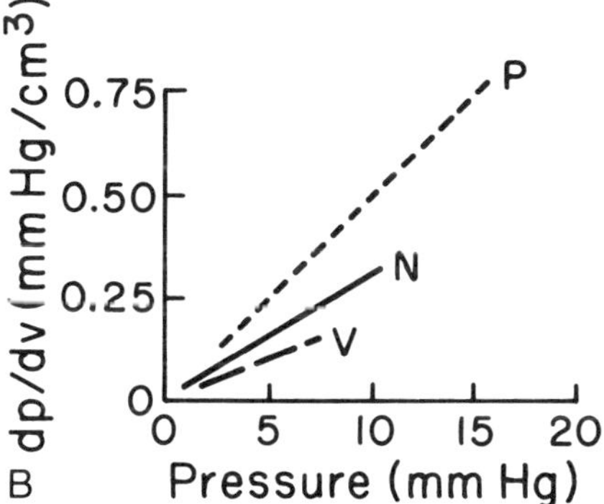

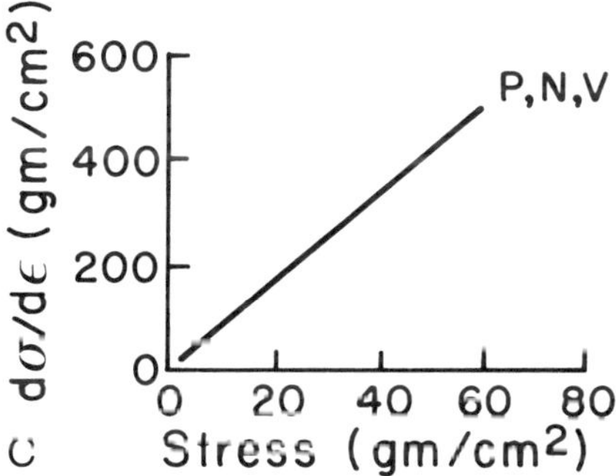

Fig. 1.8. Diastolic function of the ventricle and myocardium in asymptomatic individuals. (A) Pressure-volume relation in diastole for three groups of patients. (B) Ventricular stiffness for the pressure-volume data in (A). (C) Myocardial stiffness computed from the data in (A). Key: N, normal ventricle; P, pressure loaded ventricle; V, volume loaded ventricle; σ, circumferential wall stress; ϵ, circumferential wall strain. Curves shown are average data from Sandor and Olley.[357]

data obtained at cardiac catheterization on a child by Sandor and Olley.[357] Such data have been found to be approximately exponential in form[124,132,271], i.e.,

$$p = A + Be^{CV} \tag{1}$$

in which p is the intracavitary pressure, V is the ventricular volume corresponding to pressure p, A, B and C are constants, and e is the base of the natural logarithm. One of the implications of this formulation is the linearity of the slope of the curve, dp/dV:

$$dp/dV = C(p - A) \tag{2}$$

This slope at any pressure is the instantaneous ventricular stiffness (the inverse of the ventricular compliance); the constant C is the ventricular stiffness constant. The stiffness for the normal data of Figure 1.8A is a linear function of pressure, Figure 1.8B.

Implicit in the above discussion is that "pressure" is transmural pressure, i.e., the pressure difference across the ventricular wall.[445,176,278] Normally pericardial and pleural pressures are nearly equal.[278,426] Thus transmural pressure tends to be increased by factors which reduce intrathoracic pressure such as inspiratory resistance, and decreased by factors which raise intrathoracic pressure such as positive pressure ventilation. With acute cardiac dilatation the pericardium acts to reinforce the myocardium so that pericardial pressure exceeds that in the pleural space.[176,274]

The relationship between the ventricular diastolic pressure-volume curve and the passive behavior of the myocardial tissue is central to understanding the effects of development and disease on preload.[124,133,149,271] In Figure 1.9C the passive length-tension curve for a small linear piece of myocardium is shown, in which the tension can be viewed as the stress, i.e., the force divided by the area perpendicular to it over which it is distributed, and the length change is expressed as the strain, i.e., the change in length divided by the original length. This description allows consideration of the behavior of small elements of material independent of ventricular size or shape. Assuming the muscle acts as a homogeneous isotropic material, the myocardial stress-strain curve has also been described by an exponential expression of one or more terms analogous to Equation 1.[132,272,357] By analogy to Equation 2, the stiffness is a linear function of the stress. Papillary muscle is commonly used in animal[382,383,386] and even human[385] studies because of the relatively linear arrangement of muscle fibers.

A variety of approaches to correlating muscle stiffness with ventricular pressure-volume behavior have been tried.[133,272,279] Using a simplified analysis, Glantz and Kernoff[132] derived a pressure-volume relation of the form of Equation 1 in which the constants contained both myocardial stress-strain parameters and factors related to ventricular geometry. Their model leads to an excellent prediction of the myocardial stiffness from the pressure-volume data. More complex mathematical descriptions yield results which are qualitatively similar.[132,272] The normal strcss-strain relation shown in Figure 1.8C was calculated from the pressure-volume data in Figure 1.8A by Sandor and Olley[357] using such a simplified analysis.

The role of time-dependent properties of the myocardium in ventricular diastolic

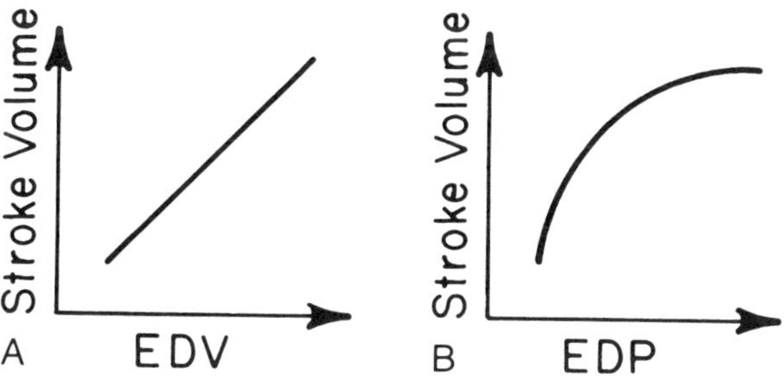

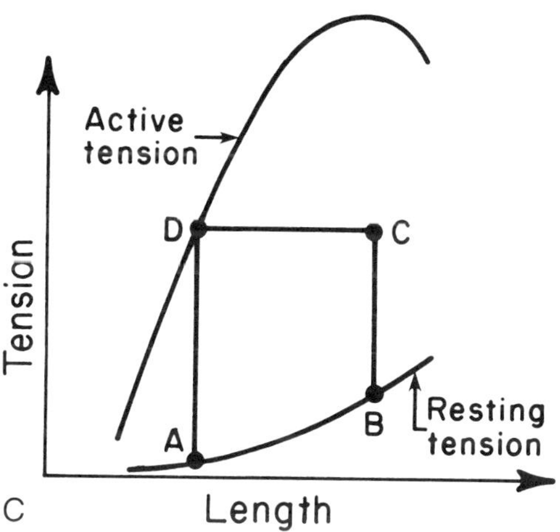

Fig. 1.9. Ventricular and myocardial function curves. (A) Effect of preload (EDV) on stroke volume for constant ejection pressure. (B) Effect of end-diastolic pressure (EDP) on stroke volume for constant ejection pressure. (C) Isometric length-tension curve for cardiac muscle. Details are discussed in the text. (Figure C is after Sonnenblick EH 1962 Implications of muscle mechanics in the heart. Federation Proceedings 21: 975–990 and Sonnenblick EH, Spotnitz HM, Spiro D 1964 Role of the sarcomere in ventricular function and the mechanism of heart failure. Circulation Research 15 (Suppl 11): 70–80, by permission of the American Heart Association, Inc.)

filling behavior remains speculative[133,149] but may be important in some pathologic settings such asymmetric septal hypertrophy.[272]

The ventricular function curve (Frank-Starling law) The linear increase in stroke volume with increased preload illustrated in Figure 1.7A can be shown for conditions of unchanged end-ejection pressure and contractility as in Figure 1.9A. Incorporating the nonlinear pressure-volume curve leads to the relation between stroke volume and end-diastolic pressure shown in Figure 1.9B. This is a ventricular function curve and illustrates the *Frank-Starling law of the heart.*[307] That is, for a given afterload and contractility, the stroke volume will increase to eject any increment in filling volume. This mechanism allows the two ventricles to maintain equal output over time despite moment-to-moment variations in the amount of blood delivered to each.[364] The increased stroke volume of a post-extrasystolic beat is due, at least in part, to this mechanism.[138] This is normally associated with function on the "steep" part of the curve (Fig. 1.9B) where increased preload is associated with little pressure change.[116]

For individual muscle strips, the effects of passive muscle stretch (preload) on contractile behavior have been examined in isometric[388], isotonic, and intermediate degree of afterload[382] experiments. The result of an isotonic experiment on cat papillary muscle is illustrated in Figure 1.9C. The resting and active tension curves are analogous to the pressure-volume and end-systolic pressure lines respectively in Figure 1.7B. The tension-length loop A–B–C–D for a specific isotonic loading corresponds to the stress-strain loop or pressure-volume loop for the whole ventricle (Fig. 1.5).

Effects of volume/pressure hypertrophy Several factors may alter the *ventricular* stiffness/compliance with or without associated changes in *myocardial* stiffness. Among these are chronic increased pressure and/or volume loading as well as normal developmental growth. Effects of volume loading exemplified by asymptomatic children with mild to moderate regurgitant lesions[357] are shown in Figure 1.8. A typical LV pressure-volume curve, Figure 1.8A, is displaced to the right of the normal curve, so that at a given pressure the volume is increased, as is the compliance (Fig. 1.8B). That is, the ventricular stiffness constant, C, is reduced in compensated volume overload. This has been shown in some animal studies.[150,303,419] In other animal studies[259] and in studies on patients[149], volume overload is associated with increased ventricular stiffness, but at supranormal filling pressure, making interpretation of ventricular behavior difficult. Of more importance is the evidence from direct measurements on myocardium[69,337] and analyses of pressure-volume data[271] that myocardial passive stress-strain properties and sarcomere length[337] do not change if volume loading is chronic and compensated. This is shown by the computed myocardial stress-strain curve in Figure 1.8C, indicating that the changes in ventricular diastolic behavior are related to changes in geometry and operating pressure but not intrinsic muscle characteristics. The pressure-volume loop for a child with compensated volume overloading due to mitral insufficiency is shown in Figure 1.6. The increased volume load is evident in the early loss of ventricular volume, owing to ejection of blood into the left atrium during the usually isovolumic phase.[138]

Hypertrophy due to pressure loading without myocardial failure is usually associated with normal[139,140,145,149] or reduced[84,143] end-diastolic volume, increased end-diastolic pressure, and elevated instantaneous ventricular stiffness.[149,124] An example is the pressure-volume loop for aortic stenosis in Figure 1.6. The chamber stiffness constant may be normal or increased, but the diastolic stress-strain behavior of the myocardium is often normal.[84,124,357,390] This is illustrated by the data for pressure overload in Figure 1.8. Some patients with severe pressure overload exhibit an increased myocardial stiffness constant[150], possibly due to fibrosis.[272]

Other factors A variety of acute events may affect diastolic-pressure relations[133,272], though probably with little effect on the myocardial stiffness constant.[237] Controversy exists as to whether sympathetic or parasympathetic stimulation alters diastolic properties of the myocardium; current evidence suggests that it does not.[149,272,275,421]

Interaction between the ventricles may also alter chamber stiffness without affecting myocardial properties. Increased end-diastolic pressure in one ventricle causes distortion of the interventricular septum with a concomitant reduction in diastolic compliance of the other.[244,445,449] The impact of elevated RVEDP on LV compliance is greater than the converse.[257] The presence of the pericardium accentuates the effect.[445] Ventricular interaction can occur in systole as well.[445] Elevated LV systolic pressure induces an increase in RV pressure. Systolic RV pressures have minimal effect on those in the LV.

Role of atrial contraction The atria serve a reservoir function during ventricular systole and a transport function during ventricular diastole and atrial systole. The effect of the atrial "kick" on stroke volume depends primarily on heart rate and ventricular function. With normal ventricular function at resting heart rates, loss of effective atrial systole reduces stroke volume approximately 5 to 30 percent.[349,156] The major impact in the normal heart is from the left atrium. Atrial systole is effective for any PR interval over the range from 0.05 to 0.20 seconds.[349] The benefit appears to derive from both the enhanced ventricular preload and reduced atrial pressure during ventricular systole, which promotes venous return.[156,239]

Developmental effects on preload Developmental changes in diastolic myocardial and ventricular behavior and their effect on cardiac output have been the subject of numerous studies. As indicated in Table 1.1, normalized end-diastolic volume is less in the newborn and infant than in the child and adult. Diastolic pressures are similar, however. In some studies ventricular stiffness constants were greater for immature animals (fetus or newborns) than for adults.[214,332,392] In others, there was little difference.[226] The results depend in part upon which ventricle is being compared[332] and the assumptions inherent in analyzing the results.[271] In individual muscle experiments, however, the fetal lamb myocardium is stiffer than that of the adult.[119] Furthermore, the sarcomere length for maximum contractility is achieved in the immature puppy heart at smaller normalized volume than in the adult dog[392], and the fetal lamb achieves little increase in stroke volume at filling pressures above 10 to 12 mmHg[207]. These findings may be explained by Friedman's observation that fetal lamb myocardium possesses approximately one-half the amount of contractile tissue per unit area of cross-section as the adult.[119] The diminished passive compliance in fetal lamb myocardium (Fig. 1.10) becomes similar to that of the adult when corrected for actual cross-sectional area of contractile tissue.

The above evidence implies that the infant heart normally functions at a relatively high preload and associated stroke volume with reduced, though still significant "preload reserve."[207] Such has been demonstrated by the diminished LV response to volume loading in neonatal lambs when compared to older infants[210,333] or adults.[333] This is considered further in the section *Contractility*.

Ventricular interaction in diastole is also age-dependent. Passive pressure-volume data for sheep hearts suggest that the effect of elevated RVEDP on LV filling is more pronounced in the newborn than the adult; the effect of elevated LVEDP on RV filling is similar at both ages.[332]

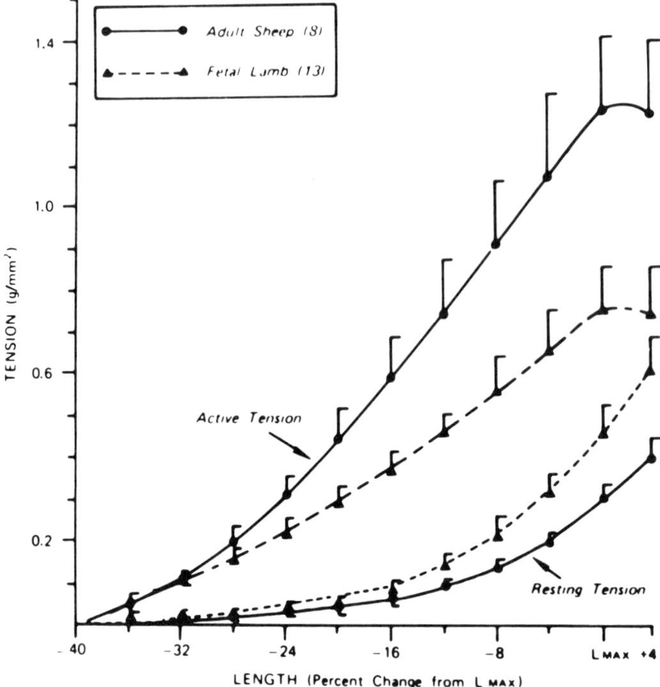

Fig. 1.10. Isometric length-tension curves for fetal lambs and adult sheep. Tension is normalized to force per unit cross-sectional area. Length is normalized to the percent change from the length producing maximum active tension. (Friedman WF 1973 The intrinsic physiologic properties of the developing heart. Progress in Cardiovascular Disease 15: 87–111, Grune & Stratton, New York, by permission.)

The transition from the immature to a more mature response to preload occurs over time. Infants under approximately 2 years of age exhibit higher ejection fraction and resting heart rate than older children and healthy adults (Tables 1.1 and 1.2). This suggests that the major changes in preload response occur before this age.

Contractility

Biochemical basis of contractility The biochemistry of myocardial contraction and its regulation have been critically reviewed briefly[6,102,280,415] and in detail.[199,251,367,404,454,455] Current understanding of this process represents the synthesis of a variety of experimental models, some of it conflicting. The somewhat speculative description which follows needs clarification in many important details.

Central to the contractile process is the presence of free Ca^{++} in the myocyte cytoplasm.[280] Excitation-contraction coupling depends upon calcium movements into and within the cell that lead to increases in $[Ca^{++}]$ at the myofilaments illustrated schematically in Figure 1.11A. During the plateau phase of the action potential, in the presence of extracellular ionized calcium, an inward Ca^{++} flux occurs across the sarcolemma, and probably the T-tubules.[364] When the intra-

Table 1.2. Resting Heart Rate for Normal Infants and Children

Age	Heart Rate (Beats/Min) Mean	5%–95%
0–24 hr	119	94–145
1–7 days	133	100–175
8–30 days	163	115–190
1–3 mo	154	124–190
3–6 mo	140	111–179
6–12 mo	140	112–177
1–3 yr	126	98–163
3–5 yr	98	65–132
5–8 yr	96	70–115
8–12 yr	79	55–107
12–16 yr	75	55–102

(Modified from Liebman J Tables of normal standards. In: Liebman J, Plonsey R, Gillette PC (eds), Pediatric Electrocardiography. © 1982 The Williams & Wilkins Co., Baltimore.)

cellular [Ca^{++}] exceeds approximately 10^{-7}M, release of intracellular stores of calcium from the sarcoplasmic reticulum (SR),[101,451] and possibly also the mitochondria,[6] is stimulated.

In resting muscle, tropomyosin and troponin inhibit interaction between the "heads" of the myosin and actin molecules. As the concentration of ionized calcium increases in the vicinity of the myofibrils, calcium binding to one subunit of the troponin causes a conformational change in the troponin and tropomyosin molecules, which promotes formation of an active complex of myosin and actin.[6,199] This complex is formed cyclically along the myofilament so that force and relative movement are accumulated. The energy for this process is derived from the hydrolysis of adenosine triphosphate (ATP) by an ATPase on the myosin head.[199,454]

The mutual affinity of myosin and actin is so high that they remain bonded in the absence of inhibitory influences. The presence of ATP promotes their separation until cleavage of the terminal phosphate which permits bonding again at a point further along the actin filament.[6,454]

In the presence of sufficient ATP, the intensity of 1c01contraction is the result of the rate of ATP hydrolysis which appears to depend in a nonlinear way on the [Ca^{++}] at the myofibril[101,280], as well as the intrinsic activity of the myosin ATPase.[455] As illustrated in Figure 1.11B contraction is initiated at concentrations exceeding approximately 5×10^{-7}M and is maximal at a concentration of approximately 10^{-5}M.[6] This is associated with saturation of the available calcium binding sites on the troponin subunit.

Relaxation occurs primarily in association with uptake of Ca^{++} by the SR using the action of an ATP-dependent calcium pump.[237,415] Extrusion of Ca^{++} from the cell also occurs by at least two sarcolemmal ATP-dependent pumps.[6,415] The reduced [Ca^{++}] leads to unbinding of calcium from the troponin subunit with

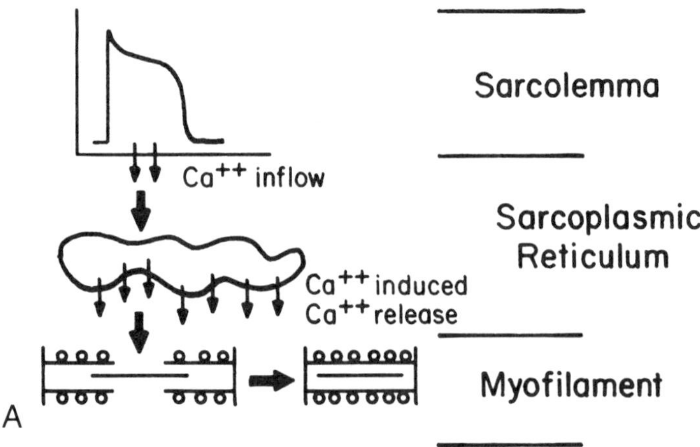

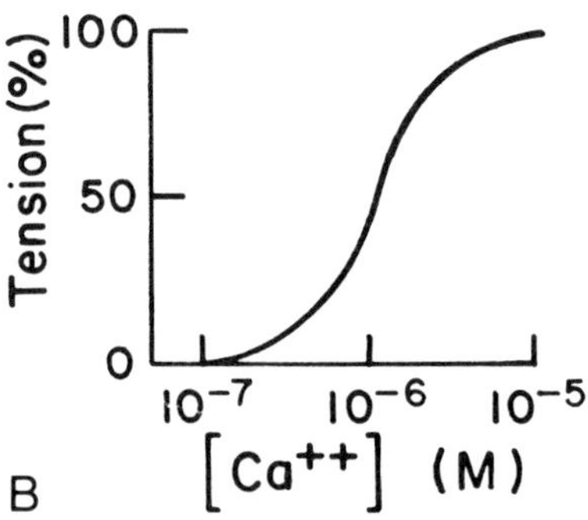

Fig. 1.11. Aspects of role of calcium in myocardial contraction. (A) Calcium movements. (Modified from Swyngedauw B, Delcayre C 1982 Biology of cardiac overload. Pathobiology Annual 12: 137.) (B) Effect of myoplasmic Ca^{++} concentration on tension development in skinned fibers of human ventricular myocardium. (Fabiato A, Fabiato F 1978 Calcium induced release of calcium from the sarcoplasmic reticulum of skinned cells from adult human, dog, cat, rabbit, rat and frog hearts and from fetal and new-born rat ventricles, Annals New York Academy of Science 307: 491. Raven Press, NY.)

conformational changes in troponin and tropomyosin which again inhibit myosin-actin interaction.

For a given sarcomere stretch (preload), short-term alteration of the intensity of contraction appears to be regulated by those factors which affect the concentration of ionized calcium at the myofilament. Most important of these is sympathetic stimulation, which acts via several mechanisms.[235,280,367] A major effect of catecholamines on the myocyte results from interaction with a membrane-bound beta-receptor (see the section *Autonomic control of cardiac function*) which stimulates membrane-bound adenyl cyclase to produce intracellular cyclic adenosine monophosphate (c-AMP). This induces at least four effects associated with increased contractility. (1) Enhanced inward flux of Ca^{++} occurs due to an increased number of active slow Ca^{++} channels, mediated by phosphorylation of sarcolemmal proteins.[251,367] There may also be increased Ca^{++} release from mitochondria,[280] though the role of c-AMP therein remains to be clarified.[183] (2) Increased Ca^{++} release from the SR leads to elevated [Ca^{++}] at the myofilaments. (3) Phosphorylation of the inhibitory subunit of troponin, mediated by c-AMP, elevates the [Ca^{++}] required for activation.[455] (4) Cyclic-AMP activates a sarcoplasmic reticulum (SR)-bound MG^{++}-dependent protein kinase which results in phosphorylation of a specific SR membrane protein involved in uptake of calcium.[404,454] The last two enhance the relaxation rate at the end of contraction, increasing available time for diastolic filling.[367] Cyclic-AMP mediated phosphorylation of myosin also occurs, but its role in myocardial contraction is obscure.[205]

Ionized calcium exerts negative feedback on the level of cyclic-AMP both by inhibiting the activity of adenyl cyclase and augmenting that of phosphodiesterase which converts cyclic-AMP to inactive 5′-adenosine monophosphate (AMP).[251] Phosphodiesterase inhibitors thus intensify the cyclic-AMP mediated effects of sympathetic stimulation.[367]

Several factors known to enhance contractility act by increasing intracellular ionized calcium without involving cyclic-AMP. These include increased extracellular Ca^{++}, alpha-adrenergic receptor stimulation (see the section *Automatic control of cardiac function)*, increased heart rate (independent of sympathetic influences) and poststimulation potentiation,[206,360] and cardiac glycosides,[49,367] the last by inhibition of the sarcolemmal Na^{+},K^{+} ATPase pump.[10,178] There is also evidence that some beta-adrenergic receptor effects can be produced without intermediary cyclic-AMP.[182,183,258]

The acid-base balance affects contractility as well. Acidosis leads to diminished contractility and response to sympathetic stimulation by unknown mechanisms.[367] Alkalosis produces opposite effects.

The biochemical bases of the negative inotropic effects of cholinergic stimulation are less well studied. Among these is a reduction in cyclic-AMP concentration, mediated at least partially by cyclic guanosine monophosphate (cyclic-GMP).[404]

Measures of contractility It is important to distinguish between measures of ventricular pump performance and myocardial *contractility*.[94] As suggested by Sonnenblick and Strobeck,[389] contractility is the intrinsic property of the myocardium which establishes the *limits* to mechanical performance. The ventricular pump performance is what the muscle actually does within these limits; it depends on the preload and afterload. Valid measures of *contractility* are independent of preload and afterload effects. The longstanding search for such measures, applicable to both experimental and clinical settings, continues to the present.

The ventricular function curve (VFC) has been proposed as an indicator of contractility.[359] A single such curve, i.e., the middle curve in Figure 1.12, can be obtained experimentally for conditions of constant afterload and contractile state. If contractility is enhanced by whatever means without a change in afterload, the VFC is displaced upward and to the left. Thus, a given preload is associated with increased stroke volume, as for the upper curve in the figure. The effect of diminished contractility is also illustrated. In addition to the practical difficulty defining the VFC in a clinical setting, other measures may be more sensitive to changes in inotropic state.[70,385]

An alternative measure is based on the observation that the velocity of contraction

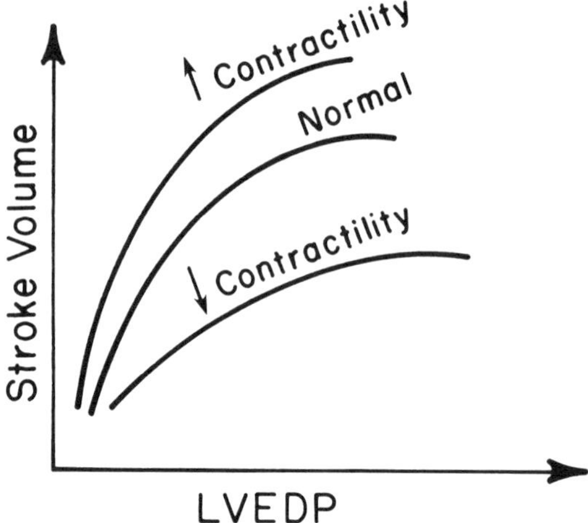

Fig. 1.12. The ventricular function curve. Left ventricular stroke volume as a function of preload, expressed as left ventricular end-diastolic pressure (LVEDP), for constant preload and contractility. Three contractile states are shown.

in isotonic experiments with isolated muscle strips is a function of the load and contractile state. When load was varied and contractile velocity measured, a characteristic *force-velocity* curve for a given preload could be generated.[382] The applicability of this relation to various loading conditions and geometries was proposed by invoking a mechanical model analogue to describe the myocardial response.[383] Based on the model proposed by Hill for skeletal muscle[169], it consists of three mechanical elements, as shown in Figure 1.13A. The model accounts qualitatively and quantitatively for important characteristics of the heart muscle.[383] The parallel elastic element (PE) represents the nonlinear resistance to preload, thought to arise largely in supporting connective tissue structures, at least at higher preload. The active tension arises from the contractile element (CE), which is freely extensible before activation. The series elastic element (SE) is stretched by the

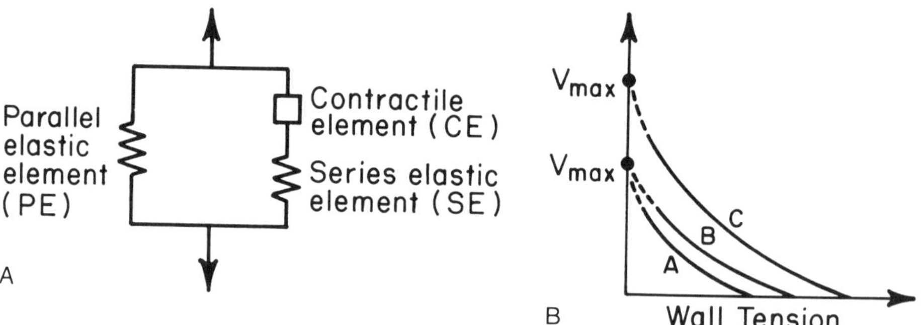

Fig. 1.13. Mechanical model representation of myocardial behavior. (A) Three-element model. (B) Velocity of contraction of the CE for the model in (A) for various loading conditions and contractile states. See text for detailed description. (Sonnenblick EH 1962 Implications of muscle mechanics in the heart. Federation Proceedings 21: 975.)

activated CE. Precise tissue correlates of these mechanical analogues have not been defined.[384]

Based on the assumption that the passive stiffness of the SE is independent of contractility, the velocity of contraction for the contractile element, V_{CE}, can be determined for isotonic and/or isometric loadings of linear muscle specimens.[383] This determination results in curves such as those illustrated in Figure 1.13B. Curve A shows V_{CE} at a given preload for various afterloads. The data have been extrapolated back to zero afterload to yield the maximum V_{CE}, V_{max}. Results of an experiment in which only preload is increased are shown as curve B.The two curves intersect at V_{max}; that is, preload does not affect it. Curve C however, represents the same myocardial tissue at the same preload as curve B but with norepinephrine added to the bathing fluid. The increase seen in V_{max} is characteristic of the effect of augmented contractility on this parameter. Results of this sort can be generated in experimental, and even clinical situations from intraventricular pressure measurements during isovolumic contraction of the intact ventricle.[70,273]

The relative sensitivity of V_{max} to alterations in contractile state and its insensitivity to preload and afterload have led to its application as a measure of myocardial contractility for experimental animals[390], adult patients,[385] and pediatric patients.[138,139] Some data suggest that V_{max} is a more suitable measure of changes in contractility than the VFC.[70] However, thoughtful critical analyses of the use of either the VFC or V_{max} have led to the conclusion that, though useful under restricted circumstances, they both lack a fundamental relationship to the innate capacity of the myocardium to convert chemical to mechanical energy.[44,389]

As described above, the end-systolic pressure-volume line (Fig. 1.7D) has been proposed as a fundamental measure of contractile state. The linearity,[147,262,254,443] independence of preload and afterload,[32,350,379,411,412] and potential for measurement in patients,[147,213,254,262] support the P-V_{es} line as such a measure. Further support comes from the apparent uniqueness of the line for a given contractile state irrespective of whether the intact ventricle or a strip of myocardium is considered,[389] whether the loading path is isometric (isovolumic), isotonic, or variably loaded,[444] or the means by which contractility is altered.[147,262,350] The P-V_{es} line does not provide direct insight into the rate of force development. Nonetheless, it appears to be the best available measure of contractility and ventricular function.[43] Other important features related to its use are discussed in the section *Myocardial oxygen consumption*.

A variety of measures of ventricular pump performance are employed clinically. Foremost among these is the ejection fraction as measured by cincangiography,[106,112,138,140,144,269,203,257,422] radionuclide angiography,[47,219,306] or as inferred from a variety of echocardiographic measurements.[22,35,97,154,159,201,217,297,395] These are discussed in detail in Chapter 2. Such parameters are often useful indicators of the ability of the heart to meet physiologic demands, and may assist in assessing the extent of reserve available. Because it is afterload dependent,[42,146] however, the ejection fraction is a less effective measure of the limiting state of the myocardium than the P-V_{es} line. This is considered further in the section *Afterload*.

Developmental effects on contractility Immature myocardium develops less tension per unit cross-sectional area than mature muscle at any preload (Fig. 1.10). The effect may derive from the fact that approximately 60 percent of the cross-sectional area of adult myocardium is contractile elements compared to 30 percent in the fetus.[119] When normalized for this factor, there is no difference in the calculated intrinsic sarcomere strength.[261] Furthermore, V_{max} is the same in both cases.[119]

Structural development of the contractile apparatus occurs throughout infancy. In the newborn myocyte there is a paucity of myofibrils which are disorganized and peripherally disposed.[230,65] There are also fewer mitochondria with variegated shape[372] and sparse cristae, implying diminished aerobic capacity.[230] The number, density, and regularity of sarcomeres increases during early infancy, and by 17 days of age in the rat[65] and 5 months in the dog[230] have achieved adult form. The mitochondria mature in shape, packing, and internal structure over the same period of time. Early differences in these structures between the two ventricles in the puppy are no longer noted by 5 months.[230] The sarcoplasmic reticulum is well developed at birth, but T-tubules develop later,[192] in the left ventricle earlier than the right.[230]

Biochemical changes in contractile proteins occur with age but may be relatively subtle. Myosin ATPase activity of fetal and neonatal lamb myocardium is approximately 20 percent less than that of older lambs and adults.[184] Age-related differences in myosin ATPase are noted in other species as well, perhaps a consequence of separate genes coding for the heavy chains of the embryonic and mature protein.[393] Altered activity may also be due to development of growth-related isoenzymes in response to the increased workload[452] as discussed in the section *Afterload*. Despite this, total myofibrillar ATPase activity[119] and [ATP][184] do not appear to change with age in lambs, though ATPase activity in rats is age-dependent.[20]

In lambs, myocardial tissue and mitochondrial creatine kinase activity increase during fetal and neonatal life to adult values at 14 days of age. Lactate dehydrogenase activity does not change.[184] Age-related activity of the Na^+,K^+ ATPase pump is species-dependent;[178,253] its significance is not clear.

Cyclic AMP-mediated effects on contractility appear to be well established before birth. Myocyte adenylate cyclase and phosphodiesterase activities are similar in newborn lambs and adult sheep[9], though not in infant and adult rabbits.[369] Myocardial tension development in fetal and adult sheep are also similarly affected by isoproterenol, either alone or in the presence of propranolol.[119] Other effects of propranol and norepinephrine which differ in immature and mature hearts are likely associated with maturation of sympathetic innervation (see the section *Autonomic control of cardiac function*) rather than myoplasmic biochemical development.

In sum, normal age-related biochemical changes in myocyte contractile function appear to be complex, relatively minor, and occur before and shortly after birth. Far more important seems to be the increase in the absolute amount as well as the proportion of contractile tissue within the myocyte that occurs during infancy. The impact of a diminished concentration of sarcomeres in the young infant is that they must operate at higher preload (see section *Preload*) and probably contractile state. The latter is supported by a variety of experimental and clinical evidence. Peak wall stress is constant from early infancy to mid-childhood (see the *Afterload*) independent of the changing proportion of contractile tissue. The rate of myocardial oxygen consumption diminishes with age (see the section *Myocardial oxygen consumption*) as does ejection fraction.[138,219,269,422] Data cited by Rudolph[344] indicate that in lambs the slope of the P-V_{es} line diminishes during the early weeks of life. Sympathomimetics augment cardiac output in infancy in both animals and humans primarily by inducing changes in heart rate,[92,344] despite adult responsiveness of isolated immature myocardial muscle strips (see *Developmental aspects* under *Autonomic control of cardiac function*). The resting tachycardia characteristic of infants (Table 1.2) is probably another manifestation of this.

The time course of these changes is unknown, though some inferences from growth data (see the sections *Morphologic development* and *Afterload*) may be warranted. These suggest that the 1- to 2-year-age period is an important transition time from infantile to more adult cardiac function.

Abnormal genetic alterations at biochemical and structural levels may alter development of contractile function in many ways, including energy transport, excitation-contraction coupling, defects in contractile proteins, structural disorganization, or infiltrative interference with myofibrils. These isues have been reviewed in detail recently.[420,424]

Afterload

The concept of afterload is straightforward when applied to one-dimensional loading of linear muscle strips. The magnitude of muscle shortening is related uniquely to the afterload for constant preload and contractile state.[388] It is not the total load which is significant, however, but the stress (force per unit cross-sectional area).

Similarly the significance of afterload in the intact ventricle is related to its effect on myocardial wall stress. The major determinants of afterload in vivo are as follows.

1. *The ventricular size*. For a thin-walled sphere with only intracavitary pressure the circumferential wall stress is given by the Laplace law:

$$\sigma = pr/2h \tag{3}$$

in which p is the pressure, r is the sphere radius, and h is the wall thickness. This relationship implies that chamber enlargement associated with increased preload, without a change in wall thickness, produces a proportional increase in afterload.

A more realistic model of the left ventricle may be that of a thick-walled ellipsoid for which a variety of simplifying assumptions have been used to evaluate the average stresses across the thickness of the wall.[148,177,270,356] Average stresses at the equator of the ellipsoid are[148,356]:

$$\sigma_m = (pb/2h)/(1 + h/2b) \tag{4}$$

$$\sigma_c = (pb/2h)[1 - b^2/2a^2(1 + h/2b)] \tag{5}$$

where σ_m is the meridional stress, σ_c is the circumferential stress, a and b are the major and minor semiaxes respectively. The circumferential stress is greater than the meridional stress throughout the cardiac cycle, but the latter is simpler to determine clinically because only the smaller chamber dimension is needed. The

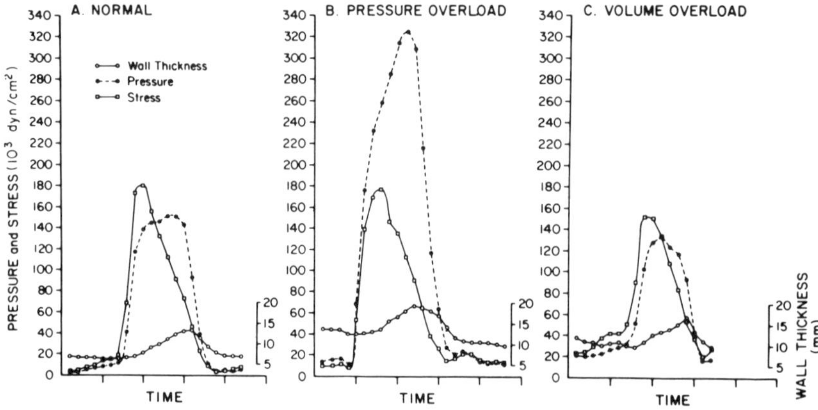

Fig. 1.14. Comparison of changes in LV pressure, wall thickness, and meridional wall stress in normal, pressure overloaded, and volume overloaded ventricles in adult patients. (Grossman W, Jones D, McLaurin LP 1975 Wall stress and patterns of hypertrophy in the human left ventrical. Journal of Clinical Investigation 56: 56, by permission of the American Society for Clinical Investigation.)

right ventricle is much more irregular in shape. Analyses of more realistic geometries are available[459] but add little to the understanding of the basic concepts.

2. *The ejection pressure*. This is the arterial pressure against which the ventricle must eject blood, systemic arterial pressure (SAP) for the left ventricle, pulmonary arterial pressure (PAP) for the right ventricle. It is not intuitively obvious at which moment in the cardiac cycle the pressure is most significant, as illustrated in Figure 1.14A. The intracavitary pressure, wall thickness, and meridional wall stress throughout one cardiac cycle are shown. The pressure increases somewhat throughout systole, but the meridional wall stress attains its peak value early and then declines as chamber size decreases and wall thickness increases. A similar result is seen for circumferential stress.[177] Borow et al[42] argue that it is the *end-systolic* stress which represents the limiting state (as, for example, in Fig. 1.5B) and end-systolic pressure is, therefore, the appropriate descriptor of the ejection pressure component of afterload.

3. *Mechanical outflow obstruction*. Outflow obstructions such as aortic or pulmonic stenosis lead to elevated intracavitary pressure during systole and increased wall stress if chamber size and thickness are constant (Equations 4 and 5). Accommodation to chronic obstruction is discussed below.

4. *Impedance of vascular beds*. Although their effects may be reflected in the ventricular ejection pressure, it is useful to consider specifically the impedances offered by the systemic and pulmonary vascular systems. Components of the impedance include aortic and pulmonary arterial *elastances*. In the pediatric population, however, these are much less important than the vascular *resistances*, arising principally from the small arteries and precapillary arterioles.[115,265] Details are considered in the sections *Components of the systemic circulation* and *Components of the pulmonary circulation*.

Acute effects of increased afterload The effect of an acutely elevated afterload is initially compensated by a sufficient increment in preload that stroke volume is maintained,[42,360] as described in Figure 1.7. Due to the higher preload, ejection

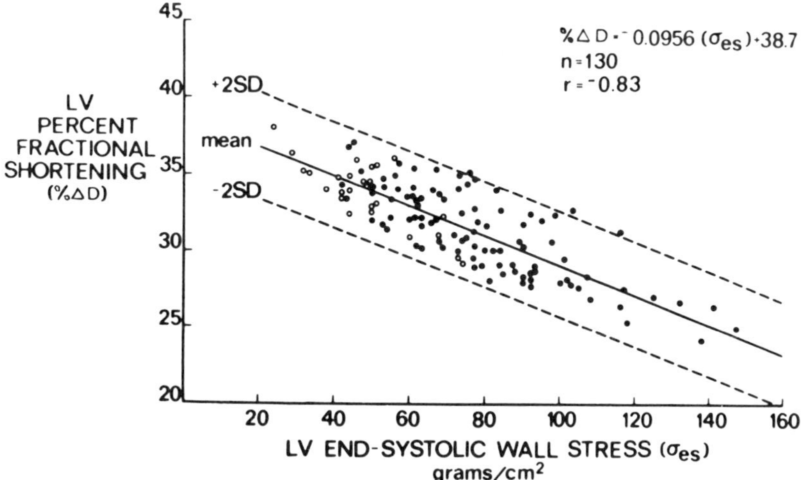

Fig. 1.15. Relation between LV end-systolic wall stress and LV percent fractional shortening in normal children and adults. ○, control values; ●, increased afterload during methoxamine infusion. (Borow KM, Green LH, Grossman W, Braunwald E 1982 Left ventricular end-systolic stress-shortening and stress-length relations in humans. American Journal of Cardiology 50: 1301.)

fraction is lower. The magnitude of the change in ejection fraction (or shortening of the ventricular cavity diameter) is directly related to the magnitude of the wall stress as shown in Figure 1.15. In some animal experiments, a gradual enhancement of contractility leads to a return of chamber dimensions toward normal,[360] though this is more difficult to demonstrate clinically.

Chronic effects of increased afterload—pressure loading Intermittent elevation of afterload by pressure loading occurs with isometric exercise such as weight lifting. Continuous pressure loading can be induced either by obstructive lesions or hypertension. All of these lead to compensatory myocardial hypertrophy as demonstrated in normal weight lifters,[37,313] and in chronically pressure loaded experimental animals[33,74,86,390] and patients.[73,84,117,139,153] Except in early infancy, the growth is entirely due to enlargement of a constant number of cells (see the section *Development at the cellular level*). Removal of the stimulus usually results in regression of some or all of the hypertrophic response,[74,417] though not always.[370,417] Many aspects of this have been reviewed recently.[106,41,146,313,324,415,452,461]

The hypertrophic response is considered to be *physiologic* so long as contractility is normal or enhanced.[313,452] The physiologic response to pressure loading is increased wall thickness relative to cavity size ("concentric" hypertrophy) such that resting systolic and diastolic stresses are maintained at the normal level[15,148,177,338] or below.[84] This is illustrated in Figure 1.14B which shows data for a well compensated pressure-overloaded ventricle. The much thicker ventricular wall, but similar stresses compared to the normal (Fig. 1.14A) can be appreciated. It has been suggested that stresses at rest are even lower in the very well compensated patient to insure equal stresses during exercise.[84] Less well compensated patients with *pathologic* hypertrophy exhibit higher resting wall stress, diminished ventricular function,[40,153] and eventually cellular degeneration.[107]

The growth in response to pressure loading occurs by addition of myofibrils in parallel to those already present, so that cell width increases preferentially.[452] This process begins within hours after the pressure increases in experimental animals: messenger ribonucleic acid (mRNA) synthesis occurs, followed by enhanced production of mitochondrial proteins and myosin, without a change in degradation rate.[280,452] In physiologic hypertrophy induced in experimental animals, an isoenzyme of myosin is produced with supernormal activity.[85,452] In humans, the proportions of myosin subtypes are altered in pressure-induced hypertrophy.[135,266] Mitochondria increase in size and number as well as in efficiency of oxidative phosphorylation.[415] Proliferation of capillaries also occurs, but does not entirely keep pace with the other elements.[452] The important implications of this observation are considered in the section *Myocardial energy supply—the coronary circulation*.

There does appear to be a limit to the size of the myocyte,[18] and very large hearts contain many polyploid cells some of which divide amitotically.[415,460] This is probably of little physiologic significance.

The precise nature of the biochemical stimulus to hypertrophic growth is unknown. It is apparent, however, that neurohumoral effects are important;[370,447] indeed hypertrophy can be produced due to adrenergic stimulation alone.[324] Furthermore, hypertrophy of one ventricle is usually associated with enlargement of the other, even without an identifiable stress-related stimulus.[106,416,277] A steroid-like cardiotropic factor, elaborated by the adrenal cortex, which exhibits cross immunoreactivity with digoxin has been found recently in experimental and possibly clinical hypertrophy.[212] Its role in normal growth is undefined.

Young patients compensate well for pressure loading of either ventricle if the load is not too severe or acute. Children with aortic stenosis or coarctation may have normal stroke volume, with reduced or normal LVEDV and elevated LV ejection fraction.[139,143] The newborn RV adapts well to systemic pressures in tetralogy of Fallot with adequate function often well into adulthood.[168,312] By contrast, adaptation of the mature RV to pressure loading is poor.[313]

Chronic effects of increased afterload—volume loading A significant increase in volume demand represents a complex type of workload associated with increased preload and hence afterload. This normally occurs intermittently in isotonic type exercise, such as long-distance running. Continuous volume loading is produced experimentally or clinically by a variety of shunt and regurgitant lesions. Hypertrophic cardiac adaptations to intermittent[37,83,318,371,414] and continuous experimental[69,259,303,335,337] and clinical[139,145,146,148,168,313] volume loading are similar: increased wall thickness and chamber size with preservation of their ratio ("eccentric" hypertrophy). Physiologic hypertrophy is associated with enhanced stroke volume, and normal contractility and systolic wall stress, though diastolic wall stress, is somewhat elevated (Fig. 1.14C).

Cell growth in response to volume loading occurs by elongation of myofibrils from addition of sarcomeres in series as well as the parallel development of new myofibrils.[452] This leads to proportional increases in cell length and width.

A hypothetical model of the relationship between the type of loading and pattern of hypertrophic ventricular growth is shown in Figure 1.16. The figure suggests

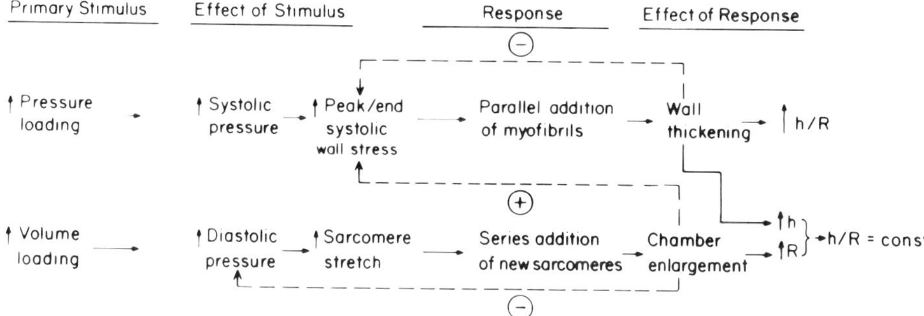

Fig. 1.16. Hypothetical model of relationship between type of loading and patterns of ventricular growth. (Modified from Grossman W 1980 Cardiac hypertrophy: Useful adaptation or pathologic process? American Journal of Medicine 69: 576.)

that the increased sarcomere stretch associated with volume loading promotes lengthening of the myofibrils leading to chamber enlargement. The resultant elevated systolic wall stress induces addition of myofibrils in parallel with consequent wall thickening, restoring normal chamber proportions.

Regression of volume loading induced physiologic hypertrophy occurs in those settings where the stimulus can be removed,[189,313,335] including detraining of athletes.[83] The situation is more complex when pathologic hypertrophy has evolved.[146]

Relationship between normal growth and volume loading Several lines of evidence suggest that normal developmental growth of the heart is primarily a physiologic hypertrophic response to the volume loading imposed by circulatory requirements of somatic growth. One approach to evaluating this concept is to examine the adaptation to hemodynamic demands different from normal. Infants with transposition of the great vessels (TGV) with intact septum may exhibit right (systemic) and left (pulmonary) ventricular growth similar to that for the normal left and right ventricles, respectively.[21] Children and young adults with congenitally corrected TGV, lacking other lesions, have normal *systemic* ventricular size and function.[144] Individuals living at high altitude where elevated pulmonary artery pressure persists normally develop RVH with normal function.[311] Following surgical repair of tricuspid atresia, pulmonary atresia, or critical pulmonary stenosis with intact ventricular septum, the right ventricle grows,[34,323] sometimes to normal proportions and function.[137]

Perhaps most significant is the striking similarity of ventricular form and function during normal growth and physiologic hypertrophy due to volume loading.[116,145,146] Thus, it appears that growth of the normal heart is not preprogrammed, but reflects the response of those tissues to increasing circulatory demands from the rest of the body. Whether biochemical stimuli play a role independent of hemodynamics is uncertain.

The additional cardiac growth resulting from endurance training is apparently not seen until adolescence. Differences in heart size between elite male endurance runners and ordinary boys were found only in those 16 years old, not in 12 to 14 year olds.[414]

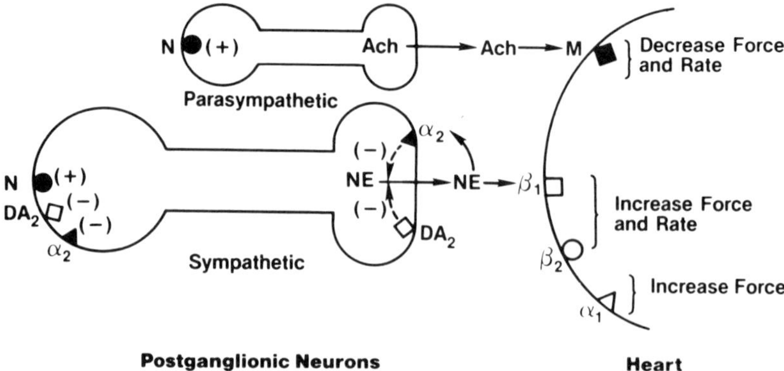

Fig. 1.17. Schematic representation of the cardiac neuroeffector junction. Shown are parasympathetic cholinergic efferent input, which inhibits rate and contractility, and sympathetic adrenergic efferent input, which enhances rate and contractility. Pre- and postsynaptic receptor types are shown. Key: α_1, alpha$_1$ adrenoceptor; α_2, alpha$_2$-adrenoceptor; β_1, beta$_1$-adrenoceptor; β_2, beta$_2$-adrenoceptor; M, muscarinic cholinergic receptor; N, nicotinic cholinergic receptor; DA_2, dopamine receptor; Ach, acetylcholine; NE, norepinephrine. (Ruffolo RR 1983 Drug, neurotransmitter and hormone receptors in the regulation of the cardiovascular system. In: Shoemaker WC, Thompson WL (eds) Critical Care: State of the Art, Vol 4. Society of Critical Care Medicine, Fullerton, CA.)

Autonomic Control of Cardiac Function

Though the heart can operate in the absence of neural control, cardiac function is normally closely regulated by the autonomic nervous system. Several recent reviews consider various aspects of this control system.[50,88,235,251,320,367] The emphasis in this section is on autonomic efferent stimulation. Integration of receptors and efferent function is considered in the section *Integrated circulatory control.*

Innervation of the heart

Sympathetic innervation The cell bodies of the part of sympathetic division of the autonomic nervous system subserving the heart lie in the upper thoracic spinal cord.[235] The short preganglionic fibers enter the paravertebral chains of ganglia bilaterally. Longer postganglionic fibers emanate from the three major cervical as well as the thoracic ganglia, and form the cardiac sympathetic nerves. These intertwine in the cardiac plexus with parasympathetic fibers before distributing ubiquitously to the cardiac tissues. Fibers from the stellate ganglia are of major importance, with those from the right side innervating primarily the right heart, especially the atrium and sino-atrial node area, and those from the left innervating the left heart, especially the ventricle.[235]

Sympathetic ganglionic neurotransmission occurs via release of acetylcholine (Ach) interacting with postsynaptic nicotinic cholinergic receptors on the postganglionic neuron.[348] This stimulates release of norepinephrine (NE) at the neuroeffector junction which, in turn, activates cardiac adrenergic receptors of the beta$_1$ type.

Recent work has demonstrated that there are a number of additional receptor types present on both postganglionic neurons and the heart itself, as shown schematically in Figure 1.17. Such receptors are characterized by their effects in response to various activators alone, or in combination with different inhibitors. The figure illustrates three kinds of adrenergic receptors found in the heart. Stimulation of the $beta_1$-adrenoceptor by neuronal NE is associated with an increase in both heart rate and contractility, an effect mediated by cyclic AMP.[48,367] Receptors in the SA node and conduction tissues promote the rate effects, while those in the atrial and ventricular myocardium produce the contractile changes.[251] Stimulation of the $alpha_1$-adrenoceptor leads to increased contractility without significant heart rate change, independent of cyclic AMP.[48,397] It has been proposed that noninnervated $beta_2$-adrenoceptors can be found at the SA node. These are activated more selectively by epinephrine (EPI) than NE.[348]

There are also a number of receptor types on the postganglionic adrenergic neuron which alter NE release.[223] Most important of these are the presynaptic autoregulatory $alpha_2$- and beta-adrenoceptors. The beta receptors, not shown in the figure, appear to facilitate NE release when stimulated by low concentrations of NE, a positive feedback mechanism.[8] The $alpha_2$ receptors exert negative feedback control by inhibiting NE release. When both are activated, the inhibitory influence predominates.[223] Also depicted are muscarinic receptors proposed to inhibit NE release when activated by Ach.[234] Other neuronal modifying receptors shown are of more pharmacologic than physiologic significance.[223]

Parasympathetic innervation The preganglionic parasympathetic neurons arise in the medulla oblongata in several areas, including the dorsal nucleus of the vagus and the nucleus ambiguus.[235] The fibers course into the thorax via the vagi and then join postganglionic sympathetic nerves during passage into or through the cardiac plexus. Ganglia occur within the heart, usually close to the structures innervated by the short postganglionic neurons. Parasympathetic nerves are distributed throughout the heart, with concentration greatest in the SA node, and diminishing in the order of AV node, right atrium, left atrium, and ventricles.[235] Both sides of the heart are subserved by fibers from both vagi, but right-sided effects predominate at the SA node, left-sided effects at the AV node.

As shown in Figure 1.17, parasympathetic neurotransmission occurs via stimulation of nicotinic cholinergic receptors on the postganglionic neuron by Ach. The consequent release of Ach at the neuroeffector junction activates cardiac muscarinic receptors. Those on the SA node, when activated, increase maximum transmembrane polarization and slow diastolic depolarization, thereby reducing heart rate.[251] Furthermore, atrioventricular conduction is slowed, and myocardial contractility is diminished. This is more significant in the atria than the ventricles.[235]

Response to autonomic stimulation

Sympathetic stimulation Stimulation of the stellate ganglia in experimental animals produces increased efflux of catecholamines from the heart, tachycardia, and enhanced contractility and ventricular function.[88,359,360] The last two are manifest by an increase in the rate of development of ventricular pressure, ejection velocity, and ejection fraction. Right stellate ganglion stimulation has the greater effect on rate; left-sided stimulation has the greater effect on contractility.[235,248]

Parasympathetic stimulation The major consequence of continuous parasympathetic stimulation is a reduction in heart rate by an amount related to the intensity of stimulation. Right vagal stimulation produces nearly twice the rate effect as the same stimulus to the left vagus.[248] Postvagal tachycardia is common, in part due to reflex baroreceptor action (see the section *Autonomic supervision*) and in part due to the Ach stimulated release of NE from chromaffin cells located in the region of the SA node.[235]

Intense vagal stimulation is associated with depression of atrial and ventricular contractility.[77] Three mechanisms have been identified: (1) stimulation of the cardiac muscarinic receptor alters the myocyte cyclic AMP level (see the section *Contractility*); (2) the Ach inhibits NE release from nearby sympathetic nerve terminals.[234]; and (3) there is a direct inhibition of adrenergic receptor activation.[235]

Parasympathetic-sympathetic interaction Interaction is suggested by the presence of sympathetic innervation of parasympathetic ganglia as well as the intimate proximity of adrenergic and cholinergic nerve terminals, even to the extent of sharing the same myelin sheath.[235]

Resting autonomic tone is present in both divisions. Their interaction is nonlinear, however, favoring the parasympathetic. That is, an increase in parasympathetic tone blunts the chronotropic effects of sympathetic stimulation; the negative chronotropy of parasympathetic stimulation is enhanced in the presence of elevated sympathetic tone.[45,247] The basis for this may be due in part to inhibition of NE release by Ach at the nerve terminal, but also appears to involve interaction at the receptor site as discussed above. This is facilitated by the close proximity of adrenergic and cholinergic nerve terminals.

Developmental aspects

Cardiac parasympathetic innervation and function in the newborn are apparently similar to those in the adult. Histochemical studies of fetal and adult sheep show no age-related differences in the density or distribution of cholinergic fibers.[119] Dose-response curves of isolated right atrial myocardium for Ach are the same for fetal and adult sheep,[119] though less effect was found for puppies than adult dogs.[428] Newborn resting vagal tone is lower than in the adult,[127] and differences in the effects of vagal stimulation between intact infant and adult hearts[247] can be explained primarily by the developmental changes in the sympathetic system and the interactions between cholinergic and adrenergic effects.

Though cardiac sympathetic nervous system function is present at birth,[89] significant postnatal development occurs in a variety of mammalian species.[88,119,121,127] Flourescent staining of NE containing tissue in fetal sheep and fetal and neonatal rabbit hearts by Friedman[119] showed large preterminal sympathetic nerve trunks with terminal varicosities which contained NE. Other studies support this paucity of sympathetic nerve fibers in the immature myocardium.[229] By contrast, the adult nerve trunks contained little NE themselves, but gave rise to a widely distributed dense network of NE containing fibers.[121]

The myocardial content of NE increases with age,[119,127] (Figure 1.18). The concentrations of myocardial enzymes associated with intraneuronal NE production and degradation also increase with age, whereas the corresponding adrenal enzymes and EPI concentrations do not.[119] Although sympathetic stimulation produces chronotropic and inotropic effects in neonates,[89] the chronotropic effect of stellate ganglion stimulation was twice as great for adult dogs as for puppies.[34]

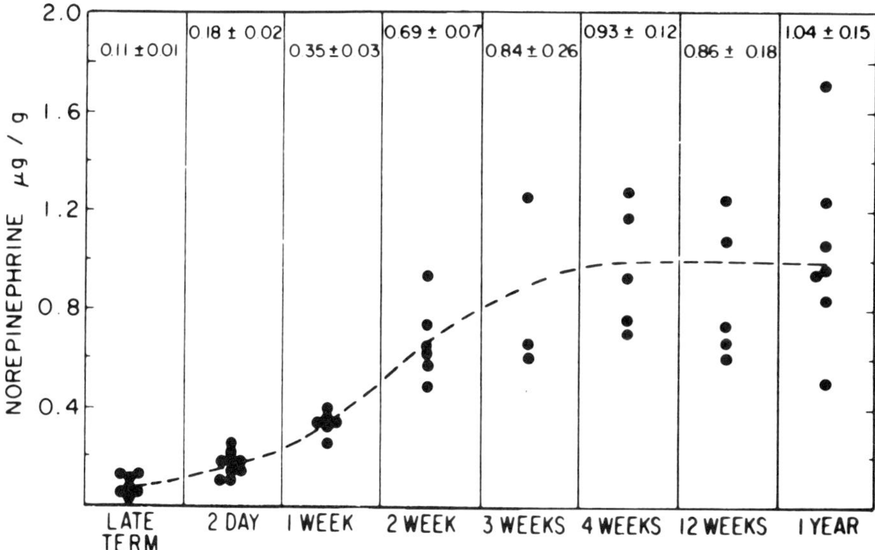

Fig. 1.18. Effect of age on myocardial norepinephrine content in rabbits. (Friedman WF, Pool PE, Jacobowitz D, Seagren BA, Braunwald E 1968 Sympathetic innervation of the developing rabbit heart—biochemical and histochemical comparisons of fetal neonatal and adult myocardium. Circulation Research 23: 25, by permission of the American Heart Association, Inc.)

Tyramine, administered to stimulate release of endogenous NE from nerve terminals, produced a similar disparity.[127] The time course shown in Figure 1.18 suggests that full innervation is achieved during later infancy, a conclusion supported by microscopic study.[229]

By contrast, cardiac adrenergic *receptors* appear to be present and fully functional before birth. The dose-response curves of myocardial tension development for isoproterenol are the same for fetal and adult sheep and are affected similarly by propranolol;[119] and yet, the neonatal cardiovascular response to exogenous NE is greater than that of older lambs[119] or adult dogs.[127] It has been suggested that this difference can be explained by the fewer sympathetic nerves available for uptake and inactivation of the NE in the newborn.[88]

Though cardiac stimulation from adrenergic nerves is limited in the young infant, circulating catecholamine levels are up to 30 times as great in the adult dog as in the newborn.[127] That this leads to a relatively elevated baseline adrenergic state is indicated by the much greater effect of propranolol on the heart rate of younger than older puppies.[458] The importance of circulating catecholamines to cardiocirculatory function is suggested by the fact that adult dogs tolerated bilateral adrenalectomy well whereas newborns suffered hypotension and cardiac slowing.[127]

Thus it appears that myocardial sympathetic innervation is incomplete at birth, and that a functional response of the infant heart involves a relatively low vagal inhibitory tone coupled with a high level of circulating catecholamines. The disparity in early postnatal cardiac sympathetic/parasympathetic development may help to explain the diminished chronotropic effects of sympathetic stimulation in the infant in the presence of parasympathetic activity.[247] The detailed time course of development to adult autonomic interactions has not been studied.

Myocardial Energetics

The heart has the unique task of supplying its own energy requirements. Because the myocardial oxygen extraction is near maximal, even at rest, the heart depends upon an efficiently regulated blood supply. Energy use of the heart in infancy is greater than either earlier or later in development, as discussed below. An overview of myocardial metabolism is in the recent review by Tripp.[424]

Myocardial oxygen consumption

The heart normally functions aerobically. Hence, its energy requirements can be assessed in terms of oxygen consumption ($M\dot{V}O_2$). The adult resting left ventricular $M\dot{V}O_2$ is approximately 8 ml/min/100 g of LV tissues,[171] about 20 times that for the entire body. Diffusion of O_2 into myocardial tissue is facilitated, probably by a myoglobin carrier.[457] Oxygen extraction is approximately 60 to 70 percent at rest, which leads to coronary sinus PO_2 of 15 to 20 mmHg with an O_2 content (C_vO_2) about 5 ml/dl,[105] similar to that for myocardial tissue.[67] Experiments with sheep have provided insight into details of myocardial energetics and how they are affected by development.

Using radioactive microspheres[166] in well-instrumented fetal lambs, 4 to 23 day old lambs, and adult sheep, Fisher et al[110] demonstrated important developmental effects shown in Table 1.3. The table indicates the expected developmental changes in arterial PO_2 and O_2 content. Heart rate increased postnatally and then diminished in the adult. Blood flow per unit weight to the whole heart was unchanged in the infant from the fetal value, but was reduced by nearly half in the adult. Of more interest was the fact that the LV blood flow was highest in the infant, whereas RV flow diminished with age.

Table 1.3. Myocardial Blood Flow and Oxygen Consumption in Resting Fetal, Infant, and Adult Sheep

		Fetus	Infant	Adult
P_aO_2 (mmHg)		24	73	90
C_aO_2 (ml/dl)		9.2	11.9	14.0
HR (beats/min)		162	210	103
Blood flow:	Hrt	145	142	77
	LVFW	162	204	106
	RVFW	213	140	62
$M\dot{V}O_2$:	Hrt	9.2	12.5	8.1
	LVFW	9.9	16.5	11.2
	RVFW	12.5	11.9	7.0

Values are means.

Oxygen consumption is computed from data of Fisher et al[108,110] using an average coronary sinus O_2 content = 3.2 ml/dl.

Blood flow and O_2 consumption units are ml/min/100 g.

Abbreviations: Hrt, entire heart; LVFW and RVFW, left and right ventricular free wall, respectively; others as in text.

In an earlier study these investigators had determined $M\dot{V}O_2$ for fetal and adult sheep.[108] They found that the coronary sinus C_vO_2 was the same for both groups. Assuming that value for all animals in the later study, their data for myocardial blood flow and oxygen delivery have been used to estimate the $M\dot{V}O_2$ values shown in the table. These results indicate that the overall $M\dot{V}O_2$ is highest for the infant. Most important however, the LV $M\dot{V}O_2$ increases by more than 50 percent from fetus to infant, and then decreases by a similar amount to the adult value. This undoubtedly reflects the myocardial adjustment to additional LV work imposed by the postnatal circulatory changes, at the same time that rapid growth to accommodate them is still occurring (see the section *Morphologic development*). Indeed, the limited capacity of the infant LV is implied by the lower O_2 consumption *per beat*, achieved at the expense of elevated total energy expenditure. Thus, as discussed in the section *Contractility*, the LV myocardium must function at an enhanced contractile state in infancy, with more limited reserve than in later life.

The fetal RV $M\dot{V}O_2$ is higher than that of the LV, consistent with the relatively greater RV output. This changes little in the infant, and then diminishes to an adult value lower than the LV $M\dot{V}O_2$. Blood flow and $M\dot{V}O_2$ of the two sides of the interventricular septum reflect the changes seen in the respective ventricular free walls.

Determinants of oxygen consumption A major focus of modern cardiovascular research has been to define and quantify the determinants of $M\dot{V}O_2$. Attention has been focussed on pressure-induced afterload of the LV as a primary determinant. Two measures of this have been employed frequently. The "tension-time index" (TTI), defined by Sarnoff et al,[358] is the area under the systolic aortic pressure curve. This is shown as the region labelled SPTI in Figure 1.19. Subsequent studies suggested that the "double product" (DP), equal to the product of systolic BP and heart rate, correlated better with $M\dot{V}O_2$ in healthy volunteers.[208,196,175]

More recent careful evaluations of the components of $M\dot{V}O_2$ have demonstrated that solely pressure-related parameters do not adequately account for the effects of external work or changes in contractility.[130,434] These are, however, incorporated in the general time-varying elastance model of the ventricle developed by Suga.[405] It was found that the myocardial O_2 consumption *per beat* could be predicted by the "pressure-volume area" (PVA), defined by the stippled region in Figure 1.20A. The PVA has been shown to predict $M\dot{V}O_2$ per beat for a wide variety of experimental conditions independent of pressure- *versus* volume-loading conditions[406,407,408,409,435] or heart rate.[410]

This concept helps to clarify the observation that pressure-loading increases $M\dot{V}O_2$ much more than volume-loading. Illustrated in Figure 1.20 are experiments performed by Suga et al.[409] Figure 1.20A shows the P-V loop for a control experiment using an isolated left ventricle. Stroke work was increased either by increasing stroke volume (Figure 1.20B) or ejection pressure (Fig. 1.20C). Though the increment in stroke work was slightly less for pressure-loading than volume-loading, the increments in both PVA and $M\dot{V}O_2$ were three times as great. Data from other investigators show similar results.[442] Thus, for a given set of loading conditions and contractility, the PVA can be used to assess their impact on myocardial oxygen consumption and the internal criteria by which cardiac function is regulated.

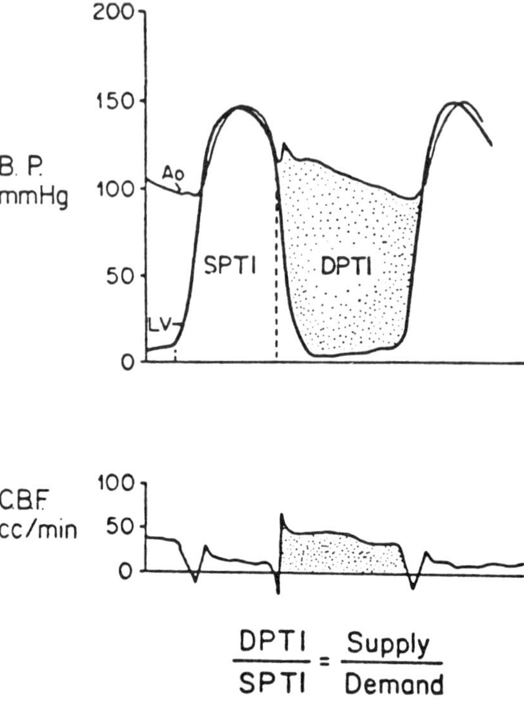

$$\frac{\text{DPTI}}{\text{SPTI}} = \frac{\text{Supply}}{\text{Demand}}$$

Fig. 1.19. Illustration of the systolic and diastolic pressure-time index ratio as a measure of the ratio of myocardial oxygen supply to demand. The upper panel shows the definitions of the systolic pressure-time index (SPTI), equal to the TTI, and diastolic pressure-time index (DPTI). The lower panel shows the coronary arterial blood flow during the phases of the cardiac cycle. The equation at the bottom of the figure suggests that the ratio of DPTI to SPTI represents a measure of the ratio of myocardial oxygen supply to demand. (Vincent WR, Buckberg GD, Hoffman JIE 1974 Left ventricular subendocardial ischemia in severe valvar and supravalvar aortic stenosis. A common mechanism. Circulation 49: 326, by permission of the American Heart Association, Inc.)

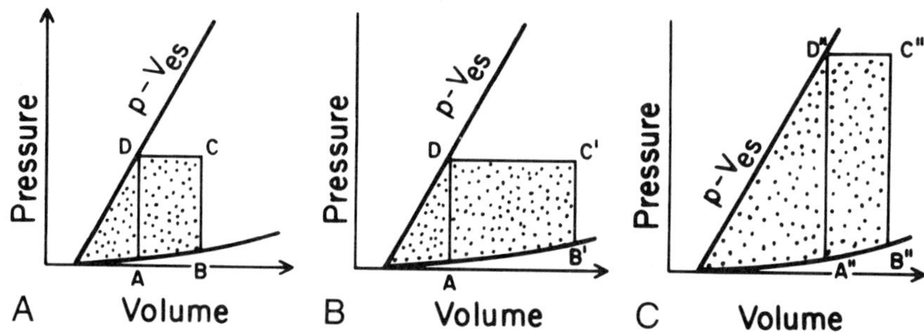

Fig. 1.20. Pressure-volume area (PVA) proposed by Suga[405] as a measure of myocardial oxygen consumption. The PVA is the stippled region bounded by the end-systolic P-V line, the end-diastolic P-V curve, and the P-V trace during systole. The graphs show data on isolated canine hearts from (Suga H, Hisano R, Hirata S, Hayashi T, Ninomiya I 1982 Mechanism of higher oxygen consumption rate: Pressure-loaded vs. volume-loaded heart. American Journal of Physiology 11: 942.) (A) Control P-V loop: PVA/beat = 805 ± 210 mmHg ml. (B) Increased stroke work with stroke volume = 2 × control, end-systolic pressure = control: PVA/beat = 1170 ± 246 mmHg ml. (C) Increased stroke work with stroke volume = control, end-systolic pressure = 1.7 × control: PVA/beat = 1854 ± 305 mmHg ml.

Distribution of myocardial oxygen consumption Circumferential wall tension is greatest at the inner surface and diminishes to a minimum at the outside.[270] Subendocardial tissue PO_2 is generally less than that of the subepicardium, despite the fact that blood flow to the inner layers is about 10 percent greater than to the outer tissues.[105] Anaerobic metabolic products accumulate more rapidly in the subendocardium when coronary flow is stopped abruptly.[93] These all suggest that the $M\dot{V}O_2$ is greatest in subendocardial tissue, placing it at increased risk of adverse effects from circulatory impairment. This is considered further in the next section.

Myocardial oxygen supply: the coronary circulation

More than for any other organ, the oxygen supply to the heart must continually match the demand. This occurs primarily by adjustment of blood supplied via the coronary circulation. Recent reviews discuss various aspects of the subject.[29,457,209,305,402]

Structural features Vascular tissue occupies about 14 percent of myocardial volume throughout life.[229] However, the structure of the coronary arteries changes continuously, from before birth through adult life.[293] In addition to lumen and medial enlargement, the intima thickens and develops fibrotic changes throughout infancy, childhood and adolescence. The inner elastic membrane, between the intima and media, undergoes the most striking changes. Near birth the homogenous circumferential layer develops localized splits which fill with infiltrating longitudinally oriented muscle fibers. This process continues until by the end of adolescence the entire layer has become a complex "musculo-elastic" structure nearly as thick as the media.[293]

The adult anatomic distribution of coronary vessels is present at birth. The epicardial arteries give rise to perpendicular branches of two types:[99] the first branch early into a fine network of arterioles which subserves the outer ¾ to ⅘ of the myocardium; the second are fewer in number, branch rarely, and reach the inner myocardium without a reduction in size. In the subendocardium the latter vessels subdivide and anastomose freely, thus forming a plexus supplied by multiple vessels. The endocardial plexus vessels are smaller in young children than adults.

The myocardial capillary lumen appears to develop by liquifaction of endothelial cell cytoplasm, both before and after birth.[229] The walls of the capillaries thin to adult proportions in the neonatal period.

Coronary flow Coronary blood flow is highly regulated; under ordinary circumstances the rate is directly proportional to $M\dot{V}O_2$.[29,208] The normal adult LV flow of approximately 80 ml/min/100 g can increase more than four times with heavy exercise.[171,175,208] Resting flow in the infant lamb is nearly twice that in the adult sheep (Table 1.3). Reduction in arterial O_2 content by hypoxemia[4,29,227] or anemia[56] leads to an increase in resting flow rate, such that coronary O_2 delivery continues to satisfy the myocardial demands.

The regulation of flow occurs by continual adjustment of vessel diameter and thereby the *resistance* to flow. A nearly constant flow rate consistent with the $M\dot{V}O_2$ is maintained, despite changes in aortic pressure over a wide range,[342] as illustrated in Figure 1.21. Each curved line in the figure corresponds to a specific $M\dot{V}O_2$.

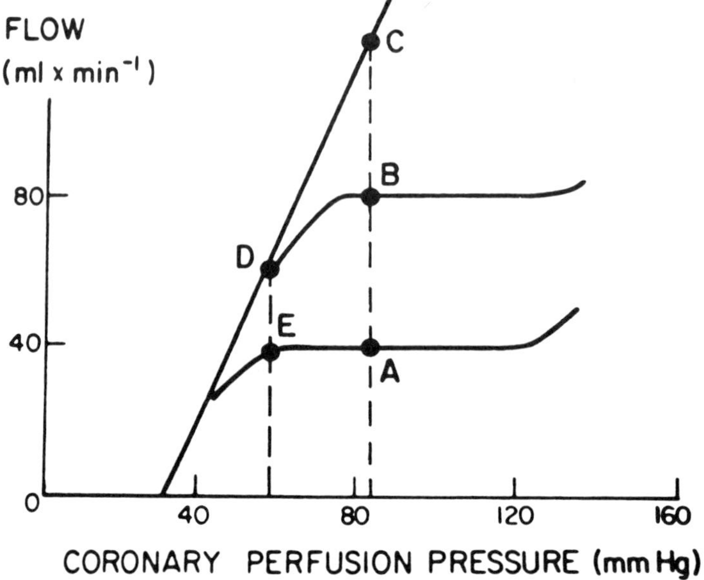

Fig. 1.21. Coronary artery pressure-flow diagram illustrating the concept of autoregulation. See text for details. (Hoffman JIE 1978 Determinants and prediction of transmural myocardial perfusion. Circulation 58: 381, by permission of the American Heart Association, Inc.)

Thus, for example, the lower curve indicates that for an aortic pressure from approximately 60 to 120 mmHg, the coronary vessel size changes to maintain a constant flow rate. At higher pressures this *autoregulation* is overcome by pressure-induced distension and the flow becomes pressure-dependent. At lower pressures, when the vessel is fully dilated, the flow again becomes pressure-dependent. This is shown by the straight inclined line which indicates the pressure-related flow for the fully dilated arteries. An increase in $M\dot{V}O_2$ induces an increased flow rate at which autoregulation occurs, indicated by the upper curve in the figure. At a given point, such as point A on the autoregulated curve, the *coronary reserve* can be visualized as the vertical distance AC to the pressure-flow line for fully dilated arteries, that is, the additional flow that can be achieved by vasodilatation at the given coronary pressure. This is a measure of the additional $M\dot{V}O_2$ which can be accommodated at that perfusion pressure, or the reduction in perfusion pressure that can be tolerated without ischemia. The coronary reserve BC for the upper curve with higher flow rate is less than for the lower curve.

The figure also demonstrates that there is a minimum coronary pressure required to initiate flow. The magnitude of this "zero-flow pressure" (P_{zf}) has been found by various investigators to be in the range of 12 to 50 mmHg.[105,302] Hypotheses for the etiology of the P_{zf} have included the magnitude of intracavitary backpressure, and the collapse of intramyocardial coronary microvessels when tissue pressures exceed intraluminal pressure.[171,427] LV myocardial tissue pressure has been measured at different locations throughout the cardiac cycle;[105] it approaches the chamber pressure near the endocardium and diminishes toward the epicardium to a magnitude of probably less than 30 percent of the chamber pressure.[19] Thus, neither hypothesis explains the P_{zf} seen during diastole, and the issue remains unresolved. The relationship of P_{zf} to the "critical closing pressure" seen in peripheral arteries (see the section *Functional description of the blood vessels*) is not defined.

Control of coronary flow Control of coronary blood flow is multifactorial and, despite major efforts to elucidate the factors, key aspects are not yet understood. At least two major mechanisms appear to be operative. The first, and probably most significant, is local vasodilatation induced by one or more tissue metabolites.[29,105,300,402,453] This conclusion is supported both by the relationship between coronary flow and $M\dot{V}O_2$, and the hyperemic response seen following temporary coronary artery occlusion.[299] Unfortunately, no single agent mediating the metabolic control has been identified. Currently, the preponderance of evidence supports adenosine as the major mediator.[28,29,300,453] As the product of dephosphorylation of AMP, adenosine production is related to the myocardial metabolic rate. Many experiments have shown it to be a powerful coronary vasodilator, but its physiologic role is still is not demonstrated unequivocally.[105] Other candidate agents include oxygen itself, CO_2, and prostacyclin (PGI_2). A role for these in normal coronary artery physiology has not yet been shown.[105,448]

The second modulator of coronary blood flow is neural control. Autonomic effects on cardiac circulation occur in response to a variety of reflex mechanisms discussed in the section *Autonomic supervision*. There are, however, complex interactions between the direct effects of autonomic stimulation on the coronary vessels and the reactive vascular response to the myocardial effects. This complexity has inhibited development of the detailed understanding of the coronary artery neuroeffector junction which has evolved for the vessels of systemic circulation (see the section *Control of vessel caliber*).

The smaller coronary arteries are innervated by both sympathetic and parasympathetic systems down to the precapillary level.[29,105,402] Parasympathetic stimulation activates coronary arterial muscarinic receptors which induce dilatation directly.[105] Sympathetic stimulation in the normal individual elicits coronary dilatation. This results from the effects of increased $M\dot{V}O_2$ overriding the constriction induced by direct stimulation of alpha$_1$-adrenoceptors on the arterioles.[105,305] There is, however, a basal sympathetic tone in the coronary arteries which modulates the response to local metabolic factors.[402] The innervation of coronary vessels matures earlier than that of the myocardium.[119] Noninnervated beta$_2$-adrenoceptors are also present; when stimulated they produce vasodilatation and may play a role in metabolic regulation of flow.[29,457]

A myogenic mechanism for autoregulation analogous to that present in systemic arterioles (see the section *Vascular smooth muscle*) has been proposed for the coronary vessels. Though a myogenic effect may play a role in reactive hyperemia,[299] it has been difficult to identify whether or not it is part of the normal regulatory response.[105,209]

Distribution of oxygen supply In order to match the nonuniform tissue distribution of $M\dot{V}O_2$, the O_2 supply increases from subepicardium to subendocardium.[105] In the autoregulated range of coronary pressure, the absolute and relative flows to individual layers of myocardium stay constant. As coronary pressure diminishes, maximum arterial dilatation occurs earliest in the inner tissues. Autoregulation is lost there while still preserved in the outer layers.[339] This concept is illustrated in Figure 1.21 in which the upper curve represents flow in subendocardial tissue for which coronary perfusion pressure at point D is not sufficient to maintain autoregulation, even though adequate for autoregulated flow in the subepicardium (point E on the lower curve). This regional disadvantage is partially compensated by greater vasodilatory capacity in the subendocardium.[209]

Another major effect on LV subendocardial O_2 supply is that produced by tissue pressure during systole. This is indicated in Figure 1.19B which shows that left coronary blood flow is markedly diminished during systole, even reversing early in the cycle. A compensatory increase occurs during diastole, so that approximately 70 to 85 percent of total LV flow is diastolic.[172] The distribution of this proportion varies from the interior where tissue pressure is high and little or no systolic flow occurs, to the exterior where there is some flow in systole.[172] By contrast, tissue pressures are much lower in the RV and perfusion there varies relatively little throughout the cardiac cycle.[106]

The implication of these observations is that subendocardial tissues are the most susceptible to ischemic injury due to a potential imbalance between their higher O_2 demand and lower supply reserve. Indeed, in both adults and children, ischemia tends to occur earliest in the subendocardium in response to either elevated $M\dot{V}O_2$ or diminished coronary perfusion.[98,172,236]

An approach to estimating the circumstances under which the subendocardium is at risk for ischemia is based on the assumptions that all subendocardial perfusion occurs during diastole, and that the subepicardium continues to be adequately perfused as subendocardial vasodilatory reserve is exhausted leading to the onset of ischemia there.[171,172] Thus subendocardial perfusion would be adequate, provided that the ratio of subendocardial to subepicardial flow (inner:outer or I:O ratio) were unchanged from its normal value of 1.1 to 1.2.[172] It has been shown that the I:O ratio could be related to an approximate estimate of the ratio of O_2 supply to demand.[171] The O_2 demand was assumed to be related to the TTI (Fig. 1.19A). The blood flow was assumed to be related to the perfusion gradient and time available for flow during diastole, as represented by the stippled area in Figure 1.19A, termed the *diastolic pressure time index* (DPTI). Despite the questionable validity of either of these measures independently, the "myocardial oxygen supply:demand ratio" ($C_aO_2 \times$ DPTI/TTI) has been successfully correlated with the I:O ratio. A myocardial oxygen supply:demand ratio less than 8 to 10 is associated with I:O ratios less than 1.0 in animal experiments,[172] and with subendocardial ischemia in adult and pediatric patients.[236,433] The pressure-loaded hypertrophied myocardium, as in aortic stenosis, is especially at risk for subendocardial ischemia.[179,236,433]

There is no direct information about the role of development in the distribution of blood supply within the myocardial wall. Studies of the response to hypoxia suggest that the coronary reserve in early infancy is similar to that later in life (see the section *Adaptation to altered oxygen supply/demand*).

Myocardial energy supply: substrate

Carbohydrates and lipids are the substrates for myocardial metabolism. Key aspects of substrate utilization and its developmental changes have been reviewed.[290,291,321,424,464] Fatty acids (FA) are the preferred substrates in normal aerobic function of the mature heart,[464] accounting for 60 to 70 percent of the energy supply.[291] The rate of fat utilization depends on both plasma concentration of FA and the energy demands of the myocytes. The in vivo intracellular rate-controlling steps are not completely defined, but differ at low and high exogenous FA concentrations.[291] Carnitine is essential to the use of fat as a substrate; it transports the acyl portion of the FA from cytosol to mitochondrion where oxidation occurs.[321] Deficiency of this vital enzyme results in myocardial dysfunction in infancy and childhood.[424,425]

The relative consumption of fats and carbohydrates is regulated in part by the dehydrogenase reaction in the citric acid cycle, as well as inhibition by FA's of several steps in glucose uptake and glycolysis.[290]

This picture contrasts sharply with the almost exclusive dependence of the fetus on carbohydrates for energy.[108] After birth there is a rapid two- to three-fold increase in activity of myocardial enzymes involved in FA metabolism,[441] with a concomitant decline in those for glycolysis.[25] Adult values are found during infancy in several species. Mitochondrial mass also doubles during this time, reflecting the increased reliance on oxidative metabolism.[263]

Adaptation to altered oxygen supply/demand

Distributional and other adaptations of the circulatory system to changes in O_2 supply and demand are considered in the section *Circulatory reserve*. Only the effects on cardiac performance are discussed here.

Increased demand—exercise The acute effect of exercise on the heart is to increase the required cardiac output and thereby the $M\dot{V}O_2$. The stimulus for the change in cardiac function appears to be both reduction in parasympathetic and increase in sympathetic signals.[432] Tachycardia occurs almost immediately at the onset of exercise, mediated by central inhibition of vagal tone.

Cardiac output increases more than 4 times in maximal exercise in humans[432] and 5 times in dogs.[431] In adults, this is achieved by increasing stroke volume about 1.5 times and heart rate about 3 times, though changes in stroke volume may be smaller at submaximal exertion.[336,432] Enhanced contractility plays a major role in maintaining or increasing stroke volume despite a shorter cycle time and elevated blood pressure.[185] That is, inducing tachycardia in normal individuals by atrial pacing alone does not alter cardiac output.[336] The essential changes in contractility are mediated by sympathetic stimulation, as demonstrated by the diminished heart rate and cardiac output in exercising dogs given propranolol.[431] The role of increased preload is minimal.[432]

Coronary blood flow increases with workload,[402] but flow redistributes somewhat, away from the subendocardium. Coronary vasodilator reserve is not exhausted however, even at maximal exercise, and the myocardial oxygen supply:demand ratio is adequate to prevent subendocardial ischemia in the normal heart.[23]

Required increases in cardiac output of infants, whatever the cause, are met largely by changes in heart rate.[344] The effect of the associated enhanced contractility is more rapid ejection with maintenance of SV. Prepubertal boys also exhibit little or no SV change at submaximal exercise.[24,245] Their adaptation is by a combination of elevated heart rate and oxygen extraction. As maximal exercise levels are approached, their heart rate increases to about 200 per minute.[245] The peak heart rate of young men is approximately 185 to 190 per minute,[37] associated with elevated stroke volume and oxygen extraction.[24] Maximal heart rate data on male adolescents demonstrate the expected transition.[414] Older prepubertal and early pubertal girls exhibit somewhat greater exercise induced changes in SV and less in oxygen extraction, similar to adult women.[24]

Adaptation of the heart to endurance training is similar to the physiologic response to chronic volume loading (see the section *Afterload*). In adults, there is a modest increase in heart size, mass, and diastolic chamber size.[37,675] These changes may occur over a few weeks.[83] Training induced enhancement of diastolic filling and stroke volume is even more significant during exercise that at rest.[329] Changes in wall thickness are small, but sufficient to maintain the normal wall to chamber ratio (see the section *Cardiac growth*). The concentric hypertrophy characteristic of isometric exercise such as weight lifting corresponds more to the physiologic response to pressure loading (see the section *Afterload*).

Many studies have attempted to document the role of altered myocardial contractility in the adaptations to endurance training from mechanical, ultrastructural, and biochemical perspectives. Studies of contractile function of muscle strips as well as isolated and in vivo hearts have produced conflicting results. Synthesis of these suggest that there is no major alteration in contractility, despite somewhat enhanced ejection rates.[37,85,363] Biochemical changes have also been difficult to document. Total contractile protein activity is not altered, though individual myosin and actomyosin ATPase activity is elevated.[85] A number of experiments suggest that calcium transport at both sarcolemmal and sarcoplasmic reticulum levels may be improved.[85] Aerobic capacity is clearly enhanced, as evidenced both by the increased density of mitochondria and the enlarged coronary vascular bed.[85] The latter occurs via increased numbers of capillaries[37] and enlargement of the coronary arteries.[216]

Resting bradycardia is characteristic of the trained individual, associated with both elevated vagal tone and diminished sympathetic tone. Heart rate at any given submaximal proportion of peak exercise is less after training than before.[37,363] Most effects of training, including moderate changes in heart size, are reversible upon cessation of regular exercise.[83] Growth of supporting tissues and coronary vessels during long-term endurance training may persist.[363]

Most studies on prepubertal children suggest that they do not exhibit changes in heart chamber size,[12,126,414] resting[126,414] or maximal[245,414] heart rate in response to endurance training, even with intensive regimens. Heart rates at submaximal exercise levels are lower after training, however.[126,245] Adolescents exhibit cardiac responses to training similar to adults.[414]

The major circulatory adjustments to endurance training are discussed in the section *Circulatory reserve*.

Reduced supply The normal delivery of O_2 to the heart can be impaired by any or a combination of three mechanisms: (1) *hypoxemia,* in which the O_2 content of the blood is reduced either by low arterial partial pressure of oxygen (P_aO_2), or impairment of oxygen carrying by hemoglobin (for example by carbon monoxide); (2) *anemia,* in which a low hemoglobin content reduces the O_2 carrying capacity of the blood; and (3) *ischemia,* in which insufficient blood supply diminishes tissue

O_2 availability irrespective of the blood O_2 content. The heart responds differently to each of these challenges.

Acute hypoxemia evokes a response which depends upon the combined effects of perfusion pressure, hemoglobin content, pH, and other factors. As P_aO_2 falls at normal pH, myocardial O_2 extraction increases until the coronary sinus PO_2 reaches a critical level of 20 mmHg, corresponding approximately to an O_2 content of 5.5 ml/dl.[29] Further hypoxemia leads to increased coronary blood flow, produced by a combination of capillary recruitment and arterial dilatation, with maintenance of tissue and coronary sinus PO_2.[105] When P_aO_2 drops to 30 to 35 mmHg in mature animals, tissue and coronary sinus PO_2 fall, despite the elevated coronary arterial flow. This may be associated with tissue lactate production.[67] Acidosis augments the hypoxia-induced increase in coronary flow.[227] Qualitatively similar increases in myocardial blood flow are seen in mature[4] and immature[68,109,227] hearts.

Acute hypoxemia induces a reactive increase in cardiac output (see the section *Circulatory reserve*), mediated in part by sympathetic efferent stimulation.[87] This occurs without impairment of ventricular performance until P_aO_2 falls to about 25 to 30 mmHg, provided pH is near normal.[68,87,90,91,227] Hypoxia and acidosis combine to depress myocardial function, probably due to the reduced affinity of hemoglobin for oxygen, leading to diminished O_2 delivery.[91,109,111] The immature heart withstands acute severe hypoxemia better than the mature heart, with a gradation from early fetus to later fetus to newborn to adult.[76] Although the mitochondria of immature hearts demonstrate increased aerobic capacity,[120] the major factor is the superior capacity of the immature myocardium for anaerobic glycolysis. This has been inferred from the fact that fetal and newborn animals survive anoxia longer than adults, and that survival time is linearly correlated with the myocardial carbohydrate concentration.[76] Direct measurements have correlated greater glycolytic activity[122] and maintainance of high-energy phosphate compounds[190] with the superior mechanical performance[191] of immature cardiac muscle strips during severe hypoxia.

Chronic hypoxia, such as at high altitude, is associated with a number of circulatory adjustments (see the sections *Circulatory reserve* and *Response to chronic hypoxia*). Adaptation of the heart depends upon whether acclimatization has occurred during development, or during adulthood. Left ventricular function, including stroke volume, heart rate, coronary blood flow, and maximal work capacity, are no different in high-altitude natives than in those raised at sea level.[123] This is due in part to higher hemoglobin concentrations at high altitude, as well as greater oxygen extraction permitted by an elevated erythrocyte concentration of 2,3-diphosphoglycerate (2,3-DPG).[231] These same mechanisms operate when chronic hypoxemia is due to cyanotic congenital heart disease.[242]

Acclimatization to high altitude hypoxia is less effective in the mature individual than during development. Differences include diminished work capacity[123] and lower stroke volume with higher heart rate at high levels of exercise work.[151]

Acute normovolemic anemia stimulates increased cardiac output with maintenance of tissue O_2 delivery.[104] In experimental animals a reduction of hematocrit to 10 to 20 is associated with resting coronary blood flow up to four times normal, unchanged $M\dot{V}O_2$, and a normal myocardial O_2 extraction ratio.[107,210] These are due largely to the combination of coronary vasodilatation and diminished blood viscosity.[104,218] Limitation in attainment of the normal ventricular function curves may occur when the coronary vessels are maximally dilated, and can be corrected in experiments by artificially increasing coronary blood flow.[56]

Chronic anemia is associated with similar increases in cardiac output and coronary blood flow, but these occur somewhat differently than in acute hemodilution. In experimental animals and patients with hematocrits as low as approximately 15, the heart rate is no different than the controls, and the increased cardiac output is mediated entirely by elevated stroke volume.[114,233] Other features of chronic anemia in experimental animals include increased heart to body weight ratio, unchanged $M\dot{V}O_2$, peak systolic stress and myocardial contractility, modestly elevated O_2 extraction ratio, and increased vascularity of the coronary circulation.[233,362] The mechanisms underlying these changes are only partly understood; recent evidence suggests that a humoral, noncatecholamine agent present in the serum of anemic patients may be responsible for a chronically enhanced contractile state.[114]

When anemia is sufficiently severe, i.e., hemoglobin less than 3.8 g/dl, heart rate and stroke volume both increase to contribute to the elevated cardiac output.[72] Exchange transfusion to normal hemoglobin levels normalizes the resting cardiac function and hemodynamics.[72]

Consideration of myocardial ischemia is beyond the scope of this chapter.

INTEGRATED SYSTEMIC CIRCULATORY FUNCTION

Components of the Systemic Circulation

The blood and vessels of the systemic circulation comprise the delivery system for the cardiac output. This transport function, illustrated in Figure 1.4, is highly regulated to meet the metabolic needs of individual tissues as well as those of the entire body. Figure 1.22 shows some important features of this system. The graph indicates the resting blood flow per unit weight to various organs (hatched areas) and the reserve flow capacity when the supplying vessels are maximally dilated (clear areas). The table shows the total tissue flows at rest and their proportion of cardiac output in a normal adult. The importance of regulated distribution is demonstrated by the unsupportable magnitude of required cardiac output if all tissue beds were simultaneously fully dilated. The actual distribution of organ flow with maximal exercise is also given. The combined mechanisms of circulatory control promote the necessary increase in cardiac output, and direct most of it to the exercising muscles. Other features are discussed below.

By necessity, only selected aspects of the circulation are considered. However, several comprehensive treatises[1,55,115,155,265] as well as more concise summaries[45,376] are available. Recent developments have been reviewed in depth in the *Handbook of Physiology*.[38,328,375]

General principles

Vascular resistance As shown schematically in Figure 1.4, the systemic cardiac output is the sum of the blood flows to the individual tissues, determined by the potential energy gradient across the tissue and its impedance to flow. This rela-

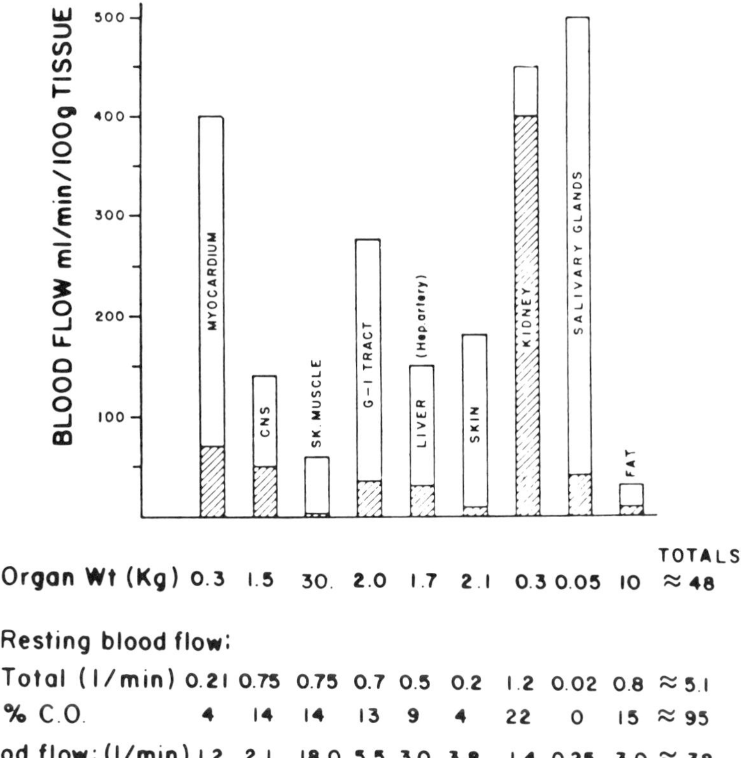

	Myocardium	CNS	Sk. muscle	G-I tract	Liver	Skin	Kidney	Salivary glands	Fat	TOTALS
Organ Wt (Kg)	0.3	1.5	30.	2.0	1.7	2.1	0.3	0.05	10	≈ 48
Resting blood flow:										
Total (l/min)	0.21	0.75	0.75	0.7	0.5	0.2	1.2	0.02	0.8	≈ 5.1
% C.O.	4	14	14	13	9	4	22	0	15	≈ 95
Max blood flow: (l/min)	1.2	2.1	18.0	5.5	3.0	3.8	1.4	0.25	3.0	≈ 38
Exercise blood flow:										
Total (l/min)	1.0	0.75	18.0	0.7	0.5	3.0	0.75	0.02	0.5	≈ 25
% C.O.	4	3	72	3	2	1.2	3	0	2	≈ 100

Fig. 1.22. Blood flows in various organs. The graph shows approximate normal resting flow/100 g of tissue (hatched area) and the corresponding flow when maximally vasodilated with a perfusion pressure of 100 mmHg (total area). The table indicates the total organ flow and its proportion of cardiac output at rest and exercise for a normal 70 kg man. The individual maximal total organ flows are shown for comparison. (Modified from Mellander S, Johansson B 1968 Control of resistance, exchange and capacitance functions in the peripheral circulation. Pharmacological Reviews 20: 117, © Am Soc Pharmacol & Exp Therapeutics, with additional data from Folkow and Neil.[115])

tionship is usefully approximated by the Poiseuille equation for steady laminar flow in a horizontal rigid circular tube[260]:

$$Q = \frac{\pi r^4 \Delta p}{8L\eta} \tag{6}$$

in which Q is the flow rate through the tube, r is the tube radius, L is the tube length, η is the viscosity of the fluid, and Δp is the mean pressure drop along the tube length. The resistance to flow, R, can then be defined as:

$$R = \frac{8L\eta}{\pi R^4} \tag{7}$$

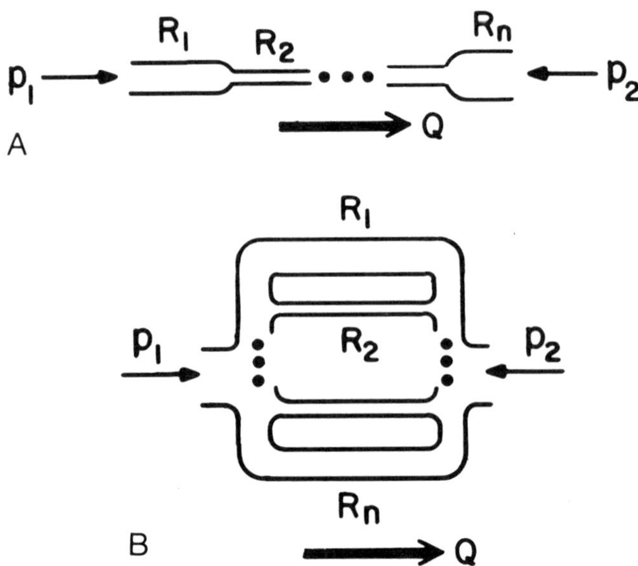

Fig. 1.23. Illustrative arrangement of flow resistances. (A) In series, (B) in parallel.

The dependence on the fourth power of the radius makes it apparent why flow through small vessels is sensitive to minute changes in their caliber.

When n vessels of varying resistance are connected in series (Fig. 1.23A) the flow through the circuit can be described in terms of an equivalent total resistance, R_{total}:

$$Q = \frac{\Delta p}{R_{total}} \tag{8}$$

in which R_{total} is the sum of the resistances:

$$R_{total} = R_1 + R_2 + \cdots + R_n \tag{9}$$

This expression demonstrates that one sufficiently high resistance can be the major determinant of the resistance of the entire circuit. Furthermore, the resistance of the group increases as the number of resistance elements increases.

A parallel arrangement of n vessels (Figure 1.23B) leads to an equivalent total resistance determined by:

$$\frac{1}{R_{total}} = \frac{1}{R_1} + \frac{1}{R_2} + \cdots + \frac{1}{R_n} \tag{10}$$

The equation illustrates how one resistance much lower than the others has a major impact on determining the R_{total}. Conversely, one resistance much higher than the others has little effect on the total flow. The other key point is that for parallel vessels with nearly equal individual resistances, the total resistance is inversely proportional to the number of vessels. The significance of this to circulatory control is considered below.

Blood flow in individual vessels is a dynamic process, varying continuously in a manner quite different from the simple steady-state assumptions leading to Equations 6 through 8. Features affecting flow in smaller resistance vessels include the interactions of vessel size,[125] hematocrit,[456,466] flow rate,[60] and the intermittent obstruction of capillaries by leukocytes.[60] Despite these complexities, direct measurement of microcirculatory flow indicate that the ratio of flow to pressure drop (R_{total}) is inversely proportional to r^4.[240]

Vascular capacitance Capacitance may be described as the volume change of a vascular bed consequent upon a unit change in transmural pressure, that is, the slope of a pressure-volume curve (cf. the diastolic ventricular pressure-volume relation, Fig. 1.8). In the case of blood vessels, complexities in the relationship due to venous collapse at low pressures, changes in vascular smooth muscle tone, and the effects of supporting tissues have made unique definition difficult.[82,338] Nonetheless, the storage function of the vascular system is essential to provide moment-to-moment adjustments to preload of the heart in response to acute alterations in *distribution* of intravascular volume, such as those induced by standing upright, as well as to compensate for volume *changes* due, for example, to hemorrhage or dehydration.[136,157,376] This is also discussed further below.

Functional description of the blood vessels

The systemic circulation consists of parallel-coupled vascular beds subserving the organs and tissues. Within each organ are series-coupled vascular sections, each more or less functionally distinct, comprised of vessels with composition and characteristics suited to their function.[115,265]

Windkessel vessels These are the distensible elastic vessels which damp the pulsatile output of the ventricle, so named for the air-filled compression chamber of eighteenth century fire engines.[292] These arteries include the aorta and its large to medium muscular branches. The approximate size and composition of the vessel walls are shown in Figure 1.24. The preponderance of elastic tissue in the aorta, largely in the medial layer,[330] implies its compliant and conductive function. This is illustrated schematically in Figure 1.25, which shows the pressure profile along the functionally differentiated vascular sections, and the maintenance of diastolic pressure with minimal resistance-induced pressure drop (Equation 8). By contrast, the large to medium muscular arteries contain most of their elastin in the internal and external elastic laminae, with the media consisting primarily of helically arranged smooth muscle cells.[330] Though they offer minimal resistance under normal circumstances, they can constrict to reduce flow to a small fraction of normal in response to severe hemorrhage[136] or the diving reflex.[36]

The pulsatile flow in these arteries is influenced by the nonlinear, time-dependent mechanical properties of the distensible walls as well as the blood itself.[82,220] Among the observed consequences is the typical change in pressure-pulse wave form from more distensible central arteries to the stiffer distal arteries (Fig. 1.26). The tracings illustrate the delay in onset of the pulse, the increased peak pressure, and the exaggeration of the dicrotic notch as the wave travels distally. Impedance analysis shows that these changes in pressure form are due to wave reflections from the less compliant distal vessels.[55,136,260]

Precapillary resistance vessels Changes in caliber of these highly muscular vessels exercise the major control over the magnitude and distribution of flow both to and

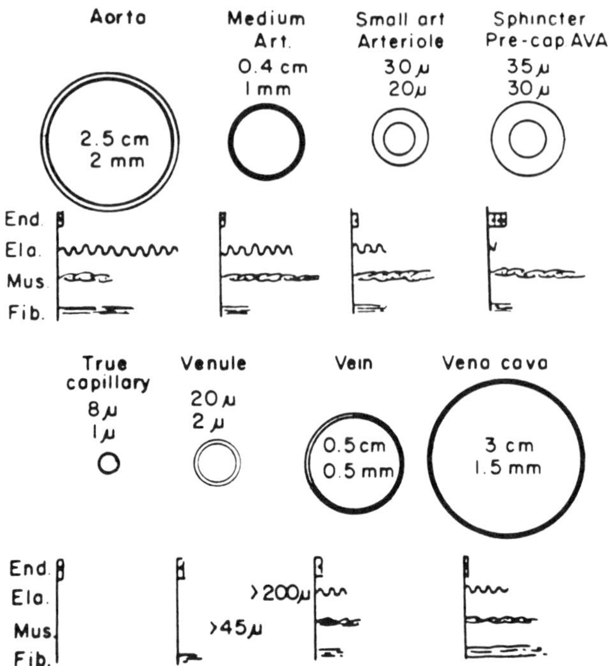

Fig. 1.24. Size and approximate composition of the wall of different blood vessels. The upper number below the name of the vessel is the lumen diameter; the lower number is the wall thickness. Abbreviations: End., endothelium; Ela., elastin; Mus., smooth muscle; Fib., fibrous connective tissue (collagen). The length of the symbol for each component corresponds to its proportion of the total thickness. (Burton AC 1951 On the physical equilibrium of small blood vessels. American Journal of Physiology 164: 319.)

within the individual organs.[265] Small arteries and arterioles (Fig. 1.24) are the chief resistance vessels at rest, providing more than 60 percent of the total vascular resistance (Fig. 1.25).[338,450] As these vessels proceed distally and become smaller, the elastic and collagen proportions diminish. The small arteries have 3 to 6 layers of smooth muscle cells arranged in helical patterns with varying pitch. Arterioles have 1 to 2 such layers.[330] Caliber changes in these vessels occur in part passively, due to alterations of transmural pressure, but primarily due to active smooth muscle constriction and relaxation. The change in diameter from full relaxation to maximal constriction may be as much as 50 to 75 percent,[136] inducing a 16 to 256 times increase in resistance.

Experimentally determined pressure-flow curves for individual organs demonstrate cessation of flow at a pressure gradient greater than zero. This has been attributed to "critical closure" as a consequence of the Laplace law,[53] but more likely is a consequence of the effect of the helical arrangement of muscle cells in the medial layer.[11]

The precapillary sphincters are probably the most distal muscular part of the terminal arteriole,[450] with smooth muscle arranged as circular rings around the vessel.[330] Their major function is to modify the number and location of perfused capillaries within the tissue at any moment.[115,265]

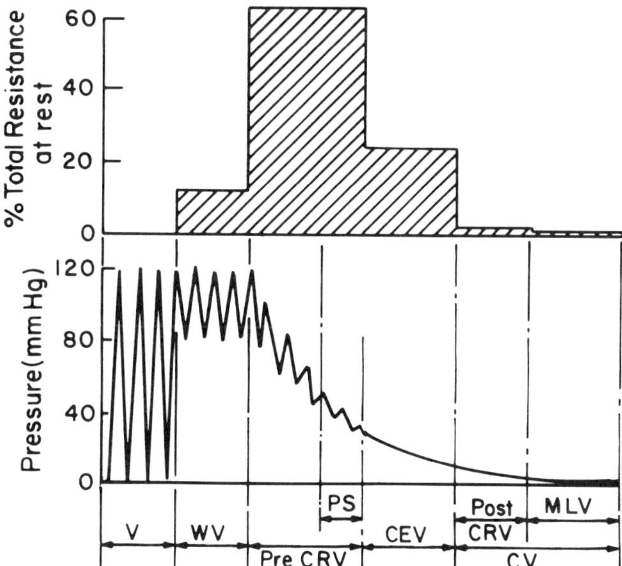

Fig. 1.25. Schematic pressure profile and approximate vascular resistance along the functionally differentiated consecutive sections of the systemic circulation. The vascular resistance shown in the upper panel is the resistance of the vessels of each type as a percentage of the total systemic vascular resistance. Symbols are: V, ventricle; WV, windkessel vessels comprising the aorta and large to medium arteries; Pre CRV, precapillary resistance vessels including small arteries, arterioles, and precapillary sphincters (PS); CEV, capillary exchange vessels; Post CRV, post-capillary resistance vessels including the postcapillary venules and small veins; MLV, medium-to-large veins; CV, capacitance vessels including the entire venous bed. (Modified from Mellander S, Johansson B 1968 Control of resistance, exchange and capacitance functions in the peripheral circulation. Pharmacological Reviews 20: 117, © Am Soc Pharmacol & Exp Therapeutics, with additional data from Rothe.[338])

Capillary exchange vessels The capillary cross-section consists of a single endothelial cell layer with some collagen around the periphery, and no smooth muscle.[330] Figure 1.24 indicates a lumen diameter of 8 μm though a recent review of many studies suggests that 4 to 7 μm may be a better estimate.[450] As shown in Figure 1.25, the resistance of the capillary bed is considerable, constituting about one quarter of the total under resting conditions, with a mean capillary pressure in the 20 to 30 mmHg range.[466] The transcapillary pressure drop depends upon the contractile state of the resistance vessels: as they relax from a constricted to dilated state, the proportion of the pressure change across the relatively constant capillary resistance increases.[115]

Postcapillary resistance vessels The smallest postcapillary venules lack a muscle layer. Venules and small veins, ranging in size from about 20 to 500 μm (Fig. 1.24) with a small amount of medial muscle[330] provide variable postcapillary resistance. Though small in magnitude, (Fig. 1.25) this resistance is important because the ratio of precapillary to postcapillary resistance determines capillary filtration pressure.[265]

Capacitance vessels The venous system consists of the venules and small veins, as well as the medium and large veins including the vena cavae. The average vein wall components are shown in Figure 1.24. The detailed arrangement varies, however, with more medial muscle in the lower body.[330]

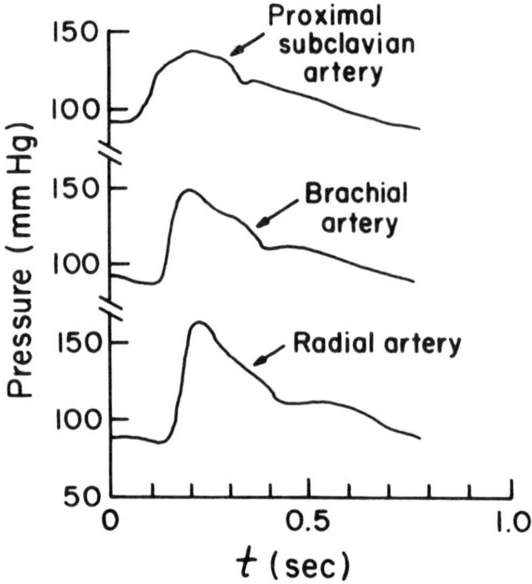

Fig. 1.26. Transformation of shape of pressure pulse wave in healthy adult from subclavian artery near the aorta to the radial artery. Pressure pulses were recorded during withdrawal of an arterial catheter (Modified from Marshall HW, Helmholz HF Jr, Wood EH 1962 Physiologic consequences of congenital heart disease. In: Hamilton WF (ed) Handbook of Physiology, Circulation, Vol 1, The Heart. American Physiological Society, Washington, DC.)

The total blood volume varies from about 80 to 90 ml/kg in infants[281,368] to 65 to 75 ml/kg in average adults.[338,377] The veins serve as the major reservoir, containing 60 to 70 percent of the blood (Table 1.4). About 80 percent of the venous blood is in the small vessels from 20 μm to 2 mm diameter.[338] Mobilization of blood from this reservoir occurs by two mechanisms:

1. Passive constriction results from a reduction in venous pressure coupled with the compliance of the vascular system. The total body compliance is about 3 ml/kg/mmHg of mean central filling pressure at approximately normal intravascular volume, of which more than 80 percent is from the systemic venous bed.[338] When venous pressures are low, volume change is enhanced by the capacity of the veins to collapse.[115] The passive transfer of volume is promoted by constriction

Table 1.4. Distribution of Blood Volume Throughout the Circulation at Rest

Vascular Bed	% of Total Blood Volume
Heart	8–11
Lungs	10–12
Systemic arteries	10–12
Capillaries	4–5
Systemic veins	
Venules/small veins	45–50
Large veins	15–20

Data from Folkow and Neil[115] and Rothe.[338]

Table 1.5. Contribution of Various Vascular Beds to the Total Blood Reservoir and Capacity to Mobilize Additional Volume in the Dog

Tissue	Resident Volume (% total blood volume)	Maximum Mobilized Volume (% resident volume)	(% total blood volume)
Liver	14	43	6
Spleen	12	75	9
Intestine	5	40	2
Skeletal muscle	14	29	4
Adipose tissue	11	36	4
Skin	2	50	1
Remainder	42	unknown	unknown
Total	100		>26

(Modified from Gow BS 1980 Circulatory correlates: Vascular impedance, resistance, and capacity. In: Bohr DR, Somlyo AP, Sparks HV Jr (eds) Handbood of Physiology, The Cardiovascular System, Vol II, Vascular Smooth Muscle. American Physiological Society, Bethesda.)

of the resistance vessels, reducing venous pressure.[136] Passive constriction accounts for approximately two-thirds of the volume which can be mobilized from the venous system.[136]

2. Active venoconstriction occurs in a number of organs. This increases venous return directly by mobilizing pooled blood, as well as by "stiffening" the veins to inhibit further pooling.[265] The active component contributes about one-third of the total volume mobilized.[136]

The venous blood pool is variably distributed among the organs (Table 1.5). With the exception of the spleen, the organs are capable of contributing about 30 to 50 percent of their blood volume with maximal sympathetic stimulation, by combined active and passive constriction. In the dog, the spleen is capable of mobilizing 75 percent of its blood into the circulation. Skeletal muscle veins contribute only by passive constriction due to the absence of adrenergic venous innervation in man and dog.[136] These combine to a potential recruitment of about one-fourth of the total blood volume (Table 1.5). The actual maximal available venous reservoir in man is about 10 percent of the total blood volume, due in part to the minimal reservoir capacity of the spleen.[136] Still less blood may be available from the venous pool than suggested above because venous tone is normally 70 percent of maximum in the erect individual.[157]

Shunt vessels Arteriovenous anastomoses permit a proportion of regional blood flow to bypass the usual nutritive function. These are found primarily in the skin where much of the blood flow subserves thermoregulation. They are similar in size and morphology to precapillary sphincters[265,330,450] (Fig. 1.24).

Lymphatic vessels These are not discussed herein. Reviews of various aspects of the lymphatic system are available.[57,291,150,166]

Vascular smooth muscle

Active control of blood vessel caliber occurs by contraction and relaxation of smooth muscle located primarily in the medial layer. As discussed below, there is considerable diversity in the primary stimuli to myocyte activity at various locations in the vascular system.[1,38]

The vascular myocyte is similar in most respects to the myocardial cell. As in myocardium, the biochemical basis of smooth muscle contraction is the interaction of elevated intracytoplasmic [Ca^{++}] and the contractile proteins forming the myofilaments.[446] Most stimuli to contraction act, at least in part, to promote transmembrane influx of extracellular Ca^{++}; they are ineffective with a calcium-free extracellular medium.[194] The exception is hypertonicity-induced contraction, which presumably results from release of intracellular Ca^{++} sequestered in sarcoplasmic reticulum and possibly mitochondria.[13]

Activation of vascular smooth muscle occurs by a variety of mechanisms. The muscles of precapillary resistance vessels exhibit pacemaker activity, associated with an action potential transmitted to local groups of cells, which induces rhythmic spontaneous contractions of the vessel. These are termed "single-unit" muscles, similar to those seen in viscera.[115] Another triggering mechanism occurs in muscles without spontaneous depolarization, but with "multi-unit" transmission of a spike-wave of depolarization initiated at a myoneural junction. Veins, larger arteries, and arteriovenous anastomoses, which are primarily under neural control, contain muscle of this type.[194]

Norepinephrine stimulates muscle contraction in those vessels possessing alpha receptors by at least two mechanisms: one, by depolarization of the membrane, the other, by an undefined action which triggers calcium influx without membrane depolarization, possibly related to altered membrane permeability to K^+ and Cl^-.[194] The latter mechanism has been termed "pharmacomechanical coupling."[380]

The primary substrate for energy generation is unknown, though both glucose and fats can be metabolized.[308] Aerobic metabolism is usual. Hypoxia impairs the contractile response to catecholamines,[81] despite the fact that significant glycolysis with lactate production occurs even under aerobic conditions.[308]

Control of vessel caliber

Multiple factors interact to control vessel caliber (Fig. 1.27). General reviews[45,115,448] as well as detailed expositions of each of the major mechanisms[31,52,54,195,286,300,352,365] are available.

Myogenic control The inherent myogenic activity of the "single-unit" type muscle maintains the precapillary resistance vessels in a partly constricted state (Fig. 1.27).[115] The extent of this basal tone is indicated by the difference between resting and fully dilated organ blood flow, shown in Figure 1.22. Those organs that require greater reserve, like myocardium and skeletal muscle, have high resting tone; those with more constant flow, such as kidney and brain, exhibit lower tone.

The regulatory capacity of intrinsic myogenic activity derives from the increased pacemaker activity and resulting muscle tone in response to stretch induced by intraluminal pressure (Fig. 1.22). This mechanism, noted first by Bayliss,[26] exerts positive feedback on the blood pressure, but tends to limit the consequent increased blood flow and capillary pressure.[195] When intraluminal pressure is persistently elevated, muscle hypertrophy ensues.[180]

Local metabolites Tissue activity, especially in muscle, induces vasodilatation opposing the intrinsic myogenic tone (Fig. 1.27). The mechanism or mechanisms for this are still unclear. Metabolites of active muscle which have been shown to

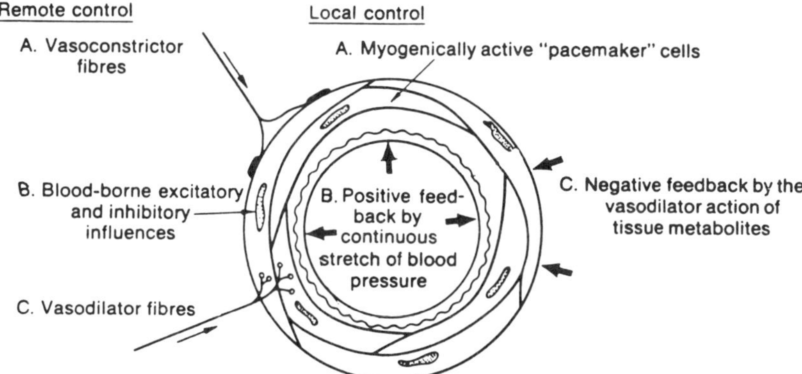

Fig. 1.27. Schematic representation of various local and remote mechanisms for control of peripheral vascular smooth muscle caliber (Folkow B, Neil E 1971 Circulation, Oxford University Press, New York.)

be vasodilators include adenosine, local hypoxemia[81,373] local hypercarbia, and elevated lactate, though to varying degrees in different tissues.[115] In skeletal muscle, vessel wall hypoxia, local hyperosmolality, and local hyperkalemia have all been proposed to act by multiple mechanisms to enhance exercise hyperemia.[391]

Endothelial cells synthesize a number of vasoactive prostaglandins from arachidonic acid.[54,448] The most important quantitatively and functionally is prostacyclin (PGI_2), a power vasodilator.[295] Prostaglandin E_2 (PGE_2), a vasodilator, and prostaglandin $F_{2\alpha}$, a constrictor in most vascular beds, are also produced in smaller amounts. A potent vasoconstrictor, thromboxane A_2 is secreted by platelets. Despite the pharmacologic importance of these compounds, they have been thought to play no significant role in adults in basal peripheral vascular tone or normal hyperemic states, such as post-exercise.[448] Recent studies suggest, however, that PGI_2 and other prostaglandins may mitigate the constrictor effect of norepinephrine in some vascular beds, especially the kidney.[54] The mechanism of action is by stimulation of adenylate cyclase leading to increased production of cyclic AMP.[295]

The prostaglandins do appear to exercise significant control on systemic circulation and patency of the ductus arteriosus (DA) during fetal life. This has been reviewed in detail.[276,286] From the perspective of postnatal systemic circulation, the most significant feature is the muscular DA. During fetal life the DA produces PGI_2[378] which, along with high circulating levels of PGE_2, is likely to be the major factor in maintenance of patency.[286] Administration of prostaglandin synthetase inhibitors to fetal animals produces closure of the DA,[400] and there is clinical evidence that cases of in utero closure of the DA have been associated with maternal ingestion of such drugs.[232]

Normal functional closure of the DA occurs by muscular contraction in the hours after birth, and is complete by 15 hours of age.[281] The stimuli for this include the direct effect of the elevated P_aO_2[167] as well as alterations in prostaglandin metabolic pathways which favor increaed levels of thromboxane A_2 relative to the dilator PG's.[317] Fibrosis and progressive obliteration of the lumen occur over sev-

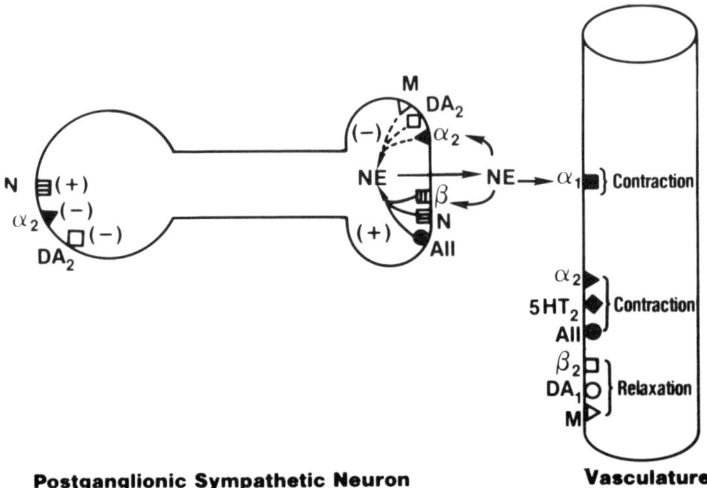

Fig. 1.28. Schematic representation of the vascular neuroeffector junction. Shown is the postganglionic sympathetic effector neuron which acts on alpha$_1$-adrenoceptors on the effector organ. Also shown are a variety of other post- and presynaptic receptors. Key: $5HT_2$, serotonin receptor; AII, angiotensin II receptor; others as shown in Figure 1.17. (Ruffolo RR 1983 Drug, neurotransmitter and hormone receptors in the regulation of the cardiovascular system. In: Shoemaker WC, Thompson WL (eds) Critical Care State of the Art, Vol 4. Society of Critical Care Medicine, Fullerton, CA.)

eral months, with complete occlusion in all but 0.04 percent of normal individuals at sea level by the end of the first year.[361] Postnatal hypoxia promotes continued patency of the DA.[284] School children residing at 15,000 feet altitude exhibit a 30 times incidence in patent ductus arteriosus over that at sea level.[311] The vasodilator PGE_1 is used to maintain patency of the DA in infants with ductal-dependent congenital heart disease.[118]

Though no single key metabolic vasodilator has been identified, it is clear that metabolic products do induce a relaxation of myogenic tone in active tissue, thereby adjusting local O_2 delivery to demand.

Neurogenic control Neurogenic signals influence vascular tone (Fig. 1.27) and the distribution of blood flow. Most important are the postganglionic sympathetic adrenergic fibers which synapse with the vessel wall at the neuroeffector junction, shown schematically in Figure 1.28, and mediate vasoconstriction. The predominant mechanism is by the action of norepinephrine (NE) released from the neuronal endplate.[348] The constrictor response is biphasic: the initial effect, within seconds, is due to activation of the postjunctional alpha$_1$-adrenoreceptor and is terminated by the efficient neuronal uptake of NE; the secondary effect, more than an order of magnitude slower, results from diffusion of NE into the vessel wall and its subsequent direct action. The relative significance of these two effects is determined in part by the size of the neuronal endplate, and the gap between the neuron and vessel. A larger endplate, as seen in large arteries, is associated with a slow-onset prolonged constriction due to a significant effect of NE diffusion. The nerves to muscular arteries and arterioles exhibit smaller endplates, and trigger a rapid, primarily receptor-mediated, action.[31]

As shown in the figure, the release of NE from the nerve terminal is modified by the effects of a variety of agents on presynaptic receptors. Most important are the inhibition of NE release by alpha$_2$-adrenoceptors and the enhancement by beta-adrenoceptors, discussed in the section *Innervation of the heart*. When NE levels are high enough to activate both receptor types, inhibition predominates.[223] Other presynaptic receptors shown exert the indicated effects on NE release. Still other inhibitory presynaptic receptors, which have been identified in some tissues, respond to prostaglandin E_1 and E_2, enkephalins, and adenosine.[223] The physiologic role of these receptors is not yet well defined.

A number of postsynaptic receptor types shown in Figure 1.28 appear to reside outside the zone of influence of neural NE and modify vascular tone primarily in response to humoral agents.[348] These are discussed below.

The density of distribution of vasoconstrictor fibers varies regionally, and longitudinally within organs, reflecting the extent to which neural regulation of blood flow occurs.[115] Thus the cerebral circulation is sparsely innervated, while that of the skin has densely distributed innervation. Within organs, the smaller arteries and arterioles possess the richest supply of nerve fibers; larger arteries and veins, and the precapillary sphincters are less well innervated.

Folkow and Neil[115] suggest that there are three major effects produced by neurogenic influences on vascular resistance. The first is promotion of redistribution of blood flow among organs in response to metabolic demands. Considerable reserve vasoconstriction is available, as evidenced by the fact that the neurogenic component of resting tone in the resistance vessels is only approximately 10 to 15 percent of the total. Second is the mobilization of tissue fluid into the vascular space as a consequence of reduced transcapillary pressure, achieved by increasing the ratio of precapillary to postcapillary resistance. The large mass of skeletal muscle serves as an important reservoir of *extravascular* fluid. This function is facilitated by the predominance of precapillary over postcapillary constrictor response characteristic of this tissue. Third, *intravascular* fluid mobilization is effected by venous capacitance vessel constriction.

Cholinergic vasodilator nerves are found in many species including man (Fig. 1.27). Sympathetic cholinergic nerves induce anticipatory increases in skeletal blood flow characteristic of the "defense reaction" seen in many animals.[3] In man, such effects are present to a lesser, and less well defined, degree.[52,115] Parasympathetic cholinergic vasodilator nerves act on the vasculature of the salivary glands, external genitalia, and other areas of functional, but not hemodynamic importance.[115]

Humoral effects Many circulating agents affect vascular caliber at sites remote from their origin (Fig. 1.27). Specific postsynaptic vascular receptors have been identified for a number of these, shown schematically in Figure 1.28. Functionally most important are the alpha$_2$- and beta$_2$-adrenoceptors, which mediate contraction and relaxation of the vessel, respectively.

The alpha$_2$-adrenoceptors, located remotely from the neuroeffector junction, respond to circulating catecholamines, EPI more so than NE.[447] They promote vascular constriction by inducing slow-channel Ca^{++} flux.[397,423] They play an important role in compensating for hypovolemia when circulating catecholamine levels are high.[39] Recent evidence suggests, however, that they may be exceptionally sensitive[224] and contribute to resting resistance vessel tone as well.[193]

Vascular $beta_2$-adrenoceptors act to stimulate adenylate cyclase production of cyclic AMP, which reduces smooth muscle tone by incompletely defined mechanisms. Those proposed include reduced phosphyorylation of myosin,[7] and enhanced sequestration and extrusion of Ca^{++}.[128] Though primarily responsive to circulating EPI[51,808] they are accessible to neurogenic NE in some tissues.[31] The distribution and density of vascular alpha- and beta-adrenoceptors, as well as receptors for other mediators of vascular tone, varies tremendously among tissues and among species. A systematic survey of this variation is needed to permit more comprehensive generalizations from individual observations.[31]

A variety of other humoral agents affect vascular tone directly, under experimental and pathological conditions. Among these are the vasoactive peptides, including angiotensin I and II, neurotensin, and vasopressin, which induce constriction, and bradykinin which produces relaxation. The effects of these and other peptides have been reviewed recently.[71,352,365] Their role in regulation of normal circulation is still speculative.

Serotonin (5-HT) induces vasoconstriction by direct action of the circulating hormone on specific vascular receptors, indirect stimulation of neural NE release, and by being taken up by the nerve terminal and released with NE.[200] Histamine dilates precapillary resistance vessels and increases capillary permeability.[115]

At least four types of opiate receptors have been identified, primarily in the central nervous system. Their role in the cardiovascular response to opiates and endogenous opioid peptides has been reviewed.[220,462] Opioids produce hypotension and bradycardia, primarily by reducing sympathetic and increasing parasympathetic efferents from the brainstem autonomic nuclei to the heart and peripheral vasculature. These effects are augmented by inhibition of adrenal medullary catecholamine release.[220] Circulating opioids increase in stress states. Plasma endorphins are elevated in neonates for more than 4 days after birth, presumably due to perinatal stress.[285,103] Opioids are believed to play a role in various types of circulatory shock,[462] and opiate antagonists have ameliorated shock in a variety of experimental models,[462] as well as human septic shock.[314] Postnatal sympathetic efferent development appears to be associated with diminished cardiovascular effects of the opioids.[221]

It is apparent from the discussion above that vessel caliber is a result of multiple local and remote factors acting on a given neuromuscular complex. These vary among tissues and longitudinally within a given vascular bed. Features of individual regional circulations are reviewed elsewhere.[115,265,375]

Coupling of the heart and circulation

The function of the heart and peripheral circulation have been considered separately in previous sections. But in fact, the output from the heart to the circulation is determined by their interaction, as suggested in Figure 1.4. The following discussion of this coupling is based upon that of Weber et al.[444]

The nature of the coupling is summarized in Figure 1.29. The left panel of Figure 1.29A depicts the effect of afterload, represented by the mean ejection pressure, on cardiac output. This relation was defined more precisely as the effect of end-systolic wall stress on the fractional shortening of the ventricular wall in the section *Afterload* and Figure 1.15. The line shown is one of a family, corre-

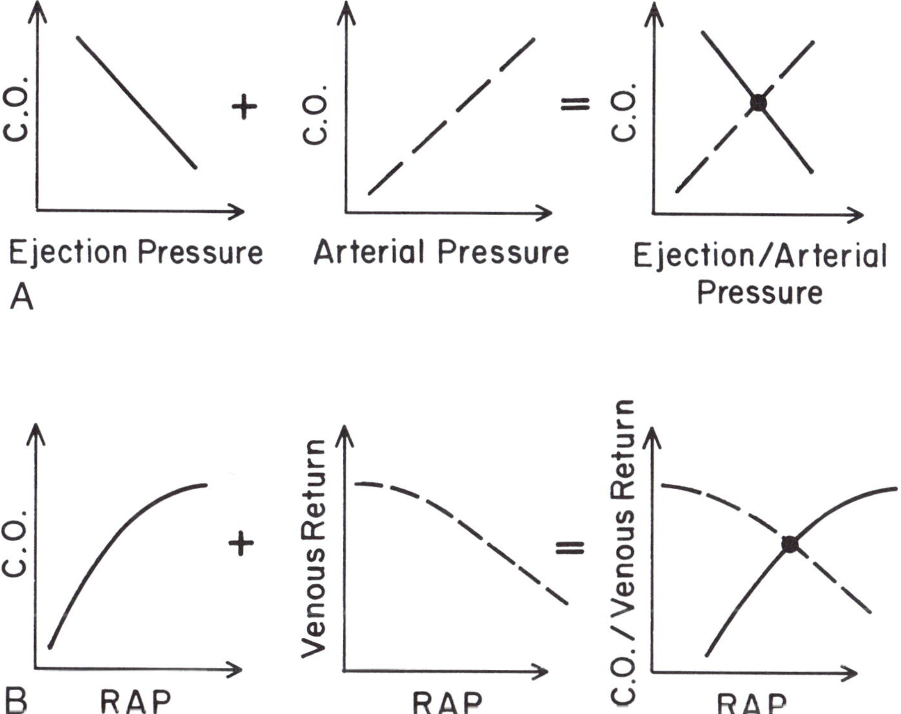

Fig. 1.29. Functional coupling of the heart to the arterial and venous circulation. (A) Arterial coupling. (B) Venous coupling. Key: Solid lines represent flow from the ventricular pump; dashed line is flow in the circulation. (Weber KT, Janicki JS, Hunter WC, Shroff S, Pearlman ES, Fishman AP 1982 The contractile behavior of the heart and its functional coupling to the circulation. Progress in Cardiovascular Disease 24: 375.)

sponding to a given preload and contractile state. The middle panel portrays the linear relation between systemic flow and mean arterial pressure, the slope of which is the total peripheral resistance. When the cardiac pump and the external load are coupled, they must be in equilibrium at the cardiac output and arterial pressure which simultaneously satisfy the two function lines, that is, where they cross. This is depicted in the right panel.

The left panel of Figure 1.29B illustrates the cardiac response to preload according to Guyton et al,[155] in which the left ventricular output is affected by the venous return to the right atrium. Assuming that flow occurs unimpeded from the right ventricle to the left atrium, this is analogous to the ventricular function curve described in the section *Preload* and in Figure 1.9B. The single curve shown corresponds to a specific diastolic compliance, afterload, and contractile state. The middle panel illustrates the dependence of venous return upon the pressure gradient, represented by the right atrial pressure. Coupling of the heart and venous circulation also requires simultaneous satisfaction of the respective function lines at their intersection, as in the right panel.

The equilibrium cardiac output must, of course, be the same for arterial and venous coupling. That is, the two right panels in the figure constitute sections

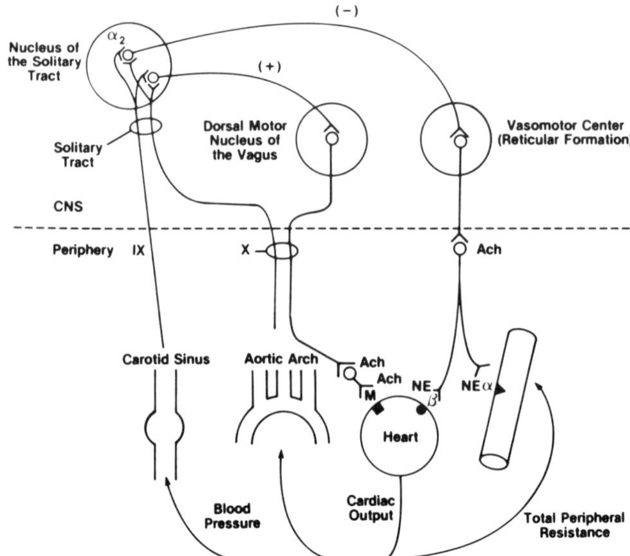

Fig. 1.30. Simplified diagram of the cardiovascular reflex loop involved in the regulation of cardiac output and blood pressure. Abbreviations are as shown in Figures 1.17 and 1.28. (Ruffolo RR 1983 Drug, neurotransmitter and hormone receptors in the regulation of the cardiovascular system. In: Shoemaker, WC, Thompson WL (eds) Critical Care State of the Art, Vol 4. Society of Critical Care Medicine, Fullerton, CA.)

through a three-dimensional surface on which the equilibrium state is one point. Different surfaces are generated for variations in intrinsic contractility. The effect of diminished venous return has a much greater effect on output of the normal heart than increased afterload; the converse is true for the failing heart.[444]

Integrated Circulatory Control

Autonomic supervision

The adequacy of circulatory function is closely monitored and supervised by a variety of reflexes which are integrated within the autonomic nervous system. Comprehensive discussions of various aspects of this system are available.[50,88,115,134,215,235,320,374,375]

Baroreflex control A schematic view of the main features of the normal cardiovascular baroreceptor reflex loop is shown in Figure 1.30. Three components comprise this closed-loop system: (1) the sensory limb, consisting of the sino-aortic baroreceptors and their afferent pathways; (2) the integrator-controller, composed of interconnected brainstem nuclei; and (3) the effector limb, activated via sympathetic efferent nerves to the heart, adrenal medulla, and peripheral circulation, and parasympathetic efferents to the heart.

The baroreceptors of major importance consist of sensory neurons located in the adventitia of the carotid sinus and aortic arch.[88] They are primarily sensitive to stretch, detecting pressure change by its effect on deformation of the vessel wall. Signals from the carotid sinus and aortic arch receptors are transmitted via the glossopharyngeal and vagus nerves, respectively, to the nucleus of the solitary tract in the medulla, Figure 1.30.[215]

Afferent activity of the carotid sinus receptors increases as mean arterial pressure increases.[88] The lower threshold for signals is a mean sinus pressure of about 60 mmHg with maximal nerve activity at about 200 mmHg.[310] In the newborn rabbit, the threshold pressure is less than 30 mmHg, consistent with the lower normal mean pressure in neonates.[88] Thus, significant afferent tone is maintained at normal blood pressure. The afferent signal at a given mean arterial pressure is affected by the magnitude of the pulse pressure. Below a mean pressure of 150 mmHg, increasing pulse pressure augments the neural flow; above that pressure, the magnitude of the pulse has no effect.[366]

The aortic baroreceptors appear to function in a similar manner to those of the carotid sinus, though the threshold for activity may be higher in some species,[310] and the effect of pulse pressure on the response to mean pressure is less.[351]

In the nucleus of the solitary tract, the baroreceptor afferents synapse with *inhibitory* neurons that act on the complex vasomotor center in the reticular formation, and with *excitatory* neurons serving the cardio-inhibitory center of the dorsal motor nucleus of the vagus (DMNV) (Fig. 1.30).[115,215]

The effector organs of central circulatory control are the heart and peripheral vessels, primarily the small arteries, arterioles, and to a lesser extent the small veins. The normal resting afferent baroreceptor signals lead to a low level of sympathetic tone in peripheral vessels, (see the section *Vascular smooth muscle*) and dominant parasympathetic tone to the heart (see the section *Response to autonomic stimulation*). Elevated blood pressure stimulates afferent baroreceptor signals, which induce depression of sympathetic efferent tone from the vasomotor center and augment parasympathetic outflow from the DMNV. These lead to bradycardia and probably a modest reduction in peripheral vascular resistance.[250]

By contrast, arterial hypotension induces diminished afferent baroreceptor signals, resulting in enhanced sympathetic efferent tone to both heart and vasculature and inhibition of parasympathetic flow to the heart. The consequences of these alterations are peripheral vasoconstriction and elevated cardiac output, leading to restoration of circulatory homeostasis.[45] Other features of this system, including the variations in effect among tissue beds, have been described in detail.[2,250,650]

Modifying factors A number of other receptors are present in the circulation and influence the output of the baroreceptor reflex loop. The most important of these are described below.

The cardiopulmonary baroreceptors are stretch receptors located in both atria and pulmonary arteries. They operate in low-pressure circuits, and at least the two types of atrial receptors are considered to sense alterations in the filling volume of the heart.[50,439] Afferent signals via fibers in the vagus nerve alter the arterial baroreflex response.[374] During hypertension and hypervolemia, both cardiopulmonary and arterial baroreceptor reflexes inhibit sympathetic and activate vagal efferents. During hypovolemia with hypotension, they both stimulate sympathetic and depress parasympathetic outflow.[2,252] The specific neurons affected by each reflex are not the same, as indicated by their different effects on heart rate and tone of individual vascular beds.[2,374]

The systemic arterial chemoreceptors are small vascular structures located above the carotid bifurcations (carotid bodies), and in the tissues between the aorta and pulmonary arteries (aortic bodies).[100,115] Afferent fibers of the glossopharyngeal and vagus nerves serve the carotid and aortic bodies, respectively. The nerve endings are sensitive to changes in chemical composition, tonicity, and temperature of their environment. Afferent signals increase in frequency when P_aO_2 or pH decrease, and when P_aCO_2, temperature, or tonicity increase.[100] The inverse changes induce a reduction in afferent activity. The efferent consequences of these signals are often difficult to predict because of the direct effects of the stimuli on cardiorespiratory function at multiple levels. For example, experimental hypoxemia in which ventilation is controlled may lead to peripheral vasoconstriction and hypertension, whereas vasodilatation is seen in the spontaneously breathing animal. The difference is likely due to the powerful vasodilatory effect of hypoxic-induced hyperventilation.[100] The major function of chemoreceptors is in regulation of respiratory function. Their role in cardiovascular regulation appears to be limited to modifying the effects of other homeostatic mechanisms.

Higher centers, including multiple areas of the cerebral cortex, hypothalamus, and cerebellum, receive and send signals to the vasomotor center.[215] They modify the integrative activities and affect efferent sympathetic tone in response, for example, to fear, rage, and the "defense reaction."[115,439]

Control of extracellular volume Renal regulation of salt and water homeostasis is beyond the scope of this chapter. However, certain features of autonomic regulation are relevant. The atrial stretch receptors, discussed above, have been shown to affect salt and water excretion. In the dog, atrial stretch produces a prompt diuresis, the atriorenal reflex. Activation of right atrial stretch receptors produces a fall in plasma renin, and presumably aldosterone; activation of left atrial receptors leads to a reduction in circulating antidiuretic hormone (ADH).[46] The effector pathways thus appear to be both neural and humoral. This powerful and rapid effect of low-pressure receptors is not seen in primates, however.[131] In detailed reviews, Gilmore[131] and Marks and Mancia[252] argue that many experiments have confounded the effects of cardiopulmonary and arterial baroreceptors. They suggest that the high-pressure receptors may be more significant in monkey and man, though the precise mode of action is undefined. Natriuresis stimulated directly by a substance released from atrial tissue has been demonstrated, but is probably not involved in acute regulation of intravascular volume.[131]

Developmental effects Autonomic control of circulation is well, but incompletely developed in the normal newborn.[134,283,286,440] The diminished heart rate and blood pressure response to baroreceptor stimulation in newborn lambs[75] is consistent with a lower level of sympathetic efferent neural output (see the section *Developmental aspects* under *Autonomic control of cardiac function*).[430] Continued maturation of peripheral sympathetic function through childhood is suggested by measurements of circulating catecholamines in response to upright posture.[16]

The precise determinant of the "setpoint" blood pressure is not known, but must undergo change during development, as indicated by Figure 1.31. The figure shows systolic blood pressure percentiles from 4 days of age through 12 years. Individuals did not necessarily "track" along the same percentile when sequential measurements were made, though a low order of tracking was found for these[62,80] and other[334,465] data. The figure suggests that blood pressure increases during the

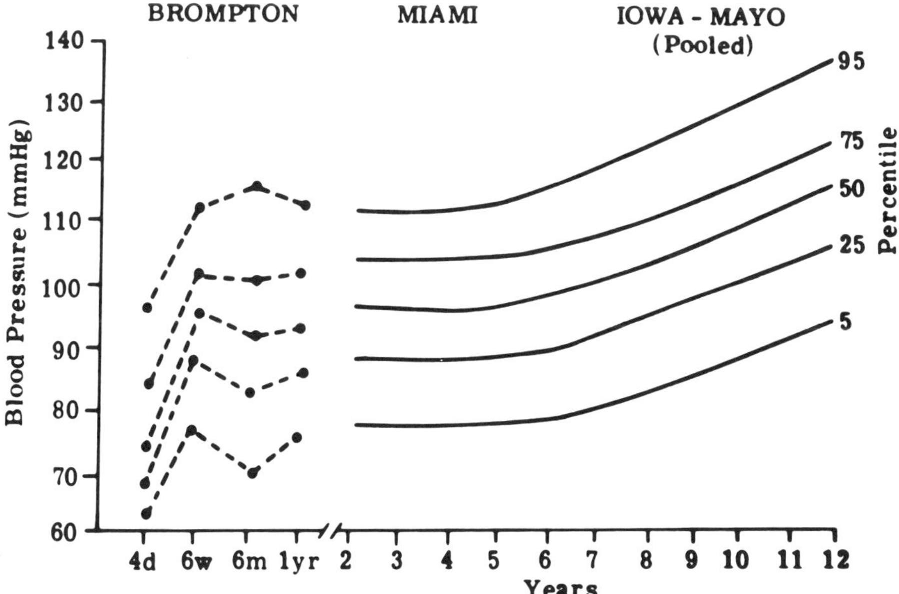

Fig. 1.31. Effect of age on percentiles of systolic blood pressure. Dashed lines show data for both sexes; solid lines show data for boys. (DeSwiet M, Fayers P, Shinebourne EA 1980 Value of repeated blood pressure measurements in children—the Brompton study. British Medical Journal 1: 1567–1569, reproduced by permission of the Authors and Editors of the British Medical Journal.)

first weeks of life, and then remains constant until about 6 years of age. It then rises gradually toward adult values. Beyond age 12, values continue to rise to a median of 128 mmHg at 18 years. The increases beyond the first decade may be in part culturally induced.[5] Among the members of a South American Indian tribe who use no salt in their diet, blood pressures do not increase beyond the second decade, remaining at about 105/67 mmHg in adult males.[298]

Circulatory reserve

The circulatory reserve is the capacity of the cardiovascular system to match oxygen supply to the demands of the individual tissues, within the hierarchical constraints imposed by the central nervous system.

Mobilization of this reserve involves the interaction of four mechanisms:

1. Increased blood flow to specific tissues occurs in response to local control (see the section *Control of vessel caliber*). This evokes a baroreflex-mediated increase in cardiac output which maintains blood pressure and flow to the other organs.[265]

2. Enhanced O_2 extraction moderates the requirement for increased blood flow. It requires reduced tissue PO_2 or a shift in the oxyhemoglobin dissociation curve to the right. In general, both increased flow and O_2 extraction are employed when O_2 supply and demand are unbalanced. The proportion of the compensation provided by each mechanism was examined by Shepherd et al[373] using a canine preparation in which all CNS efferents had been eliminated, and blood pressure could be externally controlled. The stimulus employed was a step decrease in mean blood

pressure from 100 to 50 mmHg, with varying initial O_2 extraction, O_2 consumption, and P_aO_2. In all cases, the combined effects of local vasodilatation-induced flow and increased O_2 extraction supported the tissues' O_2 requirement. With normal initial conditions, compensation for the hypotensive stimulus derived about 50 percent from increased O_2 extraction and 50 percent from augmented blood flow. When the initial (a-v)DO_2 was doubled, only 10 percent of the compensation was due to increased O_2 extraction. When initial hypoxemia was superimposed, the proportion of compensation from increased flow rose in inverse relation to the drop in arterial O_2 content.

3. The short-term work capacity of skeletal muscle exceeds the ability of its vascular bed to deliver oxygen. The difference is compensated by anaerobic metabolism of the muscle, which permits an "oxygen debt" during intense exercise that is "repaid" during an extended post-exercise hyperemia.[265]

4. The CNS can superimpose control on local regulation and redistribute blood flow accordingly. This is usually in response to one or both of two factors:

a. The heart (see the sections *Myocardial energy supply—oxygen* and *Adaptation to altered oxygen supply/demand*) and brain[30,164] must operate aerobically. Therefore, the CNS operates in concert with local factors to insure that their O_2 supply always equals demand, even at the expense of other organs. This mechanism is most apparent when the total-body delivery of oxygen is insufficient to match demand and the blood flow needed by the heart and brain is diverted from other tissues. Examples include the diving reflex,[36] hypoxia (see below), and the failing circulation (see Chapters 2 and 3).

b. Some tissues possess a vascular bed with excessive flow capacity for metabolic needs, but which subserves an additional function. Among these are the skin, which regulates heat dissipation, the kidney, which regulates salt and water excretion, and the fat, which serves as the major energy store. These vascular beds are highly innervated and fulfill their functions with significant central regulation.

These mechanisms interact to compensate for major perturbations in the balance of O_2 supply and demand. Some examples follow.

Response to increased oxygen demand—exercise The circulatory effects of exercise are illustrated in Figure 1.22. Cardiac output increases nearly five times, accompanied by elevated blood pressure and a reduction in total peripheral resistance. The majority of the incremental flow is directed to the working muscles. Flow to the heart is increased proportionally to its workload (see the section *Adaptation to altered oxygen supply/demand*). The remainder augments heat dissipation from the skin. Flow to the other organs is unchanged.

Central control is evident in many features of the response. At, or even before the onset of exercise, the heart rate and cardiac output increase, mediated by a precipitous reduction in vagal tone to the heart and an increase in sympathetic drive, overriding the normal baroreflex response.[432] Intense muscular contraction further stimulates tachycardia and hypertension, both by direct reflex input to the vasomotor center from the working muscle and by central signals.[374] The baroreflex then operates at an elevated "setpoint," moderating the hypertensive effect of the exercise[438] and regulating blood pressure around the new level.[264] In the normal individual, vascular resistance of the viscera increases just sufficiently to maintain pre-exercise flow. When compensatory mechanisms are impaired, as in anemia or heart failure, exercise leads to intense vasoconstriction of renal and mesenteric beds with significant reduction in visceral flow.[432]

Circulatory adaptations to endurance training involve primarily the heart and working muscles. Changes in cardiac form and function are discussed in the section *Adaptation to altered oxygen supply/demand*. Major effects are seen in the working muscles where the capability to reduce resistance is markedly enhanced, as is the size of the capillary bed.[37] The maximum oxygen uptake has been inversely correlated with the peripheral resistance.[63] Thus, training leads to a greater capacity for blood flow to working muscle, and an increased surface for exchange of the delivered oxygen. For example, olympic athletes exhibited maximum oxygen uptake and cardiac output more than 50 percent above that of a group of untrained college students.[37] In experiments in which one leg was trained, changes occurred only in the trained muscles.[63] The specific nature of the changes in resistance vessels and/or the mechanisms for their control are not defined.[37]

Prepubertal children show no changes in peripheral vascular function with endurance training.[245,414] During adolescence, training effects approach those of the adult.[414]

Response to reduced oxygen supply—hypoxia Acute hypoxia induces important circulatory adjustments which serve to maintain O_2 delivery to vital tissues. Provided the hypoxia is not too severe, increases occur in heart rate, ventricular contractility, cardiac output, and blood pressure. Most often peripheral vascular resistance diminishes and venoconstriction occurs. These result from the combined interactions of stimulation of the peripheral arterial chemoreceptors, direct influences of hypoxemia on the CNS, and when breathing is spontaneous, increased ventilation with hypocapnia.[100]

Adachi et al[4] used radioactive microspheres[166] to study the redistribution of blood flow due to hypoxia in anesthetized dogs. They examined the distribution with normal ventilation and inspired oxygen of 21, 10, and 5 percent. The more severe hypoxia led to reduced P_aO_2 from 83 to 24 mmHg, increased heart rate from 148 to 179 per minute, increased cardiac output from 73 to 120 ml/min/kg, and increased blood pressure from 144/120 to 171/141 mmHg. Total peripheral vascular resistance decreased 31 percent. Organ blood flow and resistance changes are shown in Table 1.6. Major increases in flow to the heart (see the section *Adaptation to altered oxygen supply/demand*) and brain[164,30] occurred, accounted for by the combined effects of reductions in locally autoregulated vascular resistance and the elevated cardiac output. All of the other organs exhibit elevated or modestly reduced resistance leading to a diminished share of the cardiac output. This presumably results from central sympathetic effects overriding local control.

Similar redistributions favoring the heart and brain occur in fetal[68] and newborn[211] lambs subjected to hypoxemia. In the fetal lamb, the heart rate decreased, characteristic of the stressed fetus,[345] and cardiac output fell. Thus, the other organs were "sacrificed" to a greater degree to meet cardiac and brain O_2 requirements. In the newborn period, the increased anaerobic capacity of the myocardium (see *Adaptation to altered oxygen supply/demand*) is partially offset by the limited reserve cardiac output (see *Contractility* and *Myocardial oxygen consumption*), and the circulatory compensation for hypoxia is probably less than later in life.[243]

Table 1.6. Effect of Severe Hypoxia on Regional Resistance and Blood Flow Distribution in the Dog

Tissue	% Δ tissue flow	% Δ fraction of CO	$\Delta R/R_0$ (%)
Heart	+285	+136	−70
Brain	+140	+46	−51
Skeletal muscle	−24	−54	+51
Kidney	+23	−25	−20
GI tract	+39	−17	−18
Liver (hepatic artery)	+54	−5	−27
Skin	0	−38	+11

Abbreviations: Δ, change; R, total peripheral vascular resistance, R_0, initial value of R.
Changes shown are induced by reducing the inspired fraction of O_2 from 0.21 to 0.05.
Additional discussion in text.
Data from Adachi et al.[4]

Response to reduced oxygen supply—anemia The responses to acute or chronic anemia promote maintenance of O_2 delivery to the tissues despite the diminished O_2 content of the blood. Thus vasodilatation, coupled with the reduced viscosity of anemic blood, enhances tissue flows (Equation 6) and O_2 delivery.[72,104,187] In chronic anemia, elevated erythrocyte 2,3-DPG levels facilitate O_2 extraction, as seen in the "physiologic anemia" of infancy.[79,301] When the O_2 carrying capacity of the blood becomes sufficiently low, central effects supervene, and flow is preferentially directed to the heart and brain at the expense of oxygen transport to other organs.[104] Adaptation of the heart to anemia is discussed in the section *Adaptation to altered oxygen supply/demand.*

THE PULMONARY CIRCULATION

The pulmonary circulation sustains a blood flow equal to the entire systemic circulation at one-fifth the pressure. The blood normally acquires oxygen for the body by flow to alveoli where the O_2 gradient saturates the hemoglobin during the red cell capillary transit time, 0.75 seconds at rest, and less than one-half of that during exercise.[152] Despite the complex functioning of the pulmonary circulation, its control appears to be regulated primarily by oxygen, without the closed-loop feedback circuitry so well developed for the systemic circulation. Grover et al,[152] Reid,[327] and Rudolph[343] have reviewed many aspects of the pulmonary circulation. This discussion is focussed primarily on those characteristics with hemodynamic significance.

Components of the Pulmonary Circulation

The pulmonary circuit consists of the right heart and pulmonary blood vessels. Cardiac function is discussed in the section *Cardiac physiology.*

Description of the vessels and their control

The pulmonary vessels Analogues for the various systemic vessels can be found in the pulmonary circuit, with similar wall components. However, it is more useful to classify them according to their position in the lung relative to the acinus (that

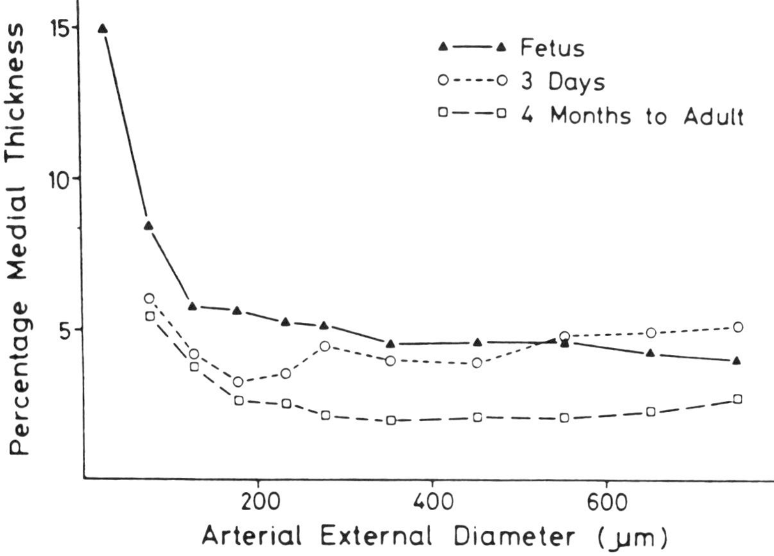

Fig. 1.32. Relation of pulmonary arterial wall thickness to arterial diameter as a function of development. (Reid, LM 1979 The pulmonary circulation: Remodeling in growth and disease. American Review of Respiratory Disease 119: 531.)

is, the gas exchange unit consisting of the respiratory bronchioles, the alveolar ducts, and the alveoli).[327] Pre-acinar vessels consist of the elastic arteries larger than 1 mm in diameter, the muscular arteries from 1 mm to 150 μm, and the corresponding veins. These lie along the airways, and have developed with them by the sixteenth week of fetal life. The intra-acinar arteries grade from highly muscular vessels into partially muscular transitional vessels, to nonmuscular arterioles which are still larger than capillaries. The extent of muscle is not directly related to size in vessels smaller than 150 μm; during childhood, much larger nonmuscular arteries are found than in either the newborn or adult. These vessels develop with the alveoli, multiplying rapidly during the first 3 years with little change in number after age 6.[170,327]

Arterial muscle undergoes major changes in two respects during development. The first is the muscle thickness which depends upon both arterial size and age. This is illustrated in Figure 1.32, which shows that the arteries smaller than approximately 150 μm are the most muscular, and that the small arteries in the fetus are more so than those in the neonate or the older infant. The reduction in muscularity of the smaller vessels, which occurs in the first 24 hours after birth,[161] is due primarily to increased compliance and dilatation resulting in thinning of the media.[170,287,437] The more delayed medial thinning for vessels larger than 200 μm, as indicated in the figure, occurs due to growth of the vessels with minimal change or even regression of the media.[61,170] In the pig, these vessels achieve functional maturity by 2 weeks of age, but remodelling continues to 6 months.[161] The second component is the extension of muscle into the respiratory unit. At birth, there are no gas exchanging airways, and arterial muscle extends only to the terminal bron-

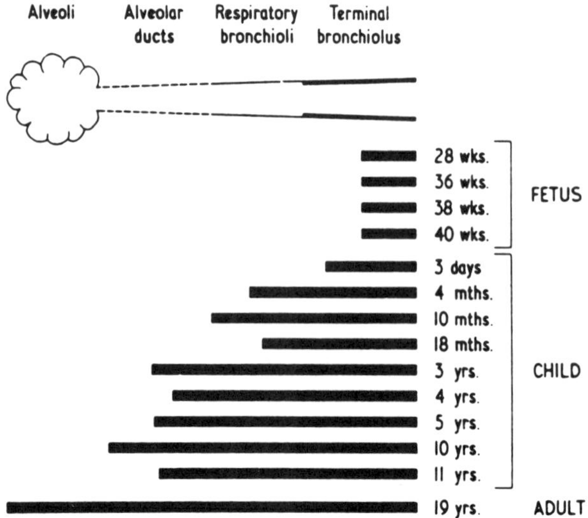

Fig. 1.33. Position within the respiratory unit at which 50 percent of the arteries are muscular. (Hislop A, Reid L 1973 Pulmonary arterial development during childhood: branching pattern and structure. Thorax 28: 129. Reproduced by permission, the Authors and Editors of Thorax.)

chiole (Fig. 1.33). The extension of muscle distally into the acinus lags behind arterial development throughout childhood.[319,327]

The main pulmonary artery (MPA) experiences important developmental changes as well.[163] In the fetus, the media of the pulmonary trunk is equal in thickness to that of the aorta. The ratio of these thicknesses falls to 0.4 to 0.7 in the adult. The elastic laminae of the normal adult aorta are composed of long, uniform circumferential fibers; those of the MPA contain short fibrils that are irregularly shaped and distributed. The fetal MPA elastica resembles that of the aorta. A transitional arrangement is seen in infancy.

Pulmonary artery pressure The rapid postnatal reduction in pulmonary artery muscle tone is reflected in a rapid fall in pulmonary artery pressure (PAP) at sea level (Fig. 1.34A).[96,325,340] The values at birth show considerable scatter, but may equal systemic pressure. The exponential decline leads to adult levels by 2 weeks of age, and the data show much less variability. The postnatal decline in hematocrit-associated reduction in viscosity may contribute to this.[241] After that time, the pulmonary arteries exhibit a low resting tone, such that, at rest, the major resistance to flow is in the capillaries and veins. The majority of the impedance, as reflected by damping of the pulse pressure, resides in the stiffer arteries.[152] Changes in resistance due to constriction arise primarily in the small highly muscular arteries.

Control of vessel caliber

The primary function of the lung is gas exchange, and the major control of pulmonary vessel caliber appears to be related to that requirement. Many different stimuli affect pulmonary vascular tone. Which of these are important in normal circumstances is not clear.

Oxygen It is now well accepted that the most powerful stimulus to pulmonary

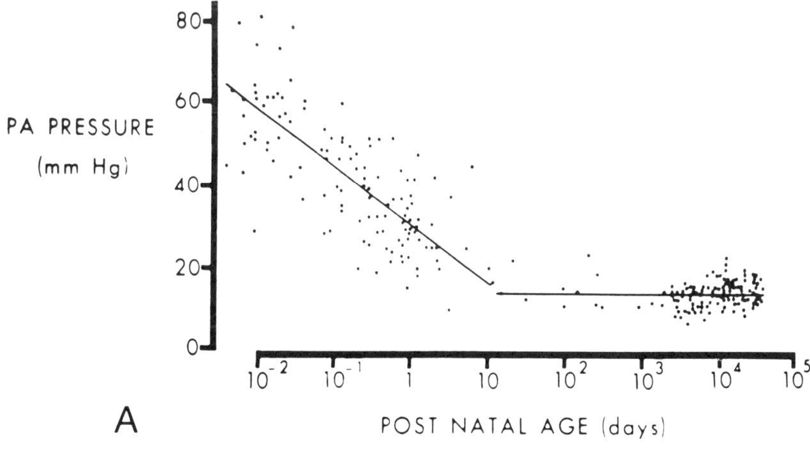

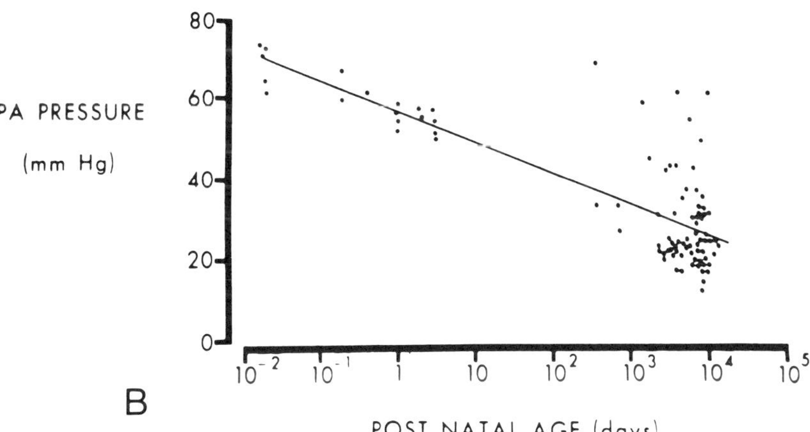

Fig. 1.34. Relationship of postnatal age to resting mean pulmonary artery pressure. (A) Residents near sea level, 257 measurements. (B) Residents at altitude 14,900 feet (4540 m), 73 measurements. (Reeves JT, Grover RF 1975 High altitude pulmonary hypertension and pulmonary edema. Progress in Cardiology 4: 99.)

arterial constriction is hypoxia.[113,152,326] Alveolar hypoxia appears to act directly on the small muscular arteries, stimulating contraction by an as yet undefined mechanism.[152] Many factors affect the intensity of this response, including the following:

1. *Degree of hypoxia.* The PAP varies inversely and linearly with the hypoxia-associated arterial saturation.[326]

2. *Age.* In animal experiments, the PAP was higher for younger than older animals, though the change in PAP for a given change in saturation was no different.[326] Newborn infants exposed to brief periods of hypoxia (inspired F_{IO_2} 0.1)

who had a patent foramen ovale or ductus arteriosus, developed right-to-left shunting consequent upon reversible, markedly elevated pulmonary artery pressures.[186]

3. *The mixed venous PO_2 (P_vO_2).* A reduction in P_vO_2 exerts a direct constrictor effect on the pulmonary arteries as well as enhancing the effect of alveolar hypoxia.[180,309] If both alveolar PO_2 and P_vO_2 are sufficiently low, the vasoconstrictor response may be blunted by functional impairment of the vascular smooth muscle.[309]

4. *Acidosis and hypercarbia.* Acidosis and hypercarbia augment hypoxia vasoconstriction. This effect is more important in newborn calves than adult cattle.[221]

5. *Intermittent or chronic hypoxia.* Exposure to intermittent or chronic hypoxia intensifies the response to acute hypoxia.[326,327]

6. *Size of the hypoxic compartment.* The intensity of constriction of a given vessel to a hypoxic stimulus is unaffected by the size of the hypoxic compartment. When the hypoxic area is small, the effect of the vasoconstriction is to divert flow to other, better oxygenated regions. When the affected area is large, then the vasoconstriction alters flow patterns minimally, but produces elevated PAP.[255,463]

Local and humoral agents Many agents affect pulmonary vascular tone including histamine, prostaglandins, and leukotrienes. Histamine is present in lung in perivascular mast cells. When resting tone is low, histamine is a modest pulmonary venoconstrictor; if resting tone is high, exogenous histamine produces vasodilation.[152] Its role in normal pulmonary vascular function is not defined.

Products of arachidonic metabolism have multiple effects on the pulmonary vascular bed. The capacity of the lung to produce and metabolize prostaglandins is very high, with enzymes present to synthesize PGI_2, PGE_2, TXA_2, $PGF_{2\alpha}$, and PGD_2.[198] Prostacyclin (PGI_2) is a powerful vasodilator in the lung.[58,198] It is a major product of pulmonary endothelium, and may assist in maintaining the normal low vascular tone. PGE_2 produces modest vasodilatation in fetal and infant lungs and mild vasoconstriction in the adult dog. $PGF_{2\alpha}$, TXA_2, and PGD_2 are powerful vasoconstrictors, but do not have a defined function in normal lung circulation. Hypoxic vasoconstriction occurs in the absence of the prostaglandins.[152]

Leukotriene D_4 has recently been shown to be a powerful pulmonary vasoconstrictor.[197] Leukotrienes C_4 and D_4 have also been found in the lung lavage fluid of newborns with persistent pulmonary hypertension.[401] However, in infant pigs, specific antagonists to both leukotrienes did not alter hypoxic vasoconstriction.[228] Thus, the issue of a physiologic role for these agents is unresolved.

Neurogenic control The pulmonary vascular bed receives generous sympathetic innervation, and contains both alpha- and beta-adrenoceptors.[152] In the fetus, sympathetic stimulation or administration of alpha-adrenergic agonists produces vasoconstriction.[343] Postnatal resting vasoconstrictor tone is low, and abolition of sympathetic innervation does not alter the hypoxic pressor response.[152] Thus the significance of neurogenic control to the pulmonary vascular bed is questionable.

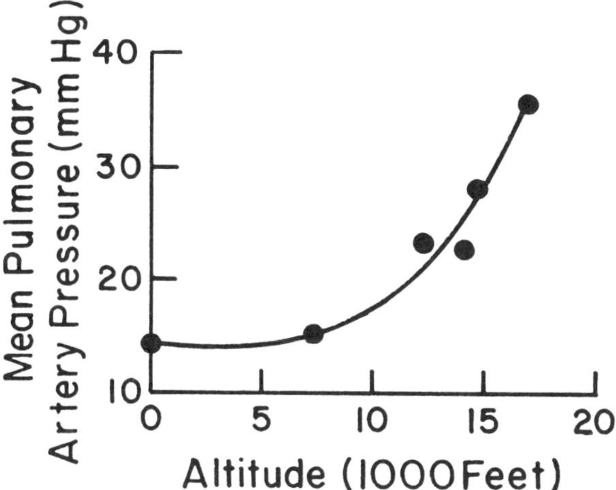

Fig. 1.35. Relationship of mean pulmonary artery pressure to altitude in residents of South America (Reeves JT 1973 Pulmonary vascular response to high altitude residence. Cardiovascular Clinics 5/1: 81.)

Response to Chronic Hypoxia

The most common challenge to the pulmonary vascular bed is exposure to chronic hypoxia associated with high altitude. Adaptation of the left ventricle and systemic circulation are discussed in the sections *Adaptation to altered oxygen supply/demand* and *Circulatory reserve*, respectively. The effect of residence at high altitude on the decline in PAP is shown in Figure 1.34B. Though the PAP of newborns is the same as at sea level (Fig. 1.34A) it changes only slowly, so that among adults the pressure is approximately twice that at sea level. The scatter among the adult measurements is much greater at high altitude than at sea level, with some very elevated pressures. Because these data were not sequential measurements, it is not clear whether some individuals had still higher PAP but did not survive to be included in the observed group. The mean PAP as a function of altitude of residence for South American natives is shown in Figure 1.35. The marked effect above 9000 feet is evident.

The mechanisms for the persistent pulmonary hypertension include retention of the fetal pattern of thick distal artery muscles, and development of new arterial muscle which extends to more distal parts of the vascular bed than at sea level.[114,132,237,288,319] The pulmonary trunk retains its fetal characteristics of medial hypertrophy and an aortic configuration of the elastica.[114,165,333,334] Adult rats exposed to chronic hypoxia and then normoxia return to normal PAP after 3 months.[319] Infant rats retained their pulmonary hypertension despite the removal of the hypoxic stress.[268] Structural abnormalities persisted in both groups.

High altitude pulmonary hypertension is associated with right ventricular hypertrophy (RVH). The magnitude of RVH is related to the history of acclimatization: the right ventricle is largest in sea level natives who have moved to high altitude, less large in native highlanders whose families have resided at high altitude for a few generations, still less large in natives who derive from many generations of highlanders, and normal for sea level residents at sea level.[326] The implication is that there is natural selection for individuals who respond to chronic hypoxia with less severe pulmonary hypertension. Such has been shown for cattle.[326]

REFERENCES

1. Abboud FM, Schmid PG, Heistad DD, Mark AL 1976 Regulation of peripheral and coronary circulation. In: Levine HJ (ed) Clinical Cardiovascular Physiology. Grune & Stratton, New York
2. Abboud FM, Thames MD 1983 Interaction of cardiovascular reflexes in circulatory control. In: Shepherd JT, Abboud FM (eds) Handbook of Physiology, Section 2: The Cardiovascular System, Vol III, Peripheral Circulation and Organ Blood Flow, Part 2. American Physiological Society, Bethesda
3. Abrahams VC, Hilton SM, Zbrozyna AW 1964 The role of active muscle vasodilatation in the alerting stage of the defence reaction. Journal of Physiology 171: 189
4. Adachi H, Strauss HW, Ochi H, Wagner HN Jr 1976 The effect of hypoxia on the regional distribution of cardiac output in the dog. Circulation Research 39: 314
5. Adams FH, Landaw EM 1981 What are healthy blood pressures for children? Pediatrics 68: 268
6. Adams RJ, Schwartz A 1980 Comparative mechanisms for contraction of cardiac and skeletal muscle. Chest 78: 123
7. Adelstein RS, Hathaway DR 1979 Role of calcium and cyclic adenosine 3′,5′-monophosphate in regulating smooth muscle contraction. American Journal of Cardiology 44: 783
8. Adler-Graschinsky E, Langer SZ 1975 Possible role of a beta-adrenoceptor in the regulation of noradrenaline release by nerve stimulation through a positive feed-back mechanism. British Journal of Pharmacology 53: 43
9. Ahumeda G, Sobel BE, Friedman WF 1976 Age-dependent mechanical and biochemical responses to glucagon. American Journal of Physiology 230: 1590
10. Akera T, Brody TM 1977 The role of Na^+, K^+-ATPase in the inotropic action of digitalis. Pharmacological Review 29: 187
11. Alexander RS 1977 Critical closure reexamined. Circulation Research 40: 531
12. Allen HD, Goldberg SJ, Sahn DJ, Schy N, Wojcik R 1977 A quantitative echocardiographic study of champion childhood swimmers. Circulation 55: 142
13. Anderson C, Hellstrand P, Johansson B, Ringberg A 1974 Contraction in venous smooth muscle induced by hypertonicity. Calcium dependence and mechanical characteristics. Acta Physiologica Scandinavica 90: 451
14. Anversa P, Olivetti G, Loud AV 1980 Morphometric study of early postnatal development in the left and right ventricular myocardium of the rat. Circulation Research 46: 495
15. Archie JP Jr, Fixier DE, Ullyot DJ, Buckberg GD, Hoffman JIE 1974 Regional myocardial blood flow in lambs with concentric right ventricular hypertrophy. Circulation Research 34: 143
16. Armando I, Levin G, Barontini M 1983 Evaluation of sympathetic nervous system and adrenomedullary activity in normal children. Journal of the Autonomic Nervous System 8: 57
17. Armour JA, Lippincott DB, Randall WC 1973 Functional anatomy of the interventricular septum. Cardiology 58: 65
18. Astorri E, Bolognesi R, Colla B, Chizzola A, Visioli O 1977 Left ventricular hypertrophy: A cytometric study on 42 human hearts. Journal of Molecular and Cellular Cardiology 9: 763
19. Baird RJ, Manktelow RT, Shah PA, Ameli FM 1970 Intramyocardial pressure. A study of its regional variations and its relationship to intraventricular pressure. Journal of Thoracic and Cardiovascular Surgery 59: 810
20. Baldwin KM, Cooke DA, Cheadle WG 1977 Enzyme alterations in neonatal heart muscle during development. Journal of Molecular and Cellular Cardiology 9: 651
21. Bano-Rodrigo A, Quero-Jimenez M, Monreno-Granado F, Gamallo-Amat C 1980 Wall thickness of ventricular chambers in transposition of the great arteries. Journal of Thoracic and Cardiovascular Surgery 79: 592
22. Barash PG, Glanz S, Katz JD, Taunt K, Talner NS 1978 Ventricular function in children during halothane anesthesia: An echocardiographic evaluation. Anesthesiology 49: 79
23. Barnard RJ, Duncan HW, Baldwin KM, Buckberg GD 1980 Effects of intensive exercise training on myocardial performance and coronary blood flow. Journal of Applied Physiology 43: 988
24. Bar-Or O, Shephard RJ, Allen CL 1971 Cardiac output of 10- to 13-year-old boys and girls during submaximal exercise. Journal of Applied Physiology 30: 219
25. Barrie SE, Harris P 1977 Myocardial enzyme activities in guinea pigs during development. American Journal of Physiology 233: H707

26. Bayliss WM 1902 On the local reaction of the arterial wall to changes of internal pressure. Journal of Physiology, London 28: 220
27. Behrman RE, Lees MH 1971 Organ blood flows of the fetal newborn and adult rhesus monkey. Biology of the Neonate 18: 330
28. Berne RM 1980 The role of adenosine in the regulation of coronary blood flow. Circulation Research 47: 803
29. Berne RM, Rubio R 1979 Coronary circulation. In: Berne RM (ed) Handbook of Physiology, Section 2: The Cardiovascular System, Vol I, The Heart. American Physiological Society, Bethesda
30. Berne RM, Winn HR, Rubio R 1981 The local regulation of cerebral blood flow. Progress in Cardiovascular Diseases 24: 243
31. Bevan JA, Bevan RD, Duckles SP 1980 Adrenergic regulation of vascular smooth muscle. In: Bohr DF, Somlyo AP, Sparks, HV Jr (eds) Handbook of Physiology, Section 2: Circulation, Vol II, Vascular Smooth Muscle. American Physiological Society, Bethesda
32. Beyar R, Sideman S 1984 A computer study of the left ventricular performance based on fiber structure, sarcomere dynamics, and transmural electrical propagation velocity. Circulation Research 55: 358
33. Beznak M, Korecky B, Thomas B 1969 Regression of cardiac hypertrophies of various origin. Canadian Journal of Physiology and Pharmacology 47: 579
34. Bjork VO, Olm CL, Bjarke BB, Thoren CA 1979 Right atrial-right ventricular anastomosis for correction of tricuspid atresia. Journal of Thoracic and Cardiovascular Surgery 77: 452
35. Bjorkhem G 1977 Echocardiographic assessment of left ventricular function. European Journal of Cardiology 6(2): 83
36. Blix AS, Folkow B 1983 Cardiovascular adjustments to diving in mammals and birds. In: Shepherd JT, Abboud FM (eds) Handbook of Physiology, The Cardiovascular System, Vol III, Peripheral Circulation and Organ Blood Flow, Part 2. American Physiological Society, Bethesda
37. Blomqvist CG 1983 Cardiovascular adaptations to physical training. Annual Review of Physiology 45: 169
38. Bohr DF, Somlyo AP, Sparks HV Jr (eds) 1980 Handbook of Physiology, The Cardiovascular System, Vol II, Vascular Smooth Muscle. American Physiological Society, Bethesda
39. Bond RF, Johnson G III 1984 Cardiovascular adrenoreceptor function during compensatory and decompensatory hemorrhagic shock. Circulatory Shock 12: 9
40. Borer JS, Jason M, Devereau RB, Fisher J, Green MV, Bacharach SL, Pickering T, Laragh JH 1983 Function of the hypertrophied left ventricle at rest and during exercise. American Journal of Medicine 75 (3A): 34
41. Borg TK, Caulfield JB 1981 The collagen matrix of the heart. In: Weber KT, Hawthorne EW (eds) Symposium on cardiac shape and structure. Federation Proceedings 40: 2037
42. Borow KM, Green LH, Grossman W, Braunwald E 1982 Left ventricular end-systolic stress-shortening and stress-length relations in humans. American Journal of Cardiology 50: 1301
43. Borow KM, Neumann A, Wynne J 1982 Sensitivity of end-systolic pressure-dimension and pressure-volume relations to inotropic state in humans. Circulation 65: 988
44. Brady AJ 1979 Mechanical properties of cardiac fibers. In: Berne RM (ed) Handbook of Physiology, Section 2: The Cardiovascular System, Vol I, The Heart. American Physiological Society, Bethesda
45. Braunwald E 1974 Regulation of the circulation. New England Journal of Medicine 290: 1124
46. Brennan LA Jr, Malvin RL, Jochim KE, Roberts DE 1971 Influence of right and left atrial receptors on plasma concentrations of ADH and renin. American Journal of Physiology 221: 273
47. Brenner JI, Moschler R, Baker K, Berman MA 1982 Evaluation of left ventricular performance in infants and children using radionuclide angiography. Pediatric Cardiology 2: 115
48. Broadley KJ 1982 Cardiac adrenoceptors. Journal of Autonomic Pharmacology 2: 119
49. Brodde OE, Motomura S, Endoh M, Schumann HJ 1978 Lack of correlation between the positive inotropic effect evoked by α-adrenoceptor stimulation and the levels of cyclic AMP and/or cyclic GMP in the isolated ventricle strip of the rabbit. Journal of Molecular and Cellular Cardiology 10: 207
50. Brown AM 1979 Cardiac reflexes. In: Berne RM (ed) Handbook of Physiology, Section 2: The Cardiovascular System, Vol 1, The Heart. American Physiological Society, Bethesda
51. Bryan LJ, Cole JJ, O'Donnel SR, Wantsall JC 1981 A study designed to explore the hypothesis that $beta_1$-adrenoceptors are "innervated" receptors and $beta_2$ adrenoceptors are "hormonal" receptors. Journal of Pharmacology and Experimental Therapeutics 216: 395
52. Burnstock G 1980 Cholinergic and purinergic regulation of blood vessels. In: Bohr DF, Somlyo AP, Sparks HV Jr (eds) Handbook of Physiology, Section 2, Circulation, Vol II, Vascular Smooth Muscle. American Physiological Society, Bethesda

53. Burton AC 1951 On the physical equilibrium of small blood vessels. American Journal of Physiology 164: 319
54. Cannon PJ 1984 Eicosanoids and the blood vessel wall. Circulation 70: 523
55. Caro CG, Pedley TJ, Seed WA 1974 Mechanics of the circulation. In: Guyton AC, Jones CE (eds) MTP International Review of Science, Physiology Series One, Vol I, Cardiovascular Physiology. University Park Press, Baltimore
56. Case RB, Berglund E, Sarnoff SJ 1955 Ventricular function: changes in coronary resistance and ventricular function resulting from acutely induced anemia and the effect thereon of coronary stenosis. American Journal of Medicine 18: 397
57. Casley-Smith JR 1977 Lymph and lymphatics. In: Kaley G, Altura BM (eds) Microcirculation, Vol. I. University Park Press, Baltimore
58. Cassin S 1980 Role of prostaglandins and thromboxanes in the control of the pulmonary circulation in the fetus and newborn. Seminars in Perinatology 4: 101
59. Cayler GG, Rudolph AM, Nadas AS 1963 Systemic blood flow in infants and children with and without heart disease. Pediatrics 32: 186
60. Chien S, Usami S 1984 Blood flow in small tubes. In: Renkin EM, Michel CC (eds) Handbook of Physiology, Section 2, The Cardiovascular System, Vol IV, Microcirculation, Part 1. American Physiological Society, Bethesda
61. Civin WH, Edwards JE 1951 The postnatal structural changes in the intrapulmonary arteries and arterioles. Archives of Pathology 51: 192
62. Clarke WR, Schrott HG, Leaverton PE, Conner WE, Lauer RM 1978 Tracking of blood lipids and blood pressure in school age children: the Muscatine study. Circulation 58: 626
63. Clausen JP 1977 Effect of physical training on cardiovascular adjustments to exercise in man. Physiological Reviews 57: 779
64. Claycomb WC 1978 Biochemical aspects of cardiac muscle differentiation. Determination of deoxyribonucleic acid template availability and 3′-hydroxyl termini in nuclei and chromatin by using exogenous deoxyribonucleic acid polymerases. Biochemical Journal 171: 289
65. Claycomb WC 1979 DNA synthesis and DNA enzymes in terminally differentiating cardiac muscle cells. Experimental Cell Research 118: 111
66. Clements IP, Brown ML, Smith HC 1981 Radionuclide measurement of left ventricular volume. Mayo Clinic Proceedings 56: 733
67. Coburn RF, Ploegmakers P, Gondrie P, Abboud R 1973 Myocardial myoglobin oxygen tensions. American Journal of Physiology 224: 870
68. Cohn HE, Sacks EJ, Heymann MA, Rudolph AM 1974 Cardiovascular responses to hypoxemia and acidemia in fetal lambs. American Journal of Obstetrics and Gynecology 120: 817
69. Cooper G IV, Puga FJ, Zujko KJ, Harrison CE, Coleman HN III 1975 Normal myocardial function and energetics in volume-overload hypertrophy in the cat. Circulation Research 32: 140
70. Covell JW, Ross J Jr, Sonnenblick EH, Braunwald E 1966 Comparison of the force-velocity relation and the ventricular function curve as measures of the contractile state of the intact heart. Circulation Research 19 (Suppl II): 364
71. Cowley AW Jr 1982 Vasopressin and cardiovascular regulation. In: Guyton AC, Hall JE (eds) Cardiovascular Physiology IV, International Review of Physiology, Vol 26. University Park Press, Baltimore
72. Cropp GJA 1969 Cardiovascular function in children with severe anemia. Circulation 39: 775
73. Culpepper WS 1983 Cardiac anatomy and function in juvenile hypertension. Current understanding and future concerns. American Journal of Medicine 75: 57
74. Cutilleta AF, Dowell RT, Rudnik M, Arcilla RA, Zak R 1975 Regression of myocardial hypertrophy, I. Experimental model, changes in heart weight, nucleic acids and collagen. Journal of Molecular and Cellular Cardiology 7: 767
75. Dawes GS, Johnston BM, Walker DW 1980 Relationship of arterial pressure and heart rate in foetal, newborn and adult sheep. Journal of Physiology, London 309: 405
76. Dawes GS, Mott JC, Shelley HJ 1959 The importance of cardiac glycogen for the maintenance of life in foetal lambs and newborn animals during anoxia. Journal of Physiology, London 146: 516
77. DeGeest H, Levy MN, Zieske H, Lipman RI 1965 Depression of ventricular contractility by stimulation of the vagus nerves. Circulation Research 17: 222
78. de la Cruz MV, Anselmi G, Romero A, Monroy G 1960 A qualitative and quantitative study of the ventricles and great vessels of normal children. American Heart Journal 60: 675
79. Delivoria-Papadopoulos M, Roncevic NP, Oski FA 1971 Post-natal changes in oxygen transport of term, premature and sick infants: The role of red cell 2,3-diphosphoglycerate and adult hemoglobin. Pediatric Research 5: 235

80. DeSwiet M, Fayers P, Shinebourne EA 1980 Systolic blood pressure in a population of infants in the first year of life—the Brompton study. Pediatrics 65:1028
81. Detar R, Bohr DF 1968 Oxygen and vascular smooth muscle contraction. American Journal of Physiology 214: 241
82. Dobrin PB 1983 Vascular mechanics. In: Shepherd JT, Abboud FM (eds) Handbook of Physiology, The Cardiovascular System, Vol III Peripheral Circulation and Organ Blood Flow, Part I. American Physiological Society, Bethesda
83. Dock DS, Kraus WL, McGuire LB, Hyland JW, Haynes W, Dexter L 1961 The pulmonary blood volume in man. Journal of Clinical Investigation 40: 317
84. Donner R, Carabello BA, Black I, Spann JF 1983 Left ventricular wall stress in compensated aortic stenosis in children. American Journal of Cardiology 51: 946
85. Dowell RT 1983 Cardiac adaptations to exercise. Exercise and Sport Sciences Reviews 11: 99
86. Dowell RT, McManus RE III 1978 Pressure-induced cardiac enlargement in neonatal and adult rats. Circulation Research 42: 303
87. Downing SE 1972 Neural regulation of circulation during hypoxia and acidosis with special reference to the newborn. Federation Proceedings 31: 1209
88. Downing SE 1979 Baroreceptor regulation of the heart. In: Berne RM (ed) Handbook of Physiology, Section 2: The Cardiovascular System, Vol. I, The Heart. American Physiological Society, Bethesda
89. Downing SE, Talner NS, Campbell AGM, Halloran KH, Wax HB 1969 Influence of sympathetic nerve stimulation on ventricular function in the newborn lamb. Circulation Research 25: 417
90. Downing SE, Talner NS, Gardner TH 1966 Influences of hypoxemia and acidemia on left ventricular function. American Journal of Physiology 210: 1327
91. Downing SE, Talner NS, Gardner TH 1966 Influences of arterial oxygen tension and pH on cardiac function in the newborn lamb. American Journal of Physiology 211: 1203
92. Driscoll DJ, Gilette PC, Lewis RM, Hartley CJ, Schwartz A 1979 Comparative hemodynamic effects of isoproterenol, dopamine and dobutamine in the newborn dog. Pediatric Research 13: 1006
93. Dunn RB, Griggs DM Jr 1975 Transmural gradients in ventricular tissue metabolites produced by stopping coronary blood flow in the dog. Circulation Research 37: 438
94. Elzinga G, Westerhof N 1979 How to quantify pump function of the heart. The value of variables derived from measurements on isolated muscle. Circulation Research 44: 303
95. Emery JL, Mithal A 1961 Weights of cardiac ventricles at and after birth. British Heart Journal 23: 313
96. Emmanouilides GC, Moss AJ, Duffie ER Jr, Adams FH 1964 Pulmonary arterial pressure changes in human newborn infants from birth to 3 days of age. Journal of Pediatrics 65: 327
97. Epstein ML, Goldberg SJ, Allen HD, Konecke L, Wood J 1975 Great vessel, cardiac chamber, and wall growth patterns in normal children. Circulation 51: 1124
98. Esterly JR, Oppenheimer EH 1967 Some aspects of pathology in infancy and childhood, IV, Myocardial and coronary lesions in cardiac malformations. Pediatrics 39: 896
99. Estes EH Jr, Entman ML, Dixon HB II, Hackel DB 1966 The vascular supply of the left ventricular wall. Anatomic observations, plus a hypothesis regarding acute events in coronary artery disease. American Heart Journal 71: 58
100. Eyzaguirre C, Fitzgerald RS, Lahiri S, Zapata P 1983 Arterial chemoreceptors. In: Shepherd JT, Abboud FM (eds) Handbook of Physiology, Section 2: The Cardiovascular System, Vol III, Peripheral Circulation and Organ Blood Flow, Part 2. American Physiological Society, Bethesda
101. Fabiato A, Fabiato F 1978 Calcium induced release of calcium from the sarcoplasmic reticulum of skinned cells from adult human, dog, cat, rabbit, rat and frog hearts and from fetal and newborn rat ventricles. Annals New York Academy of Science 307: 491
102. Fabiato A, Fabiato F 1979 Calcium and cardiac excitation-contraction coupling. Annual Review of Physiology 41: 473
103. Facchinetti F, Bagnoli F, Bracci R, Genazzani AR 1982 Plasma opioids in the first hours of life. Pediatric Research 16: 95
104. Fan, F-C, Chen, RYZ, Schuessler GB, Chien S 1980 Effects of hematocrit variations on regional hemodynamics and oxygen transport in the dog. American Journal of Physiology 238: H545
105. Feigl EO 1983 Coronary physiology. Physiological Reviews 63: 1–205
106. Ferlinz J 1982 Right ventricular function in adult cardiovascular disease. Progress in Cardiovascular Diseases 25: 225
107. Ferrans VJ 1978 Myocardial ultrastructure in human cardiac hypertrophy. In: Kaltenbach M, Loogen F, Olsen EGJ (eds) Cardiomyopathy and Myocardial Biopsy. Springer-Verlag, Berlin
108. Fisher DJ, Heymann MA, Rudolph AM 1980 Myocardial oxygen and carbohydrate consumption in fetal lambs in utero and in adult sheep. American Journal of Physiology 238: H399

109. Fisher DJ, Heymann MA, Rudolph AM 1982 Fetal myocardial oxygen and carbohydrate consumption during acutely induced hypoxemia. American Journal of Physiology 242: 657
110. Fisher DJ, Heymann MA, Rudolph AM 1982 Regional myocardial blood flow and oxygen delivery in fetal, newborn, and adult sheep. American Journal of Physiology 243: 729
111. Fisher DJ, Heymann MA, Rudolph AM 1982 Fetal myocardial oxygen and carbohydrate metabolism in sustained hypoxemia in utero. American Journal of Physiology 243: 959
112. Fisher EA, DuBrow IW, Hastreiter AR 1975 Right ventricular volume in congenital heart disease. American Journal of Cardiology 36: 67
113. Fishman AP 1976 Hypoxia on the pulmonary circulation: how and where it acts. Circulation Research 38: 221
114. Florenzano F, Diaz G, Regonesi C, Escobar E 1984 Left ventricular function in chronic anemia: Evidence of noncatecholamine positive inotropic factor in the serum. American Journal of Cardiology 54: 638
115. Folkow B, Neil E 1971 Circulation. Oxford University Press, New York
116. Ford LE 1976 Heart size. Circulation Research 39: 297
117. Frank O 1895 Zur dynamik des herzmuskels. Zeitschrift fur Biologie 32: 370 Translated by Chapman CB, Wasserman E 1959, as: On the dynamics of cardiac muscle. American Heart Journal 58: 282, 467
118. Freed MD, Heymann MA, Lewis AB, Roehl SL, Kensey RC 1981 Prostaglandin E_1 in infants with ductus arteriosus-dependent congenital heart disease. Circulation 64: 899
119. Friedman WF 1973 The intrinsic physiologic properties of the developing heart. In: Friedman WF, Lesch M, Sonneblick EH (eds) Neonatal Heart Disease. Grune & Stratton, New York
120. Friedman WF, Kirkpatrick SE 1977 Fetal cardiovascular adaptation to asphyxia. In: Gluck L (ed) Intrauterine Asphyxia and the Developing Fetal Brain. Year Book, Chicago
121. Friedman WF, Pool PE, Jacobowitz D, Seagren BA, Braunwald E 1968 Sympathetic innervation of the developing rabbit heart—biochemical and histochemical comparisons of fetal neonatal and adult myocardium. Circulation Research 23: 25
122. Friedman WF, Su JY 1973 Comparison of the responses of fetal and adult cardiac muscle to hypoxia. American Journal of Physiology 224: 1249
123. Frisancho AR 1975 Functional adaptation to high altitude hypoxia. Science 187: 313
124. Gaasch WH, Levine HJ, Quinones MA, Alexander JK 1976 Left ventricular compliance: Mechanisms and clinical implications. American Journal of Cardiology 38: 645
125. Gaehtgens P 1980 Flow of blood through narrow capillaries: Rheological mechanisms determining capillary hematocrit and apparent viscosity. Biorheology 17: 183
126. Geenen DL, Gilliam TB, Crowley D, Moorehead-Steffens C, Rosenthal A 1982 Echocardiographic measures in 6 to 7 year old children after an 8 month exercise program. American Journal of Cardiology 49: 1990
127. Geis WP, Tatooles CJ, Priola DV, Friedman WF 1975 Factors influencing neurohumoral control of the heart in the newborn dog. American Journal of Physiology 228: 1685
128. Gerthoffer WT, Trevethick MA, Murphy RA 1984 Myosin phosphorylation and cyclic adenosine 3′,5′-monophosphate in relaxation of arterial smooth muscle by vasodilators. Circulation Research 54: 83
129. Ghani QP, Hollenberg M 1978 Poly(adenosine diphosphate ribose) metabolism and regulation of myocardial cell growth by oxygen. Biochemical Journal 170: 387
130. Gibbs CL, Chapman JB 1979 Cardiac energetics In: Berne RM (ed) Handbook of Physiology. Section 2: The Cardiovascular System, Vol I, The Heart. American Physiological Society, Bethesda
131. Gilmore JP 1983 Neural control of extracellular volume in the human and nonhuman primate. In: Shepherd JT, Abboud FM (eds), Handbook of Physiology, The Cardiovascular System, Vol III, Part 2. American Physiological Society, Bethesda
132. Glantz SA, Kernoff RS 1975 Muscle stiffness determined from canine left ventricular pressure-volume curves. Circulation Research 37: 787
133. Glantz SA, Parmley WW 1975 Factors which affect the diastolic pressure-volume curve. Circulation Research 42: 171
134. Gootman PM, Buckley NM, Gootman N 1979 Postnatal maturation of neural control of the circulation. Reviews in Perinatal Medicine 3: 1
135. Gorza L, Mercadier JJ, Schwartz K, Thornell LE, Sartoe S, Schiaffino S 1984 Myosin types in the human heart. Circulation Research 54: 694
136. Gow BS 1980 Circulatory correlates: Vascular impedance, resistance, and capacity. In: Bohr DR, Somlyo AP, Sparks HV Jr (eds) Handbook of Physiology, The Cardiovascular System, Vol II, Vascular Smooth Muscle. American Physiological Society, Bethesda
137. Graham TP Jr, Bender HW, Atwood GF, Page DL, Sell CGR 1974 Increase in right ventricular

volume following valvulotomy for pulmonary atresia or stenosis with intact ventricular septum. Circulation 50 (Suppl II): 69

138. Graham TP Jr, Jarmakani JM 1971 Evaluation of ventricular function in infants and children. Pediatric Clinics of North America 18: 1109
139. Graham TP Jr, Jarmakani JM 1973 Hemodynamic investigation of congenital heart disease in infancy and childhood. In: Friedman WF, Lesch M, Sonnenblick EH (eds) Neonatal Heart Disease. Grune & Stratton, New York
140. Graham TP Jr, Jarmakani JM, Atwood GF, Canent RV 1973 Right ventricular volume determinations in children. Normal values and observations with volume or pressure overload. Circulation 47: 144
141. Graham TP Jr, Jarmakani JM, Canent RV Jr, Capp MP, Spach MS 1968 Characterization of left heart volumes and mass in normal children and in infants with intrinsic myocardial disease. Circulation 38: 826
142. Graham TP Jr, Jarmakani JM, Canet RV Jr, Morrow MN 1971 Left heart volume estimation in infancy and childhood, reevaluation of methodology and normal values. Circulation 43: 895
143. Graham TP Jr, Lewis BW, Jarmakani JM, Canent RV, Capp MP 1970 Left heart volume and mass quantification in children with left ventricular pressure overload. Circulation 41: 203
144. Graham TP Jr, Parrish MD, Boucek RJ Jr, Boerth RC, Breitweser JA, Thompson S, Robertson RM, Morgan JR, Friesinger GC 1983 Assessment of ventricular size and function in congenitally corrected transposition of the great arteries. American Journal of Cardiology 51: 244
145. Grant C, Greene DG, Bunnell IL 1965 Left ventricular enlargement and hypertrophy. A clinical angiocardiographic study. American Journal of Medicine 39: 895
146. Grossman W 1980 Cardiac hypertrophy: Useful adaptation or pathologic process? American Journal of Medicine 69: 576
147. Grossman W, Braunwald E, Mann T, McLaurin LP, Green LH 1977 Contractile state of the left ventricle in man as evaluated from the end-systolic pressure-volume relation. Circulation 56: 845
148. Grossman W, Jones D, McLaurin LP 1975 Wall stress and patterns of hypertrophy in the human left ventricle. Journal of Clinical Investigation 56: 56
149. Grossman W, McLaurin LP 1976 Diastolic properties of the left ventricle. Annals of Internal Medicine 84: 316
150. Grossman W, McLaurin LP, Stafadouros MA 1974 Left ventricular stiffness associated with chronic pressure and volume overload. Circulation Research 35: 793
151. Grover RF, Lufschanowski R, Alexander JK 1976 Alterations in the coronary circulation of man following ascent to 3100 m altitude. Journal of Applied Physiology 41: 832
152. Grover RF, Wagner WW Jr, McMurtry IF, Reeves JT 1983 Pulmonary circulation. In: Shepherd JT, Abboud FM (eds) Handbook of Physiology, The Cardiovascular System, Vol III, Part 1. American Physiological Society, Bethesda
153. Gunther S, Grossman W 1979 Determinants of ventricular function in pressure-loaded hypertrophy in man. Circulation 59: 679
154. Gutgesell HP, Paquet M, Duff DF, McNamara DG 1977 Evaluation of left ventricular size and function by echocardiography. Results in normal children. Circulation 56: 457
155. Guyton AC, Jones CE, Coleman TG 1973 Circulatory physiology: cardiac output and its regulation. Saunders, Philadelphia
156. Guyton RA, Andrews MJ, Hickey PR 1976 The contribution of atrial contraction to right heart function before and after right ventriculotomy. Journal of Thoracic and Cardiovascular Surgery 71: 1
157. Hainsworth R, Linden RJ 1983 Reflex control of vascular capacitance. In: Guyton AC, Young DB (eds) Cardiovascular Physiology III, International Review of Physiology, Vol 18. University Park Press, Baltimore
158. Hales JRS 1973 Radioactive microsphere measurements of cardiac output and regional tissue blood flow in the sheep. Pfluegers Archives 344: 119
159. Halon DA, Amital N, Gotsman MS, Lewis BS 1979 Serial echocardiography during the first 3 months of life in normal neonates. European Journal of Cardiology 9: 393
160. Haworth SG 1983 Pulmonary vascular disease in secundum atrial septal defect in childhood. American Journal of Cardiology 51: 265
161. Haworth SG, Hislop AA 1981 Adaptation of the pulmonary circulation to extra-uterine life in the pig and its relevance to the human infant. Cardiovascular Research 15: 108
162. Heath D, Edwards JE 1958 The pathology of hypertensive pulmonary vascular disease: a description of six grades of structural changes in the pulmonary arteries with special reference to congenital cardiac septal defects. Circulation 18: 533
163. Heath D, Wood EH, DuShane JW, Edwards JE 1959 The structure of the pulmonary trunk at

different ages and in cases of pulmonary hypertension and pulmonary stenosis. Journal of Pathology and Bacteriology 77: 443
164. Heistad DD, Kontos HA 1983 Cerebral circulation. In: Shepherd JT, Abboud FM (eds) Handbook of Physiology, Section 2: The Cardiovascular System, Vol III, Peripheral Circulation and Organ Blood Flow, Part 1. American Physiological Society, Bethesda
165. Henry WL, Ware J, Gardin JM, Hepner SI, McKay J, Weiner M 1978 Echocardiographic measurements in normal subjects—growth-related changes that occur between infancy and early adulthood. Circulation 57: 278
166. Heymann MA, Payne BD, Hoffman JIE, Rudolph AM 1977 Blood flow measurements with radionuclide-labeled particles. Progress in Cardiovascular Diseases 20: 55
167. Heymann MA, Rudolph AM 1975 Control of the ductus arteriosus. Physiological Review 55: 62
168. Higgins CB, Mulder DG 1972 Tetralogy of Fallot in the adult. American Journal of Cardiology 29: 837
169. Hill AV 1938 The heat of shortening and the dynamic constants of muscle. Proceedings, The Royal Society of London, Series B 216: 136
170. Hislop A, Reid L 1973 Pulmonary arterial development during childhood: branching pattern and structure. Thorax 28: 129
171. Hoffman JIE 1978 Determinants and prediction of transmural myocardial perfusion. Circulation 58: 381
172. Hoffman JIE, Buckberg GD 1976 Transmural variations in myocardial perfusion. Progress in Cardiology 5: 37
173. Hoffman JIE, Rudolph AM 1970 The natural history of isolated ventricular septal defect with special reference to selection of patients for surgery. Advances in Pediatrics 17: 57
174. Hoffman JIE, Rudolph AM, Heymann MA 1981 Pulmonary vascular disease with congenital heart lesions: Pathologic features and causes. Circulation 64: 873
175. Holmberg S, Serzysko W, Varnauskas E 1971 Coronary circulation during heavy exercise in control subjects and patients with coronary heart disease. Acta Medica Scandinavica 190: 465
176. Holt JP, Rhode EA, Kines H 1960 Pericardial and ventricular pressures. Circulation Research 8: 1171
177. Hood WP, Rackley CE, Rolett EL 1968 Wall stress in the normal and hypertrophied human left ventricle. American Journal of Cardiology 22: 550
178. Houden TJ, Friedman WF 1982 Age-related effects of digoxin on myocardial contractility and Na-K pump in sheep. American Journal of Physiology 243: H517
179. Huber D, Grimm J, Koch R, Krayenbuehl HP 1981 Determinants of ejection performance in aortic stenosis. Circulation 64: 126
180. Hughes JD, Rubin LJ 1984 Relation between mixed venous oxygen tension and pulmonary vascular tone during normoxic, hyperoxic and hypoxic ventilation in dogs. American Journal of Cardiology 54: 1118
181. Hume WR 1980 Structural response of the blood vessel wall to sustained rise in wall tension. In: Bevin JA, Godfraind T, Maxwell RA, Vanhoutte PM (eds) Vascular Neuroeffector Mechanisms. Raven Press, New York
182. Ingebretsen WR Jr, Becker E, Friedman WF, Mayer SE 1977 Contractile and biochemical response of cardiac and skeletal muscle to isoproterenol covalently linked to glass beads. Circulation Research 40: 474
183. Ingebretsen WR Jr, Friedman WF, Mayer SE 1981 Isoproterenol-induced restoration of contraction in K^+-depolarized hearts: relationship to c-AMP. American Journal of Physiology 241: H187
184. Ingwall JS, Kramer MF, Woodman D, Friedman WF 1981 Maturation of energy metabolism in the lamb: changes in myosin ATPase and creative kinase activities. Pediatric Research 15: 1128
185. James FW, Kaplan S, Glueck CJ, Tsay JY, Knight MJ, Sarwar CJ 1980 Responses of normal children and young adults to controlled bicycle exercise. Circulation 61: 902
186. James LS, Rowe RD 1957 The pattern of response of pulmonary and systemic arterial pressures in newborn and older infants to short periods of hypoxia. Journal of Pediatrics 51: 5
187. Jan, K-M, Chien S 1977 Effect of hematocrit variations on coronary hemodynamics and oxygen utilization. American Journal of Physiology 233: 106
188. Jarmakani MM, Edwards SB, Spach MS, Canent RV Jr, Capp MP, Hagan MJ, Barr RC, Jain V 1968 Left-ventricular pressure-volume characteristics in congenital heart disease. Circulation 37: 879
189. Jarmakani JM, Graham TP Jr, Canent RV Jr 1982 Left ventricular contractile state in children with successfully corrected ventricular septal defect. Circulation 45 & 46 (Suppl I): 102
190. Jarmakani JM, Nagatomo T, Nakazawa M, Langer GA 1978 Effect of hypoxia on myocardial high energy phosphates in neonatal mammalian heart. American Journal of Physiology 235: H475

191. Jarmakani JM, Nakazawa M, Nagamoto T, Langer GA 1978 Effect of hypoxia on mechanical function in the neonatal mammalian heart. American Journal of Physiology 235: 469
192. Jewitt PH, Sommer JR 1972 The sarcoplasmic reticulum: ultrastructural differentiation in newborn dog and cat papillary muscle. Circulation 43, 44 (Suppl II): 11
193. Jie K, Van Brummelen P, Vermey P, Timmermans P, Van Zwieten PA 1984 Identification of vascular postsynaptic $alpha_1$- and $alpha_2$-adrenoceptors in man. Circulation Research 54: 447
194. Johansson B, Somlyo AP 1980 Electrophysiology and excitation-contraction coupling. In: Bohn DF, Somlyo AP, Sparks HV Jr (eds) Handbook of Physiology, Section 2, Circulation, Vol II, Vascular Smooth Muscle. American Physiological Society, Bethesda
195. Johnson PC 1980 The myogenic response. In: Bohr DF, Somlyo AP, Sparks HV Jr (eds) Handbook of Physiology, Section 2, Circulation, Vol II. Vascular Smooth Muscle. American Physiological Society, Bethesda
196. Jorgensen CR, Wang K, Wang Y, Gobel FL, Nelson RR, Taylor H 1973 Effect of propranolol on myocardial oxygen consumption and its hemodynamic correlates during upright exercise. Circulation 48: 1173
197. Kadowitz PJ, Hyman AL 1984 Analysis of responses to leukotriene D_4 in the pulmonary vascular bed. Circulation Research 55: 707
198. Kadowitz PJ, Lippton HL, McNamara DB, Spannhake EW, Hyman AL 1982 Action and metabolism of prostaglandins in the pulmonary circulation. In: Oates JA (ed) Prostaglandins and the Cardiovascular System. Raven Press, New York
199. Katz AM 1970 Contractile proteins of the heart. Physiological Reviews 50: 63
200. Kawasaki H, Takasaki K 1984 Vasoconstrictor response induced by 5-hydroxytryptamine released from vascular adrenergic nerves by periarterial nerve stimulation. Journal of Pharmacology and Experimental Therapeutics 229: 816
201. Kaye HH, Tynan M, Hunter S 1975 Validity of echocardiographic estimates of left ventricular size and performance in infants and children. British Heart Journal 37: 371
202. Keen EN 1955 The postnatal development of the human cardiac ventricles. Journal of Anatomy 89: 484
203. Kennedy JW, Baxter WA, Figley MM, Dodge HT, Blackmon JR 1966 Quantitative angiography. I, The normal left ventricle in man. Circulation 34: 272
204. Kennedy T, Summer W 1982 Inhibition of hypoxic pulmonary vasoconstriction by Nifedipine. American Journal of Cardiology 50: 864
205. Kerrick WGL, Hoar PE, Cassidy PS 1980 Calcium-activated tension: The role of myosin light chain phosphorylation. Federation Proceedings 39: 1558
206. Kirkpatrick SE, Naliboff J, Pitlick PT, Friedman WF 1975 Influence of poststimulation potentiation and heart rate on the fetal lamb heart. American Journal of Physiology 229: 318
207. Kirkpatrick SE, Pitlick PT, Naliboff J, Friedman WF 1976 Frank-Starling relationship as an important determinant of fetal cardiac output. American Journal of Physiology 231: 495
208. Kitamura K, Jorgensen CR, Gobel FL, Taylor HL, Wang Y 1972 Hemodynamic correlates of myocardial oxygen consumption during upright exercise. Journal of Applied Physiology 32: 516
209. Klocke FJ, Ellis AK 1980 Control of coronary blood flow. Annual Review of Medicine 31: 489
210. Klopfenstein HS, Rudolph AM 1978 Postnatal changes in the circulation and responses to volume loading in sheep. Circulation Research 42: 839
211. Koehler RC, Jones MD Jr, Traystman RJ 1982 Cerebral circulatory response to carbon monoxide and hypoxic hypoxia in the lamb. American Journal of Physiology 243: H27
212. Kolbel F, Schreiber V 1983 Biochemical regulator in cardiac hypertrophy. Basic Research in Cardiology 78: 351
213. Kono A, Maughan WL, Sunagawa K, Hamilton K, Sagawa K, Weisfeldt ML 1984 The use of left ventricular end-ejection pressure and peak pressure in the estimation of the end-systolic pressure-volume relationship. Circulation 70: 1057
214. Korecky B, Bernath P, Rosengarten M, Taichman GC 1974 Effect of age on the passive stress-strain relationship of the rat heart. Federal Proceedings 33: 321
215. Korner PI 1979 Central nervous control of autonomic cardiovascular function. In: Berne RM (ed) Handbook of Physiology, Section 2: The Cardiovascular System, Vol I, The Heart. American Physiological Society, Bethesda
216. Kramsch DM, Aspen AJ, Abramowitz BM, Kreimendahl T, Hood WB Jr 1981 Reduction of coronary atherosclerosis by moderate conditioning exercise in monkeys on atherogenic diet. New England Journal of Medicine 305: 1483
217. Krovetz LJ, McLaughlin TG, Mitchell MB, Schiebler GL 1967 Hemodynamic findings in normal children. Pediatric Research 1: 122
218. Kuramoto K, Matsushita S, Matsuda T, Mifune J, Sakai M, Iwasaki T, Shinagawa T, Moroki

N, Murakami M 1980 Effect of hematocrit and viscosity on coronary circulation and myocardial oxygen utilization. Japanese Circulation Journal 44: 443

219. Kurtz D, Ahnberg DS, Freed M, LaFarge CG, Treves S 1976 Quantitative radionuclide angiocardiography. Determination of left ventricular ejection fraction in children. British Heart Journal 38: 966
220. LaGamma EF 1984 Endogenous opiates and cardiopulmonary function. Advances in Pediatrics 31: 1
221. LaGamma EF, Itskovitz J, Rudolph AM 1983 Maturation of circulatory responses to methionine-enkephalin. Pediatric Research 17: 162
222. Laks MM, Morady F, Swan HJC 1973 Myocardial hypertrophy produced by subhypertensive doses of norepinephrine in the dog. Chest 64: 75
223. Langer SZ 1977 Presynaptic receptors and their role in the regulation of transmitter release. British Journal of Pharmacology 60: 481
224. Langer SZ, Shepperson NB 1982 Postjunctional $alpha_1$- and $alpha_2$-adrenoceptors: Preferential innervation of $alpha_1$-adrenoceptors and the role of neuronal uptake. Journal of Cardiovascular Pharmacology 4: S8
225. Leake CD 1962 The historical development of cardiovascular physiology. In: Hamilton WF (ed) Handbook of Physiology, Circulation, Vol. 1, The Heart. American Physiological Society, Washington, DC
226. Lee JC, Downing SE 1974 Left ventricular distensibility in newborn piglets, adult swine, young kittens and adult cats. American Journal of Physiology 226: 1484
227. Lee JC, Halloran KH, Taylor JFN, Downing SE 1973 Coronary flow and myocardial metabolism in newborn lambs: Effects of hypoxia and acidemia. American Journal of Physiology 224: 1381
228. Leffler CW, Mitchell JA, Green RS 1984 Cardiovascular effects of leukotrienes in neonatal piglets. Circulation Research 55: 780
229. Legato MJ 1979 Cellular mechanisms of normal growth in the mammalian heart. I. Qualitative and quantitative features of ventricular architecture in the dog from birth to five months of age. Circulation Research 44: 250
230. Legato MJ 1979 Cellular mechanisms of normal growth in the mammalian heart II. A quantitative and qualitative comparison between the right and left ventricular myocytes in the dog from birth to five months of age. Circulation Research 44: 263
231. Lenfant C, Torrance JD, Reynafarje C 1971 Shift of the O_2-Hb dissociation curve at altitude; mechanism and effect. Journal of Applied Physiology 30: 625
232. Levin DL 1980 Effects of inhibition of prostaglandin synthesis on fetal development, oxygenation, and the fetal circulation. Seminars in Perinatology 4: 35
233. Levine HJ, Wolk MJ, Keefe, JF, Bing OHL, Snow JA, Messer JV 1977 Myocardial mechanics and energetics in experimental iron-deficiency anemia. American Journal of Physiology 232: 470
234. Levy MN, Blattberg B 1976 Effect of vagal stimulation on the overflow of norepinephrine into the coronary sinus during cardiac sympathetic nerve stimulation in the dog. Circulation Research 38: 81
235. Levy MN, Martin PJ 1979 Neural control of the heart. In: Berne RM (ed), Handbook of Physiology, Section 2: The Cardiovascular System, Vol I, The Heart. American Physiological Society, Bethesda
236. Lewis AB, Heymann MA, Stanger P, Hoffman JIE, Rudolph AM 1974 Evaluation of subendocardial ischemia in valvar aortic stenosis in children. Circulation 49: 978
237. Lewis BS, Gotsman MS 1980 Current concepts of left ventricular relaxation and compliance. American Heart Journal 99: 101
238. Liebman J 1982 Tables of normal standards. In: Liebman J, Plonsey R, Gillette PC (eds), Pediatric Electrocardiography. Williams & Wilkins, Baltimore
239. Linden RJ, Mitchell JH 1960 Relation between left ventricular diastolic pressure and myocardial segment length and observations on the contribution of atrial systole. Circulation Research 8: 1092
240. Lipowsky HH, Kovalchek S, Zweifach BW 1978 The distribution of blood rheological parameters in the microcirculation of cat mesentery. Circulation Research 43: 738
241. Lister G, Hellenbrand WE, Kleinman CS, Talner NS 1982 Physiologic effects of increasing hemoglobin concentration in left-to-right shunting in infants with ventricular septal defects. New England Journal of Medicine 306: 502
242. Lister G, Talner NS 1981 Oxygen Transport in Congenital Heart Disease. Cardiovascular Clinics 11/2: 129
243. Lister G, Walter TK, Versmold HT, Dallman PR, Rudolph AM 1979 Oxygen delivery in lambs: Cardiovascular and hematological development. American Journal of Physiology 237: 668
244. Little WC, Badke FR, O'Rourke RA 1984 Effect of right ventricular pressure on the end-diastolic

left ventricular pressure-volume relationship before and after chronic right ventricular pressure overload in dogs without pericardia. Circulation Research 54: 719

245. Lussier L, Buskirk ER 1977 Effects of an endurance training regimen on assessment of work capacity in prepubertal children. Annals of the New York Academy of Sciences 301: 734
246. Lynch JJ, Schuchard GH, Gross, CM, Wann LS 1984 Prevalence of right-to-left atrial shunting in a healthy population: detection by Valsava maneuver contrast echocardiography. American Journal of Cardiology 53: 1478
247. Mace SE, Levy MN 1983 Autonomic nervous control of heart rate: sympathetic-parasympathetic interactions and age related differences. Cardiovascular Research 17: 547
248. Mace SE, Levy MN 1983 Neural control of heart rate: A comparison between puppies and adult animals. Pediatric Research 17: 491
249. Manasek FJ 1979 Organization, interactions, and environment of heart cells during myocardial ontogeny. In: Berne RM (ed) Handbook of Physiology, Section 2: The Cardiovascular System, Vol I, The Heart. American Physiological Society, Bethesda
250. Mancia G, Mark AL 1983 Arterial baroreflexes in humans. In: Shepherd JT, Abboud FM (eds) Handbook of Physiology, Section 2: The Cardiovascular System, Vol III, Peripheral Circulation and Organ Blood Flow, Part 2. American Physiological Society, Bethesda
251. Manger WM 1982 Catecholamines in normal and abnormal cardiac function. Advances in Cardiology 30: 1
252. Mark AL, Mancia G 1983 Cardiopulmonary baroreflexes in humans. In: Shepherd JT, Abboud FM (eds), Handbook of Physiology, The Cardiovascular System, Vol III, Part 2. American Physiological Society, Bethesda
253. Marsh AJ, Lloyd BL, Taylor RR 1981 Age dependence of myocardial Na^+-K^+-ATPase activity and digitalis intoxication in dog and guinea pig. Circulation Research 48: 329
254. Marsh JD, Green LH, Wynne J, Cohn PF, Grossman W 1979 Left ventricular end-systolic pressure-dimension and stress-length relations in normal human subjects. American Journal of Cardiology 44: 1311
255. Marshall BE, Marshall C, Benumof JL, Saidman LJ 1981 Hypoxic pulmonary vasoconstriction in dogs: Effects of lung segment size and oxygen tension. Journal of Applied Physiology: Respiratory, Environmental and Exercise Physiology 51: 1543
256. Marshall HW, Helmholz HF Jr, Wood EH 1962 Physiologic consequences of congenital heart disease. In: Hamilton WF (ed) Handbook of Physiology, Circulation, Vol I, The Heart. American Physiological Society, Washington, DC
257. Matthew R, Thilenius, OG, Arcilla RA 1976 Comparative response of right and left ventricles to volume overload. American Journal of Cardiology 38: 209
258. Mayer SE, Dobson JG Jr, Ingebretsen WR Jr, Becker E, Brown JH, Friedman WF, Ross J Jr 1978 Ionic regulation of signal transfer from adrenergic receptors in cardiac muscle. Advances in Cyclic Nucleotide Research 9: 305
259. McCullagh WH, Covell JW, Ross J Jr 1972 Left ventricular dilatation and diastolic compliance changes during chronic volume overloading. Circulation 45: 943
260. McDonald DA 1960 Blood Flow in Arteries. Arnold, London
261. McPherson RA, Kramer MF, Covell JW, Friedman WF 1976 A comparison of the active stiffness of fetal and adult cardiac muscle. Pediatric Research 10: 660
262. Mehmel HC, Stockins B, Ruffmann K, v.Olshausen K, Schuler G, Kubler W 1981 The linearity of the end-systolic pressure-volume relationship in man and its sensitivity for assessment of left ventricular function. Circulation 63: 1216
263. Mela L, Delivoria-Papadopoulos M, Miller LD 1978 Fetal and neonatal mitochondrial electron transfer chain. In: Longo LD, Reneau DD (eds) Fetal and Newborn Cardiovascular Physiology, Vol 2. Garland Publishing, New York
264. Melcher A, Donald DE 1981 Maintained ability of carotid baroreflex to regulate arterial pressure during exercise. American Journal of Physiology 241: 838
265. Mellander S, Johansson B 1968 Control of resistance, exchange and capacitance functions in the peripheral circulation. Pharmacological Reviews 20: 117
266. Mercadier JJ, Bouvert P, Gorza L, Schiaffino S, Chizzonile RA, Zak R, Swynghedauw B, Schwartz K 1983 Myosin isoenzymes in normal and hypertrophied human ventricular myocardium. Circulation Research 53: 52
267. Messer JV, Wagman RJ, Levine HF, Neill WA, Kasnow N, Gorlin R 1962 Patterns of human myocardial oxygen extraction during rest and exercise. Journal of Clinical Investigation 41: 725
268. Meyrick B, Reid L 1978 The effect of continued hypoxia on rat pulmonary arterial circulation. An ultrastructural study. Laboratory Investigation 38: 188
269. Miller GAH, Swan HJC 1964 Effect of chronic pressure and volume overload on left heart volume in subjects with congenital heart diseases. Circulation 30: 205

270. Mirsky I 1969 Left ventricular stress in the intact heart. Biophysical Journal 9: 189
271. Mirsky I 1976 Assessment of passive elastic stiffness of cardiac muscle: Mathematical concepts, physiologic and clinical considerations, directions of future research. Progress in Cardiovascular Diseases 18: 277
272. Mirsky I 1979 Elastic properties of the myocardium: A quantitative approach with physiological and clinical applications. In: Berne RM (ed) Handbook of Physiology, Section 2. The Cardiovascular System, Vol I, The Heart. American Physiological Society, Bethesda
273. Mirsky I, Ellison RC, Hugenholtz PG 1971 Assessment of myocardial contractility in children and young adults from ventricular pressure recordings. American Journal of Cardiology 27: 359
274. Mirsky I, Rankin JS 1979 The effects of geometry, elasticity and external pressures on the diastolic pressure-volume and stiffness-strain relations. How important is the pericardium? Circulation Research 44: 601
275. Mitchell JH, Linden RJ, Sarnoff SJ 1960 Influence of cardiac sympathetic and vagal nerve stimulation on the relation between left ventricular diastolic pressure and myocardial segment length. Circulation Research 8: 1100
276. Mitchell MD 1982 Prostaglandin synthesis, metabolism and function in the fetus. In: James CT (ed) Biochemical Development of the Fetus and Neonate. Elsevier, Amsterdam
277. Mitchell RS, Stanford RE, Silvers GW, Dart G 1976 The right ventricle in chronic airway obstruction: A clinopathologic study. American Review of Respiratory Disease 114: 147
278. Morgan BC, Guntheroth WC, Dinard DH 1965 Relationship of pericardial to pleural pressure during quiet respiration and cardiac tamponade. Circulation Research 16: 493
279. Moriarty TF 1980 The law of LaPlace. Its limitations as a relation for diastolic pressure, volume, or wall stress of the left ventricle. Circulation Research 46: 321
280. Morkin E, LaRaia PJ 1974 Biochemical studies on the regulation of myocardial contractility. New England Journal of Medicine 290: 445
281. Morse M, Cassels DE, Schlutz FW 1947 Blood volumes of normal children. American Journal of Physiology 151: 448
282. Morthy SS, Losasso AM, Gibbs PS 1978 Acquired right-to-left intracardiac shunts and severe hypoxemia. Critical Care Medicine 6: 28
283. Moss AJ, Duffie ER Jr, Emmanouilides GC 1963 Blood pressure and vasomotor reflexes in the newborn infant. Pediatrics 32: 175
284. Moss AJ, Emmanouilides GC, Duffie ER Jr 1961 Closure of the ductus arteriosus in the newborn infant. Pediatrics 52: 25
285. Moss IR, Conner H, Yee WFH, Iorio P, Scarpelli EM 1982 Human beta-endorphin-like immunoreactivity in the perinatal/neonatal period. Journal of Pediatrics 101: 443
286. Mott JC, Walker DW 1983 Neural and endocrine regulation of circulation in the fetus and newborn. In: Shepherd JT, Abboud FM (eds) Handbook of Physiology, The Cardiovascular System, Vol III, Peripheral Circulation and Organ Blood Flow, Part II. American Physiological Society, Bethesda
287. Naeye RL 1966 Development of systemic and pulmonary arteries from birth through early childhood. Biologia Neonatorum 10: 8
288. Naeye RL, Letts HW 1962 The effects of prolonged neonatal hypoxemia on the pulmonary vascular bed and heart. Pediatrics 30: 902
289. Navarathnam V 1965 The ontogenesis of cholinesterase activity within the heart and cardiac ganglia in man, rat, rabbit and guinea-pig. Journal of Anatomy 99: 459
290. Neeley JR, Morgan HE 1974 Relationship between carbohydrate and lipid metabolism and energy balance of heart muscle. Annual Review of Physiology 36: 413
291. Neeley JR, Rovetto MJ, Oram JF 1972 Myocardial utilization of carbohydrate and lipids. Progress in Cardiovascular Diseases 15: 289
292. Neil E 1983 Peripheral circulation: historical aspects. In: Shepherd JT, Abboud FM (eds) Handbook of Physiology, The Cardiovascular System, Vol III, Peripheral Circulation and Organ Blood Flow, Part I. American Physiological Society. Bethesda
293. Neufeld HH, Wagenvoort CA, Edwards JE 1962 Coronary arteries in fetuses, infants, juveniles and young adults. Laboratory Investigation 11: 837
294. Nicoll PA, Taylor AE 1977 Lymph formation and flow. Annual Review of Physiology 39: 73
295. Nukamp FP 1982 Prostacyclin and the cardiovascular system. Netherlands Journal of Medicine 25: 15
296. Oberhansli I, Brandon G, Friedli B 1981 Echocardiographic growth patterns of intracardiac dimensions and determination of function indices during the first year of life. Helvetia Paediatrica Acta 36: 325
297. Oberhansli I, Brandon G, Lacourt G, Friedli B 1980 Growth patterns of cardiac structures and

changes in systolic time intervals in the newborn and infant. Acta Paediatrica Scandinavica 69: 239
298. Oliver WJ, Cohen EL, Neel JV 1975 Blood pressure, sodium intake, and sodium related hormones in the Yanomamo Indians, a "no salt" culture. Circulation 52: 146
299. Olsson RA 1975 Myocardial reactive hyperemia. Circulation Research 37: 263
300. Olsson RA 1981 Local factors regulating cardiac and skeletal muscle blood flow. Annual Review of Physiology 43: 385
301. Oski FA 1973 Designation of anemia on a functional basis. Journal of Pediatrics 83: 353
302. Pantley GA, Ladley HD, Bristow JD 1984 Low zero-flow pressure and minimal capacitance effect on diastolic coronary arterial pressure-flow relationships during maximum vasodilation in swine. Circulation 70: 485
303. Papadimitriou JM, Hopkins BE, Taylor RR 1974 Regression of left ventricular dilation and hypertrophy after removal of volume overload: Morphological and ultrastructural study. Circulation Research 35: 127
304. Parmley WW, Talbot L 1979 Heart as a pump. In: Berne RM (ed) Handbook of Physiology, Section 2: The Cardiovascular System, Vol I, The Heart. American Physiological Society, Bethesda
305. Parratt JR 1980 Effects of adrenergic activators and inhibitors on the coronary circulation. In: Szekeres L (ed) Handbook of Experimental Pharmacology, Adrenergic Activators and Inhibitors, Vol 54 Part I. Springer-Verlag, Berlin
306. Parrish MD, Graham TP Jr, Born ML, Jones J 1982 Radionuclide evaluation of right and left ventricular function in children: validation of methodology. American Journal of Cardiology 49: 1241
307. Patterson SW, Starling EH 1914 On the mechanical factors which determine the output of the ventricles. Journal of Physiology 48: 357
308. Paul RJ 1980 Chemical energetics of vascular smooth muscle. In: Bohr DF, Somlyo AP, Sparks HV Jr (eds) Handbook of Physiology, Section 2. Circulation, Vol II, Vascular Smooth Muscle. American Physiological Society, Bethesda
309. Pease RD, Benumof JL, Trousdale FR 1982 P_AO_2 and P_vO_2 interaction on hypoxic pulmonary vasoconstriction. Journal of Applied Physiology: Respiratory, Environmental and Exercise Physiology 53: 134
310. Pelletier CL, Clement DL, Shepherd JT 1972 Comparison of afferent activity of canine aortic and sinus nerves. Circulation Research 31: 557
311. Penaloza D, Arias-Stella J, Sime F, Recauarreu S, Marticorena E 1964 The heart and pulmonary circulation in children at high altitudes: Physiological, anatomical, and clinical observations. Pediatrics 34: 568
312. Perloff JK 1978 The clinical recognition of congenital heart disease. WB Saunders, Philadelphia
313. Perloff JK 1982 Development and regression of increased ventricular mass. American Journal of Cardiology 50: 605
314. Peters WP, Friedman PA, Johnson MW 1981 Pressor effects of naloxone in septic shock. Lancet 1: 529
315. Poole PE, Averill KH, Vogel JHK 1962 Effect of ligation of left pulmonary artery at birth on maturation of pulmonary vascular bed. Medicina Thoracalis 19: 362
316. Pool PE, Vogel JHK, Blount SG Jr 1962 Congenital unilateral absence of a pulmonary artery. The importance of blood flow in pulmonary hypertension. American Journal of Cardiology 10: 706
317. Printz MP, Skidgel RA, Friedman WF 1984 Studies of pulmonary prostaglandin biosynthesis and catabolic enzymes as factors in ductus arteriosus patency and closure. Evidence for a shift in products with gestational age. Pediatric Research 18: 19
318. Purfurst WD, Gunther KH, Drescher E, Austenat J, Hujer W 1982 The relationship of left ventricular function and mass in arterial hypertension—an echo and apexcardiographic comparison with sportsmen and controls. European Heart Journal 3 (Suppl A): 119
319. Rabinovitch M, Reid LM 1981 Quantitative structural analysis of the pulmonary vascular bed in congenital heart defects. Cardiovascular Clinics 11/2: 149
320. Randall, WC (ed) 1977 Neural Regulation of the Heart. Oxford University Press, New York
321. Randle PJ, Tubbs PK 1979 Carbohydrate and fatty acid metabolism. In: Berne RM (ed) Handbook of Physiology, Section 2: The Cardiovascular System, Vol I, The Heart. American Physiological Society, Bethesda
322. Rankin JS, McHale PA, Arentzen CE, Ling D, Greenfield DC Jr, Anderson RW 1976 The three-dimensional dynamic geometry of the left ventricle in the conscious dog. Circulation Research 39: 304
323. Rao PS, Liebman JL, Borkat G 1976 Right ventricular growth in a case of pulmonic stenosis with intact ventricular septum and hypoplastic right ventricle. Circulation 53: 389

324. Rapaport E 1982 Pathophysiological basis of ventricular hypertrophy. European Heart Journal 3 (Suppl A): 29
325. Reeves JT, Grover RF 1975 High altitude pulmonary, hypertension and pulmonary edema. Progress in Cardiology 4: 99
326. Reeves JT, Wagner WW Jr, McMurtry IF, Grover RF 1979 Physiologic effects of high altitude on the pulmonary circulation. In: Robertshaw D (ed) Environmental Physiology III, International Review of Physiology, Vol 20. University Park Press, Baltimore
327. Reid LM 1979 The pulmonary circulation: Remodeling in growth and disease. American Review of Respiratory Disease 119: 531
328. Renkin EM, Michel CC (eds) 1984 Handbook of Physiology, The Cardiovascular System, Vol IV, Microcirculation, Parts 1 and 2. American Physiological Society, Bethesda
329. Rerych SK, Scholz PM, Sabiston DC, Jones RH 1980 Effects of exercise training on left ventricular function in normal subjects: A longitudinal study by radionuclide angiography. American Journal of Cardiology 45: 244
330. Rhodin JAG 1980 Architecture of the vessel wall. In: Bohr DF, Somlyo AB, Sparks HV Jr (eds) Handbook of Physiology, The Cardiovascular System, Vol II, Vascular Smooth Muscle. American Physiological Society, Bethesda
331. Roge CLL, Silverman NH, Hart PA, Ray RM 1978 Cardiac structure growth pattern determined by echocardiography. Circulation 57: 285
332. Romero T, Covell JW, Friedman WF 1972 A comparison of pressure-volume relations of the fetal, newborn and adult heart. American Journal of Physiology 222: 1285
333. Romero TE, Friedman WF 1979 Limited left ventricular response to volume overload in the neonatal period: A comparative study with the adult animal. Pediatric Research 13: 910
334. Rosner B, Hennekens CH, Kass EH, Miall WE 1977 Age specific correlation analysis of longitudinal blood pressure data. American Journal of Epidemiology 106: 306
335. Ross J Jr 1974 Adaptations of the left ventricle to chronic overload. Circulation Research 34–35 (Suppl II): 1164
336. Ross J Jr, Linhart JW, Braunwald E 1965 Effects of changing heart rate in man by electrical stimulation of the right atrium: Studies at rest, during exercise, and with isoproterenol. Circulation 32: 549
337. Ross J Jr, McCullagh WH 1972 Nature of enhanced performance of the dilated left ventricle in the dog during chronic volume overloading. Circulation Research 30: 549
338. Rothe CF 1983 Venous system: Physiology of the capacitance vessels. In: Shepherd JT, Abboud FM (eds) Handbook of Physiology, The Cardiovascular System, Vol III, Peripheral Circulation and Organ Blood Flow, Part I. American Physiological Society, Bethesda
339. Rouleau J, Boerboom LE, Surjadhana A, Hoffman JIE 1979 The role of autoregulation and tissue diastolic pressures in the transmural distribution of left ventricular blood flow in anesthetized dogs. Circulation Research 45: 804
340. Rowe RD, James LS 1957 The normal pulmonary arterial pressure during the first year of life. Journal of Pediatrics 51: 1
341. Rowlatt UF, Rimoldi HJA, Lev M 1963 The quantitative anatomy of the normal child's heart. Pediatric Clinics of North America 10: 499
342. Rubio R, Berne RM 1975 Regulation of coronary blood flow. Progress in Cardiovascular Disease 18: 105
343. Rudolph AM 1979 Fetal and neonatal pulmonary circulation. Annual Review of Physiology 41: 383
344. Rudolph AM 1983 Circulatory changes during the perinatal period. Pediatric Cardiology 4 (Suppl II): 17
345. Rudolph AM, Itskovitz J, Iwamoto H, Reuss ML, Heymann MA 1981 Fetal cardiovascular responses to stress. Seminars in Perinatology 5: 109
346. Rudolph AM, Neuhauser EDB, Golinko RJ, Auld PAM 1961 Effects of pneumonectomy on pulmonary circulation in adult and young animals. Circulation Research 9: 856
347. Rudolph AM, Yuan S 1966 Responses of the pulmonary vasculature to hypoxia and H^+ ion concentration changes. Journal of Clinical Investigation 45: 399
348. Ruffolo RR 1983 Drug, neurotransmitter and hormone receptors in the regulation of the cardiovascular system. In: Shoemaker WC, Thompson WL (eds) Critical Care State of the Art, Vol 4. Society of Critical Care Medicine, Fullerton, CA
349. Ruskin JP, McHale PA, Harley A, Greenfield JC Jr 1970 Pressure-flow studies in man: Effect of atrial systole on left ventricular function. Journal of Clinical Investigation 49: 478
350. Sagawa K 1981 The end-systolic pressure-volume relation of the ventricle: Definition, modifications and clinical use. Circulation 63: 1223
351. Sagawa K 1983 Baroreflex control of systemic arterial pressure and vascular bed. In: Shepherd

JT, Abboud FM (eds) Handbook of Physiology, The Cardiovascular System Vol III. Peripheral Circulation and Organ Blood Flow, Part II. American Physiological Society, Bethesda
352. Said SI 1983 Vasoactive Peptides: State-of-the-art review. Hypertension 5 (Supp I): 17
353. Saldana M, Arias-Stella J 1963 Studies on the structure of the pulmonary trunk—II. The evolution of the elastic configuration of the pulmonary trunk in people native to high altitudes. Circulation 27: 1094
354. Saldana M, Arias-Stella J 1963 Studies on the structure of the pulmonary trunk—III. The thickness of the media of the pulmonary trunk and ascending aorta in high altitude natives. Circulation 27: 1101
355. Sandler H, Alderman E 1974 Determination of left ventricular size and shape. Circulation Research 34: 1
356. Sandler H, Dodge HT 1963 Left ventricular tension and stress in man. Circulation Research 13: 91
357. Sandor GGS, Olley PM 1982 Determination of left ventricular diastolic chamber stiffness and myocardial stiffness in patients with congenital heart disease. American Journal of Cardiology 49: 771
358. Sarnoff SJ, Braunwald E, Welch GH Jr, Case RB, Stainsby WN, Macruz R 1958 Hemodynamic determinants of oxygen consumption of the heart with special reference to the tension-time index. American Journal of Physiology 192: 148
359. Sarnoff SJ, Brockman SK, Gilmore JP, Gilmore MS, Linden RJ, Mitchell JH 1960 Regulation of ventricular contraction-influence of cardiac sympathetic and vagal nerve stimulation on atrial and ventricular dynamics. Circulation Research 8: 1108
360. Sarnoff SJ, Mitchell JH 1962 The control of the function of the heart. In: Handbook of Physiology Vol I. Circulation. American Physiological Society, Washington, DC
361. Scammon RE, Norris EH 1918 On the time of the postnatal obliteration of the fetal blood passages (foramen ovale, ductus arteriosus, ductus venosus). Anatomical Record 15: 165
362. Scheel KW, Brody DA, Ingram LS, Keller F 1976 Effects of chronic anemia on the coronary and coronary collateral vasculature in dogs. Circulation Research 38: 553
363. Scheuer J, Tipton CM 1977 Cardiovascular adaptations to physical training. Annual Reviews of Physiology 39: 221
364. Schlant RC, Sonnenblick EH, Gorlin R 1982 Normal physiology of the cardiovascular system. In: Hurst JW (ed) The Heart. McGraw-Hill, New York
365. Schmid PG, Sharabi FM, Phillips MI 1983 Peptides and blood vessels. In: Shepherd JT, Abboud FM (eds) Handbook of Physiology, The Cardiovascular System, Vol III. Peripheral Circulation and Organ Blood Flow, Part II. American Physiological Society, Bethesda
366. Schmidt RM, Kumada M, Sagawa K 1972 Cardiovascular responses to various pulsatile pressures in the carotid sinus. American Journal of Physiology 223: 1–7
367. Scholz H 1980 Effects of beta- and alpha-adrenoceptor activators and adrenergic transmitter releasing agents on the mechanical activity of the heart. In: Szekeres L (ed) Handbook of Experimental Pharmacology, Vol 54, Part 1. Springer-Verlag, Berlin
368. Schulman J, Smith CH, Stern GS 1954 Studies on the anemia of prematurity. American Journal of Diseases in Children 88: 567
369. Schumacher WA, Sheppard JR, Mirkin BL 1982 Biological maturation and beta-adrenergic effectors: Pre- and postnatal development of the adenylate cyclase system in the rabbit heart. Journal of Pharmacology and Experimental Therapeutics 223: 587
370. Sen S 1983 Regression of cardiac hypertrophy, experimental animal model. American Journal of Medicine 75: 87
371. Shapiro LM, Smith RG 1983 Effect of training on left ventricular structure and function. An echocardiographic study. British Heart Journal 50: 534
372. Sheldon CA, Friedman WF, Sybers HD 1976 Scanning electron microscopy of fetal and neonatal lamb cardiac cells. Journal of Molecular and Cellular Cardiology 8: 853
373. Shepherd AP, Granger HJ, Smith EE, Guyton AC 1973 Local control of tissue oxygen delivery and its contribution to the regulation of cardiac output. American Journal of Physiology 225: 747
374. Shepherd JT 1982 Reflex control of arterial blood pressure. Cardiovascular Research 16: 357
375. Shepherd JT, Abboud FM (eds) Handbook of Physiology, The Cardiovascular System, Vol III, Peripheral Circulation and Organ Blood Flow, Parts 1 and 2. American Physiological Society, Bethesda
376. Shepherd JT, Vanhoutte PM 1978 Role of the venous system in circulatory control. Mayo Clinic Proceedings 53: 247
377. Sjostrand T 1962 Blood volume. In: Hamilton WF (ed) Handbook of Physiology, Section 2: Circulation, Vol I. American Physiological Society, Washington, DC

378. Skidgel RA, Friedman WF, Printz MP 1984 Prostaglandin biosynthetic activities of isolated fetal lamb ductus arteriosus, other blood vessels and lung tissue. Pediatric Research 18: 12
379. Sodums MT, Badke FR, Starling MR, Little WC, O'Rourke RA 1984 Evaluation of left ventricular contractile performance utilizing end-systolic pressure-volume relationships in conscious dogs. Circulation Research 54: 731
380. Somlyo AV, Somlyo AP 1968 Electromechanical and pharmacomechanical coupling in vascular smooth muscle. Journal of Pharmacology and Experimental Therapeutics 159: 129
381. Sommer JR, Johnson EA 1979 Ultrastructure of cardial muscle. In: Berne RM (ed) Handbook of Physiology, Section 2: The Cardiovascular System, Vol I. The Heart. American Physiological Society, Bethesda
382. Sonnenblick EH 1962 Force-velocity relations in mammalian heart muscle. American Journal of Physiology 202: 931
383. Sonnenblick EH 1962 Implications of muscle mechanics in the heart. Federation Proceedings 21: 975
384. Sonnenblick EH 1964 Series elastic and contractile elements in heart muscle: Changes in muscle length. American Journal of Physiology 207: 1330
385. Sonnenblick EH, Braunwald E, Morrow AG 1965 The contractile properties of human muscle: Studies on myocardial mechanics of surgically excised papillary muscles. Journal of Clinical Investigation 44: 966
386. Sonnenblick EH, Ross J Jr, Covell JW, Spotnitz HM, Spiro D 1967 The ultrastructure of the heart in systole and diastole. Changes in sarcomere length. Circulation Research 21: 423
387. Sonnenblick EH, Skelton CL 1974 Reconsideration of the ultrastructural basis of cardiac length-tension relations. Circulation Research 35: 517
388. Sonnenblick EH, Spotnitz HM, Spiro D 1964 Role of the sarcomere in ventricular function and the mechanism of heart failure. Circulation Research 15 (Suppl II): 70
389. Sonnenblick EH, Strobeck JE 1977 Derived indices of ventricular and myocardial function. New England Journal of Medicine 296: 978
390. Spann JF Jr, Buccino RA, Sonnenblick EH, Braunwald E 1967 Contractile state of cardiac muscle obtained from cats with experimentally produced ventricular hypertrophy and heart failure. Circulation Research 21: 341
391. Sparks HV Jr 1980 Effect of local metabolic factors on vascular smooth muscle. In: Bohr DF, Somlyo AP, Sparks, HV Jr (eds) Handbook of Physiology, Section 2: The Cardiovascular System. Vol II. Vascular Smooth Muscle. American Physiological Society, Bethesda
392. Spotnitz WD, Spotnitz HM, Truccone NJ, Cottrell TS, Gersony W, Malm JR, Sonnenblick EH 1979 Relation of ultrastructure and function. Sarcomere dimensions, pressure-volume curves, and geometry of the intact left ventricle of the immature canine heart. Circulation Research 44: 679
393. Sreter FA, Balint M, Gergely J 1975 Structural and functional changes of myosin during development. Comparison with adult fast, slow and cardiac myosin. Developmental Biology 46: 317
394. St John Sutton MG, Gewitz MH, Shah B, Cohen A, Reichek N, Gabbe S, Huff DS 1984 Quantitative assessment of growth and function of the cardiac chambers in the normal human fetus: A prospective longitudinal echocardiographic study. Circulation 69: 645
395. St John Sutton MG, Marier DL, Oldershaw PJ, Sacchetti R, Gibson DG 1982 Effect of age related changes in chamber size, wall thickness, and heart rate on left ventricular function in normal children. British Heart Journal 48: 342
396. St John Sutton MG, Raichlen JS, Reichek N, Huff DS 1984 Quantitative assessment of right and left ventricular growth in the human fetal heart: A pathoanatomic study. Circulation 70: 935
397. Starke K, Docherty JR 1982 Types and functions of peripheral alpha-adrenoceptors. Journal of Cardiovascular Pharmacology 4: S3
398. Starling EH 1915 Principles of human physiology, 2nd edn. Lea & Febiger, Philadelphia
399. Starling EH 1918 The 1915 Linacre lecture: The law of the heart. In: Chapman CB, Mitchell JH (eds) 1965 Starling On The Heart. Dawsons of Pall Mall, London
400. Starling MB, Elliot RB 1974 The effects of prostaglandins, prostaglandin inhibitors, and oxygen on the closure of the ductus arteriosus, pulmonary arteries and umbilical vessels in vitro. Prostaglandins 8: 187
401. Stenmark KR, James SL, Voelkel NF, Toews WH, Reeves JT, Murphy RC 1983 Leukotriene C_4 and D_4 in neonates with hypoxemia and pulmonary hypertension. New England Journal of Medicine 309: 77
402. Stone HL 1983 Control of the coronary circulation during exercise. Annual Review of Physiology 45: 213
403. Streeter DD Jr 1979 Gross morphology and fiber geometry of the heart. In: Berne RM (ed) Handbook of Physiology, Section 2: The Cardiovascular System, Vol I. The Heart. American Physiological Society, Bethesda

404. Stull JT, Mayer SE 1979 Biochemical mechanisms of adrenergic and cholinergic regulation of myocardial contractility. In: Berne RM (ed) Handbook of Physiology, Section 2: The Cardiovascular System, Vol I. The Heart. American Physiological Society, Bethesda
405. Suga H 1979 Total mechanical energy of a ventricle model and cardiac energy consumption. American Journal of Physiology 236: H498
406. Suga H, Goto Y, Yamada O, Igarashi Y 1984 Independence of myocardial oxygen consumption from pressure-volume trajectory during diastole in canine left ventricle. Circulation Research 55: 734
407. Suga H, Hayashi T, Shirahata M 1981 Ventricular systolic pressure-volume area as predictor of cardiac oxygen consumption. American Journal of Physiology 240: H39
408. Suga H, Hayashi T, Suehiro S, Hisano R, Shirahata M, Ninomiya I 1981 Equal oxygen consumption rates of isovolumic and ejecting contractions with equal systolic pressure-volume areas in canine left ventricle. Circulation Research 49: 1082
409. Suga H, Hisano R, Hirata S, Hayashi T, Ninomiya I 1982 Mechanisms of higher oxygen consumption rate: Pressure-loaded vs. volume-loaded heart. American Journal of Physiology 11: 942
410. Suga H, Hisano R, Hirata S, Hayashi T, Yamada O, Ninomiya I 1983 Heart rate-independent energetics and systolic pressure-volume area in dog heart. American Journal of Physiology 244: 206
411. Suga H, Sagawa K 1972 Mathematical relationship between instantaneous ventricular pressure-volume ratio and myocardial force-velocity relation. Annals of Biomedical Engineering 1: 160
412. Suga H, Sagawa K, Kostiuk DP 1976 Controls of ventricular contractility assessed by pressure-volume ratio, E_{max}. Cardiovascular Research 10: 582
413. Suga H, Sagawa K, Shoukas AA 1973 Load-independence of the instantaneous pressure-volume ratio of the canine left ventricle and effects of epinephrine and heart rate on the ratio. Circulation Research 32: 314
414. Sundberg S, Elovainio R 1982 Cardiorespiratory function in competitive endurance runners aged 12–16 years compared with ordinary boys. Acta Paediatrica Scandinavica 71: 987
415. Swynghedauw B, Delcayre C 1982 Biology of cardiac overload. Pathobiology Annual 12:137
416. Tadokoro M, Arai S 1972 Myocardial cell in right ventricular hypertrophy. Tohoku Journal of Experimental Medicine 106: 5
417. Tarazi RC 1983 Regression of left ventricular hypertrophy by medical treatment: Present status and possible implications. American Journal of Medicine 75: 80
418. Tarazi RC, Sen S, Saragoca M, Khairallah P 1982 The multifactorial role of catecholamines in hypertensive cardiac hypertrophy. European Heart Journal 3 (Suppl A): 103
419. Taylor RR, Hopkins BE 1972 Left ventricular response to experimentally induced chronic aortic regurgitation. Cardiovascular Research 6: 404
420. Taylor WJ 1983 Genetic aspects of the cardiomyopathies. Progress of Medical Genetics 5: 163
421. Templeton GH, Ecker RR, Mitchell JH 1972 Left ventricular stiffness during systole and diastole: The influence of changes in volume and inotropic state. Cardiovascular Research 6: 95
422. Thilenius OG, Arcilla RA 1974 Angiographic right and left ventricular volume determination in normal infants and children. Pediatric Research 8: 67
423. Timmermans PBMWM, van Zwieten PA 1982 $Alpha_2$-adrenoceptors: Classification, localization, mechanisms and targets for drugs. Journal of Medicinal Chemistry 25: 1390
424. Tripp ME 1984 Congestive cardiomyopathy of childhood. Advances in Pediatrics 31: 179
425. Tripp ME, Katcher ML, Peters HA, Gilbert EF, Arya S, Hodach RJ, Shug AL 1981 Systemic carnitine deficiency presenting as familial endocardial fibroelastosis. New England Journal of Medicine 305: 385
426. Tyson GS, Maier GW, Olsen CO, Davis JW, Rankin JS 1984 Pericardial influences on ventricular filling in the conscious dog. Circulation Research 54: 173
427. Uhlig PN, Baer RW, Vlahakes GJ, Hanley FL, Messina LM, Hoffman JIE 1984 Arterial and venous coronary pressure-flow relations in anesthetized dogs. Circulation Research 55: 238
428. Urthaler F, Walker AA, James TN 1980 Changing negative inotopic effect of acetylcholine in maturing canine cardiac muscle. American Journal of Physiology 238: H1
429. Van Meirop LHS 1979 Morphological development of the heart. In: Berne RM (ed) Handbook of Physiology, Section 2: The Cardiovascular System, Vol I, The Heart. American Physiological Society, Bethesda
430. Vapaavouri EK, Shinebourne EA, Williams RL, Heymann MA, Rudolph AM 1973 Development of cardiovascular responses to autonomic blockade in intact fetal and neonatal lambs. Biology of the Neonate 22: 177
431. Vatner SF, Franklin D, Higgins CB, Patrick T, Braunwald E 1972 Left ventricular response to severe exertion in untethered dogs. Journal of Clinical Investigation 51: 3052

432. Vatner SF, Pagani M 1976 Cardiovascular adjustments to exercise: Hemodynamics and mechanisms. Progress in Cardiovascular Disease 19: 91
433. Vincent WR, Buckberg GD, Hoffman JIE 1974 Left ventricular subendocardial ischemia in severe valvar and supravalvar aortic stenosis. A common mechanism. Circulation 49: 326
434. Vinten-Johansen J, Barnard RJ, Buckberg GD, Becker H, Duncan HW, Robertson JM 1982 Left ventricular O_2 requirements of pressure and volume loading in the normal canine heart and inaccuracy of pressure-derived indices of O_2 demand. Cardiovascular Research 16: 439
435. Vinten-Johansen J, Dunean HW, Finkenberg JG, Hume MC, Robertson JM, Barnard RJ, Buckberg GD 1982 Prediction of myocardial O_2 requirements by indirect indices. American Journal of Physiology 12: H862
436. Virmani R, Roberts WC 1979 Pulmonary arteries in congenital heart disease: A structure-function analysis. Cardiovascular Clinics 10: 455
437. Wagenvoort CA, Wagenvoort N 1977 Pathology of Pulmonary Hypertension. Wiley, New York
438. Walgenbach SC, Donald DE 1983 Inhibition by carotid baroreflex of exercise-induced increases in arterial pressure. Circulation Research 52: 253
439. Walgenbach SC, Shepherd JT 1984 Role of arterial and cardiopulmonary mechanoreceptors in the regulation of arterial pressure during rest and exercise in conscious dogs. Mayo Clinic Proceedings 59: 467
440. Wallgren G, Hanson JS, Lind J 1967 Quantitative studies of the human neonatal circulation. III. Observations on the newborn infant's central circulatory responses to moderate hypovolemia. Acta Paediatrica Scandinavica Supplement 179: 44
441. Warshaw JB 1972 Cellular energy metabolism during fetal development: IV. Fatty acid activation, acyl transfer and fatty acid oxidation during development of the chick and rat. Developmental Biology 28: 537
442. Weber KT, Janicki JS 1977 Myocardial oxygen consumption: The role of wall force and shortening. American Journal of Physiology 233: H421
443. Weber KT, Janicki JS, Hefner LL 1976 Left ventricular force-length relations of isovolumic and ejecting contractions. American Journal of Physiology 231: 337
444. Weber KT, Janicki JS, Hunter WC, Shroff S, Pearlman ES, Fishman AP 1982 The contractile behavior of the heart and its functional coupling to the circulation. Progress in Cardiovascular Disease 24: 375
445. Weber KT, Janicki JS, Shroff MS, Fishman AP 1981 Contractile mechanics and interaction of the right and left ventricles. American Journal of Cardiology 47: 686
446. Weiss GB 1977 Calcium and contractility in vascular smooth muscle. Advances in General and Cellular Pharmacology 2: 71
447. Wilffert B, Timmermans PEMWM, van Zwieten PA 1982 Extrasynaptic location of alpha$_2$- and noninnervated beta$_2$-adrenoceptors in the vascular system of the pithed normotensive rat. Journal of Pharmacology and Experimental Therapetucs 221: 762
448. Wennmalm A 1982 Participation of prostaglandins in the regulation of peripheral vascular resistance. Advances in Prostaglandin, Thromboxane and Leukotriene Research 10: 303
449. Weyman AE, Wann S, Feigenbaum H, Dillon JC 1976 Mechanism of abnormal septal motion in patients with right ventricular volume overload. Circulation 54: 179
450. Wiedeman MP 1984 Architecture. In: Renkin EM, Michel CC (eds) Handbook of Physiology, Section 2, The Cardiovascular System, Vol IV, Microcirculation, Part 1. American Physiological Society, Bethesda
451. Wier WG 1980 Calcium transients during excitation-contraction coupling in mammalian heart: Aequorin signals of canine Purkinje fibers. Science 207: 1085
452. Wikman-Coffelt J, Parmley WW, Mason DT 1979 The cardiac hypertrophy process—analyses of factors determining pathological vs physiological development. Circulation Research 45: 697
453. Wilcken DEL 1983 Local factors controlling coronary circulation. American Journal of Cardiology 52: 8A
454. Winegrad S 1982 Mechanism of contraction in cardiac muscle. In: Guyton AC, Hall JE (eds) Cardiovascular Physiology IV, International Review of Physiology, Vol 26. University Park Press, Baltimore
455. Winegrad S 1984 Regulation of cardiac contractile proteins; correlations between physiology and biochemistry. Circulation Research 55: 565
456. Whittaker SRF, Winton FR 1933 The apparent viscosity of blood flowing in the isolated hindlimb of the dog and its variation with corpuscular concentration. Journal of Physiology, London 78: 339
457. Wittenberg JB 1970 Myoglobin-facilitated oxygen diffusion: Role of myoglobin in oxygen entry into muscle. Physiological Reviews 50: 559

458. Woods WT, Urthaler F, James TN 1978 Progressive postnatal changes in sinus node response to atropine and propranolol. American Journal of Physiology 234: 412
459. Yettram AL, Vinson CA, Gibson DG 1982 Computer modeling of the human left ventricle. Transactions of the American Society of Mechanical Engineers 104: 148
460. Zak R 1974 Development and proliferative capacity of cardiac muscle cells. Circulation Research 34–35 (Suppl II): 17
461. Zak R, Kizu A, Bugaisky L 1979 Cardiac hypertrophy: its characteristic as a growth process. American Journal of Cardiology 44: 941
462. Zaloga GP, Hostinsky C, Chernow B 1984 Endogenous opioid peptides: Critical care implications. Heart & Lung 13(4): 421
463. Zasslow MA, Benumof JL, Trousdale FR 1982 Hypoxic pulmonary vasoconstriction and the size of hypoxic compartment. Journal of Applied Physiology: Respiratory, Environmental and Exercise Physiology 53: 626
464. Zierler KL 1976 Free fatty acids as substrates for heart and skeletal muscle. Circulation Research 38: 459
465. Zinner SH, Martin LF, Sacks F, Rosner B, Kass EH 1974 Longitudinal study of blood pressure in childhood. American Journal of Epidemiology 100: 437
466. Zwelfach BW, Lipowsky HH 1984 Pressure-flow relations in blood and lymph microcirculation. In: Renkin EM, Michel CC (eds), Handbook of Physiology, Section 2, The Cardiovascular System, Vol. IV, Microcirculation, Part 1. American Physiological Society, Bethesda

2
Noninvasive Recognition and Assessment of the Failing Circulation

Richard A. Schieber

Over the past decade the number of new techniques available to assess and monitor the patient with circulatory failure has increased dramatically. Some of these techniques are widely available, inexpensive, portable, and simple to use. Others are available only in a few centers, require expensive, stationary equipment and trained technicians, or present special hazards, such as radiation to the young patient. Nevertheless, information is given here on both commonplace and unusual techniques because of the strong efforts underway by researchers, clinicians, and equipment manufacturers to improve the noninvasive assessment of the cardiovascular system.

Techniques used to evaluate the child with congenital heart disease are not emphasized, since references abound[1,78,117] and the diagnosis and management are now relatively straightforward. The goal instead is to describe devices and methods presently or potentially useful in the assessment of the child with a structurally normal heart but a failing circulation. Table 2.1 summarizes the techniques available for each cardiovascular function.

Validation studies comparing a noninvasive method to an accepted standard are emphasized, using data on infants and children when available. The true utility of these noninvasive methods depends on their accuracy. Special attention is thus paid to comparisons between a noninvasive technique and its accepted standard, and the systematic errors of both types of measurements. A correlation coefficient (r) or linear regression analysis equation is provided whenever possible. The correlation coefficient, when squared, represents the variation in one (dependent) variable explained by the other (independent) variable. A p value associated with the correlation coefficient describes the likelihood that the coefficient could erroneously be at least as large as stated due to chance alone, when in truth no correlation exists at all. Although statistical analysis summarizes data compactly and describes the *mean* value well, it does not adequately deal with the problem of the individual patient who falls outside the usual confidence limits. When a measurement is critical in making a decision, the results of several independent techniques may need to be compared to be sure that the patient is not one of the rare outliers whose noninvasive test would correlate poorly with an invasive study. Special mention is made when a validation study shows a substantial number of outliers. In such a study, an unacceptably large difference between noninvasive

Table 2.1. Noninvasive Techniques

- Recognition of circulatory failure
  - Physical examination
  - Chest roentgenogram
- Assessment of circulatory failure
  - Physiologic evaluation
    - Electrocardiogram
    - Blood pressure
      - Auscultation
      - Palpation
      - Doppler ultrasound
      - Oscillometry
    - Ventricular performance
      - Ventricular volume
        - Echo: M-Mode and 2D
        - Radionuclide angiography (First-pass, MUGA)
        - Nuclear probe
      - Cardiac output
        - Echo: M-Mode and 2D
        - Doppler
        - Acetylene
        - Microcavitations
        - Radiodensitometry
      - LVEDP
        - M-Mode echo
      - Contractility (stroke volume and ejection fraction)
        - Echo: M-Mode and 2D
        - Radionuclide angiography (First-pass, MUGA)
        - Nuclear probe
      - Regional wall motion disorders
        - 2D echo
        - MUGA
      - Pulmonary hypertension
        - M-Mode echo
        - Doppler ultrasound
      - Intravascular blood volume
        - RBC volume
        - Plasma volume
  - Anatomic evaluation
    - Intracardiac shunts
      - Echo: M-Mode and 2D
      - Doppler ultrasound
      - Radionuclide angiography
    - Ischemia and infarct imaging
      - "Hot" and "cold" spot scintigraphy
      - Thallium-201: resting and exercise
      - PET
      - Isoenzyme analysis
      - MRI
    - Other
      - Computed tomography
      - Dynamic spatial reconstructor

measurements and their standard values may exist for many data pairs, even though the correlation coefficient is quite high.

To compare the measurements of any patient to those obtained in a validation study, that patient must have the same characteristics of the study population, and all study criteria should be met. If this is not strictly possible, as is usually the case, an in-house validation study should be performed first, so that the individual will be compared more accurately with a similar group. A regression analysis on the in-house study group should then be applied to the measurements from the patient to reestablish the relationship in that patient between the noninvasive test and the standard.

RECOGNITION OF THE FAILING CIRCULATION

Physical Examination

Recognition of the young patient with congestive heart failure or circulatory collapse depends on the physical examination.[22,67,154] Dyspnea, tachycardia, cardiomegaly, and hepatomegaly are the four cardinal signs and symptoms seen most often in infants and children with congestive heart failure. However, the patient with circulatory collapse may have signs of shock.

The child has a marked change in central and peripheral color, respiratory pattern and rate, and level of motor activity. Peripheral cyanosis of only the skin, with pink nailbeds, indicates regional vasoconstriction of nonvital organs. Central cyanosis of the lips, tongue, and buccal mucosa reflects a low arterial oxygen saturation (generally less than 85 percent) due to a right-to-left intracardiac shunt, pulmonary ventilation-perfusion mismatch, or hemoglobinopathy. Peripheral pallor is a cause for alarm, since either the patient is severely anemic or has such a low cardiac output that the compensatory vasoconstrictor response has reduced skin perfusion to a critically low level. A grayish cast or mottling of the skin often accompanies such states, and is a marker of metabolic acidemia. The respiratory pattern may confirm this impression: Kussmaul's pattern of tachypnea and hyperpnea is the respiratory compensation for metabolic acidemia. Bradypnea or apnea signify impending cardiopulmonary arrest, due to cerebral hypoxia, ischemia, or exhaustion of the respiratory muscles. Finally, a reduction of spontaneous motor activity indicates severely reduced cardiac output.

The observer should feel the temperature of the hands and feet, as well as check the character, rate, and regularity of the central and distal pulses. Distal extremity coolness is an early sign of circulatory inadequacy.[76] An advancing or receding level of demarcation between proximal warmth and distal coolness with changes in therapy is a very useful gross estimate of total cardiac output and regional perfusion. Faint and rapid distal pulses imply hypotension, and palpable pulsus paradoxus (reduction in systolic blood pressure with inspiration) may indicate the presence of constrictive pericardial disease, restrictive cardiomyopathy, severe left ventricular (LV) dysfunction, or obstructive pulmonary disease.[22] A weak central pulse is a sure sign of hypotension if no LV outflow tract obstruction is present. Special attention should be paid to the character of the femoral and axillary pulses, since the carotid arterial pulse may be difficult to feel in infants with naturally short necks, and the brachial pulse may be as faint as the radial or ulnar pulse in low-flow states. Bounding pulses occasionally occur in children with congestive heart failure caused by a large central or peripheral run-off of blood into a low-pressure vascular bed, such as a patent ductus arteriosus, arteriovenous malformation, aortic regurgitation, or occasionally a ventricular septal defect. Early ("warm") shock, a hyperdynamic circulatory state also causing bounding pulses, is often missed in children, because its physical signs (e.g., tachypnea and tachycardia) may be erroneously attributed to other causes, or because its progression to "cold" shock may be very rapid.

Physical evidence of increased central venous pressure may be subtle. Distention of the neck veins is difficult to appreciate in infants and young children, although engorgement of the scalp and hand veins is readily seen. Kussmaul's sign (increased venous pressure with inspiration) is found in patients with constrictive pericardial disease, including tamponade, and restrictive cardiomyopathy.

Rales or wheezes signify either increased interstitial lung water caused by increased pulmonary capillary hydrostatic pressure or permeability, or reduced plasma oncotic pressure. Hepatosplenomegaly is a cardinal sign of congestive heart failure. The congested liver should have a round edge, but one displaced by a depressed hemidiaphragm or enlarged from hepatocellular disease should have a sharp edge.

Finally, the cardiac examination may define the origin of circulatory depression. The presence of a pericardial friction rub or knock indicates pericardial effusion or constrictive pericarditis, respectively. However, a pericardial effusion may not be the source of the failing circulation: for example, the child with uremic pericarditis may have congestive heart failure due to fluid overload rather than inadequate cardiac filling due to pericardial restriction. Faint or soft heart tones (subtle signs) or a prominent apical or left parasternal S_3 indicates myocardial dysfunction.

Chest Roentgenography

Although circulatory congestion or failure is usually evident by physical examination, occasionally the chest roentgenogram (CXR) is needed to differentiate cardiac from pulmonary disease. The CXR is especially useful in assessing cardiac size, pulmonary vascular markings, and the presence of any pulmonary parenchymal or pleural disease. The transverse cardiac diameter is the distance between the extreme left and right heart borders, while the transverse thoracic diameter is the distance between pleural surfaces at the level of the dome of the right hemidiaphragm.[30] Their ratio, the cardiothoracic (CT) index, should be less than .65 during the first year of life, less than .60 in the second year, less than approximately .52 between 3 and 6 years, and less than .51 beyond that. Comparison measurements of patients in the intensive care unit (ICU) require a full inspiratory effort. Established normal values may underestimate the CT index of supine ICU patients older than 3 years of age, since these standards were established using erect views.[93]

Pulmonary vascular markings are important in the assessment of pulmonary venous congestion, demonstrated by fine interstitial peripheral lung markings, large central hilar markings with indistinct borders, and alveolar opacification indicative of pulmonary edema. The presence of air, fluid, or blood in the mediastinal, pleural, or pericardial cavity may also detected by CXR.

ASSESSMENT OF THE FAILING CIRCULATION

Once the clinician identifies the presence of hemodynamic abnormality, further testing is needed to define its etiology, severity, and progress. One should choose a test based on its usefulness and local availability. The following techniques are described in approximate descending order of usual availability.

Electrocardiography

Electrocardiography (ECG) remains useful for diagnosis and continuous monitoring of the patient with circulatory failure. Diagnostic (12-lead) ECG is warranted for most patients with circulatory failure, particularly if due to congenital or acquired cardiac disease. The presence of a congenital heart malformation may be identified by physical examination (increased precordial impulse, single S_2, cardiac murmur, or abnormal pulses), chest roentgenography (cardiomegaly, abnormal pulmonary vascular markings, or abnormal situs) and diagnostic electrocardiography (abnormal QRS axis, increased or decreased ventricular or atrial forces). Certain congenital malformations are associated with reduced cardiac output, either due to the abnormal physiologic state caused by the malformation (e.g., hypoplastic left heart syndrome with a restrictive ductus arteriosus) or due to complications of the malformation (e.g., bacterial endocarditis of a bicuspid aortic valve with massive aortic regurgitation). Some malformations involve the conduction system directly, and may be associated with rhythm disturbances which can reduce cardiac output. Examples include the patient with Ebstein's malformation of the tricuspid valve with supraventricular tachycardia, congenitally corrected transposition of the great vessels with congenital complete heart block, and mitral valve prolapse with atrial or ventricular tachycardia.

A few types of acquired heart disease may be associated with reduced cardiac output. Kawasaki disease may cause an acute myocardial infarction due to thrombosis of a coronary artery aneurysm, and viral myocarditis may result in a hypocontractile left ventricle. The patient with myocardial ischemia will have characteristic ST segment and T wave abnormalities, with pathologic Q waves if infarction has occurred. Patients with acute pericarditis initially have ST segment elevations in many leads, but lack pathologic Q waves. Later, the ST segment returns to the isoelectric level, but widespread T wave inversion is seen with low voltage QRS complexes.

Continuous ECG monitoring is part of routine pediatric intensive care. Secure attachment of leads and skin electrodes with proper grounding of all electrical equipment is needed to avoid artifacts which may be misinterpreted as dysrhythmias. Disorders of rate and rhythm and their changes with treatment are particularly important to recognize. The patient with a heart rate which is inappropriately rapid for age (sinus tachycardia) should be assessed to determine whether the rate is appropriate for his physiologic state. For instance, the hypovolemic patient may maintain a normal cardiac output by increasing the heart rate via an increased release of endogenous catecholamines and suppression of parasympathetic tone. However, a normal heart rate in a child with hypovolemic shock is distinctly ominous, since the patient may have progressed midway from tachycardia to bradycardia and may subsequently suffer cardiac arrest if slowing continues. On the other hand, a reduction in heart rate toward normal in such a child receiving appropriate fluid therapy is encouraging. A tachycardia originating from a focus other than the sinus node is usually supraventricular in origin in a child, and may be recognized by its abrupt appearance and disappearance, a typically narrow QRS complex with a fast and very regular rate, and unrecognizable or absent P waves. Ventricular tachycardia, although rare in children, may occur spontaneously or in association with ventricular surgery or cardiopulmonary arrest from other causes.[115]

Special mention should be made of the ECG changes by severe, life-threatening hyperkalemia.[142] The earliest changes are seen in patients with a serum potassium (K^+) concentration between 5.5 and 6.0 mEq/L due to an increased rate of repolarization: the T wave becomes premature, symmetric, and narrow-based. The amplitude may initially be normal, not tall. At a serum K^+ concentration approximately 6.5 mEq/L, the PR interval lengthens and the QRS interval increases due to a reduction in membrane responsiveness and conduction velocity. When K^+ concentration reaches about 7.0 mEq/L, intraatrial conduction slows, and the P wave becomes broad and low, with eventual sinoatrial arrest occurring when the K^+ concentration reaches about 8.8 mEq/L. The QRS interval increases further and blends into the peaked T wave, mimicking a sine wave. Although each ECG change may be seen at a spectrum of K^+ concentrations, the change should never be ignored. Acidemia, hyponatremia, and hypocalcemia augment the changes seen. Although the ECG changes may simulate ventricular tachycardia, the appropriate emergency treatment consists of pharmacologic reestablishment of a normal extracellular potassium concentration, not electrical cardioversion.

Bradyarrhythmias other than sinus bradycardia are usually caused by second-degree (Mobitz type II, or dropped beats) or third-degree atrioventricular block. If cardiac output is low, emergency institution of temporary transvenous pacemaker therapy is indicated. These problems may occur in children predisposed to spontaneous deterioration of the conduction system (e.g., corrected transposition of the great vessels or single ventricle) or in the postoperative patient (e.g., following repair of a ventricular septal defect, tetralogy of Fallot, or atrioventricular canal). The child with a structurally normal heart who suffers a cardiopulmonary arrest usually develops sinus tachycardia prior to arrest, followed by sinus bradycardia, idiojunctional or idioventricular rhythm with progressive slowing, and finally asystole, electromechanical dissociation with wide and bizarre QRS complexes, or ventricular fibrillation.

Blood Pressure Measurement

Although systemic arterial hypotension is a late finding in patients with shock, blood pressure (BP) measurements remain an indispensable monitor of the hemodynamic response to therapy. Several types of devices are now available to obtain BP noninvasively. To categorize these, Ramsey[108] has described six fundamental features of these instruments; (1) an inflatable cuff, (2) a means of inflating the cuff, (3) a means of deflating the cuff, (4) a pressure sensor and indicator, (5) a signal sensor or detector, (6) a determination strategy and algorithm.

The four major classes of noninvasive devices use the auscultatory, palpatory, Doppler ultrasonic, and oscillometric methods (Fig. 2.1). These can be subdivided into: (1) manual types requiring no electrical power, (2) semiautomatic devices which are manually inflated but electronically determine the pressure, and (3) fully automatic devices which inflate and deflate the cuff and determine the pressure.

Traditional BP monitoring uses stethoscope auscultation of the first and fourth (muffling) Korotkoff sounds to define the systolic (P_s) and diastolic (P_d) pressures, respectively. The pressure sensor is a mercury manometer or aneroid gauge. Its advantages are its ease of use and low cost. However, too small a cuff may overestimate the pressure by inadequately compressing the vessel, whereas too rapid

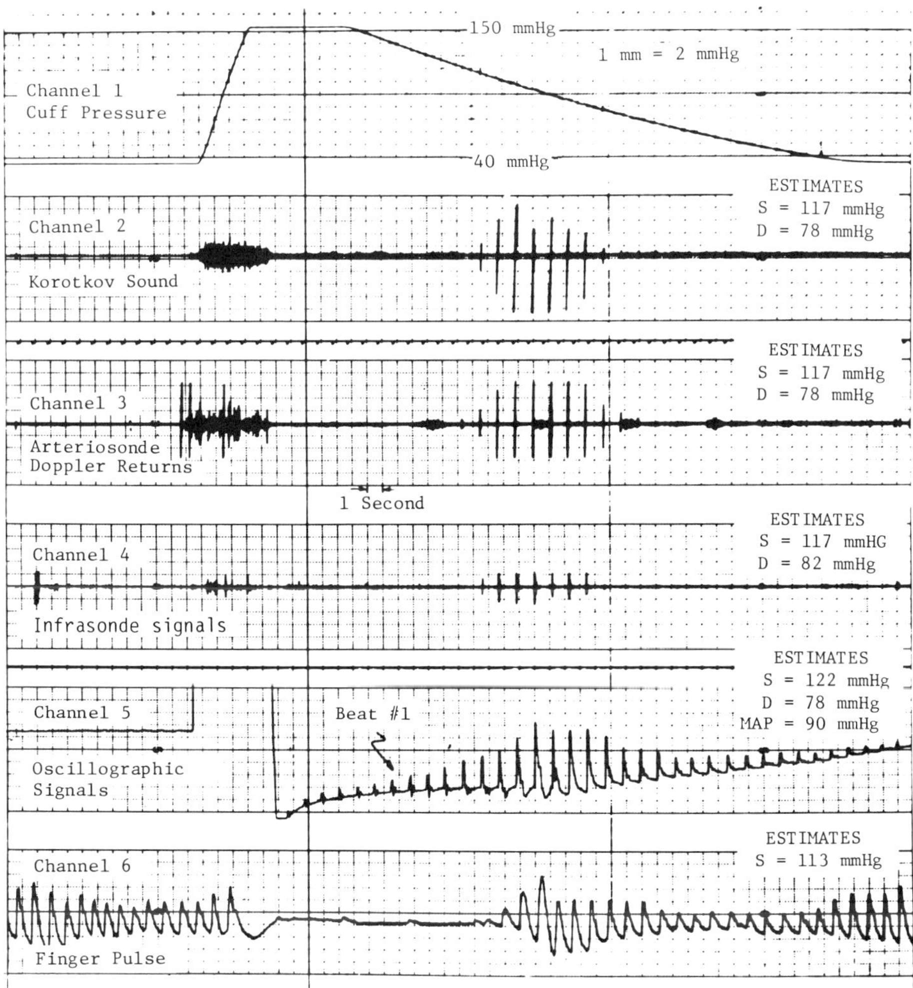

Fig. 2.1. Simultaneous demonstration of auscultatory, oscillographic, and palpatory occlusive blood pressure measurements. Estimates are human interpretation of strip charts. An Arteriosonde 1225, Infrasonde 3000, Dinamapp 845, and Datascope 865 finger pulse sensor were used. (Apple HP 1980 Automatic noninvasive blood pressure monitors: What is available. In: Gravenstein JS (ed) Essential Noninvasive Monitoring in Anesthesia. Grune & Stratton, New York, by permission.)

deflation may underestimate both phasic pressures, since the accuracy of the system is only as great as the millimeters of mercury deflated per beat.[97] Also, the Korotkoff sounds are often inaudible in shock states.[32]

Using the palpatory method, the technician places two fingers or a pulse transducer over an artery distal to the inflated cuff. Inflation and deflation are performed manually, and a mercury or aneroid gauge senses the pressure. Although the system is simple and inexpensive, it has the same disadvantages as the auscultatory method. Also, diastolic BP cannot yet be accurately measured with pulse transducer devices.[6]

Doppler ultrasound technique is a substantial improvement over these methods. Ultrasonic waves are produced in response to an electrical signal at 2 to 8 MHz by a transducer which contains two lead zirconate titanate crystals.[132] One crystal transmits waves through the skin into an artery distal to an occluded cuff, and one receives the reflected wave. The difference in the transmitted and reflected frequencies is compared, and the change is proportional to the velocity of arterial wall motion. If the cuff is inflated above P_s, arterial wall velocity remains less than .5 cm/sec, the frequency of transmitted sound does not change, and no Doppler shift is heard. When the cuff is deflated to P_s, the arterial wall snaps open. Once amplified, the change in frequency is heard as the characteristic short, relatively high-frequency (200 to 500 Hz) sound during opening, and a longer, low-frequency signal (30 to 100 Hz) during closing of the artery. As P_d is approached, the signal due to closure occurs later and later in the cycle. Once P_d is reached, the closing sound merges with the opening sound of the subsequent beat, causing the rumbling closing signal to disappear and the opening signal to become soft and faint. P_d is thus a more subjective end-point than P_s. The pressure sensor is a mercury or aneroid gauge. Detection of the Doppler shift depends on proper positioning of the transducer over the artery.

One such device, the Arteriosonde 1225 (Roche Medical Electronics, Inc., Cranbury, NJ), manually inflates the cuff and automatically deflates it at an adjustable, linear bleed rate between 2 and 5 mmHg/sec. The deflation time depends on heart rate, since two beats are compared at each pressure during deflation to reduce the likelihood of motion artifact producing an erroneous BP. This technique is also hindered by external electrical interference. The unit is available for approximately $5,000. The Infrasonde 3000 (Marion Scientific Corp., Costa Mesa, CA) detects subaudible frequencies (10 to 40 Hz) to determine systolic and diastolic pressures. The cuff is inflated manually, but deflated automatically at a 3 mmHg/sec linear bleed rate. The technique is more resistant to motion artifacts (frequency $\leq$10Hz) and electrical interference (60 Hz), and costs approximately $800.[6]

Oscillometry was initially used to determine only the mean BP (P_m), although manufacturers of later-model equipment claimed it could also be used to accurately detect P_s and P_d. The amplitude of small variations (oscillations) in cuff pressure present with each heart beat changes at different pressures. A cuff encloses separate pressure and pulse amplitude detectors. At suprasystolic cuff pressures, low-amplitude oscillations are detected. At P_s, the amplitude increases abruptly. As cuff pressure is reduced further, the amplitude continues to increase until a plateau is reached. The mean pressure occurs at the lowest pressure at which maximum oscillations are detected.[54,106] As the cuff deflates further, a large, abrupt decrease in oscillations will be detected at P_d. Since an electrical pump automatically inflates the cuff, unrecognized runaway or prolonged inflation may cause ischemic nerve damage.[124,136] Deflation occurs in 3 mmHg decrements, and two beats are compared for oscillatory amplitude at each pressure level. Although this improves the precision to within 3 mmHg, long deflation and cycle times are required with this technique. The internal pressure sensor, a solid-state transducer, is more resistant to overshoot than a mercury manometer. Since the cuff itself detects the oscillations, careful positioning of a sensor over the artery is not necessary. However, a loose fit or residual air in the cuff severely attenuates the signal, and motion renders the technique useless. Partial occlusion of the release valve results in residual air and pressure in the cuff, which increases the automatic "zero" calibration value and causes erroneously low BP values.[116] One such unit, the Dinamapp 845 (Critikon, Inc., Tampa, FL), costs approximately $1,800.

Many studies have attempted to validate each technique. A major problem with all studies is the potential inaccuracy of intraarterial pressure measurements, the standard with which these techniques are compared. As discussed in the next chapter, errors arise due to the improper and/or undocumented resonant frequency and damping factor of the catheter-tubing-transducer system. "Whip" artifact, kinetic energy of blood flow, and augmentation of systolic pressure in peripheral arteries due to reflectance waves and arterial compression by a cuff inflated beyond the site of cannulation also yield erroneous values.[27,150] Ideally, the accuracy of a noninvasive system should be within 3 mmHg of the standard, since this is the usual precision of most transducer-pressure module assemblies in current use. With these caveats in mind, the relative merits of the four noninvasive techniques can be compared (Table 2.2).

Cohn et al[32] demonstrated the gross inaccuracy of auscultation and palpation in hypotensive adults with increased peripheral resistance. Stegall et al.[132] noted that two patients in shock had normal intraarterial pressures although no Korotkoff sounds were audible. Auscultation and palpation are thus unreliable methods in monitoring critically ill patients.

Results of validation studies using the Doppler technique vary. P_s measured by Doppler is often close in value to the directly-measured pressure. However, identical numbers should not be expected, since errors greater than 10 mmHg for any single determination were found in approximately half of the studies listed in Table 2.2[41,54,68,106] P_s may be either underestimated or overestimated by Doppler, and errors in both directions may occur in the same patient within minutes.[68] P_d is often unreliably estimated by Doppler technique.

Automated oscillometry yields values which approximate P_m, although any individual reading may have an error similar in magnitude to Doppler technique. Several studies[107,151] have demonstrated that invasive and oscillometric measurements of P_m generally move in the same direction during spontaneous changes in blood pressure; the trend capability is satisfactory even if the absolute numbers are not equal.

At present, it is difficult to conclude which method is universally most accurate. However, the Pedisphyg manual Doppler system (CAS, Inc., Upper Montclair, NJ) stands out in this summary as the most accurate technique on the basis of studies of normotensive children by Reder et al.[110]

If potentially inaccurate, of what value are automated or electronically assisted BP determinations? First, indirect systolic pressure provides an approximate measure of the true systolic pressure in the patient in whom no Korotkoff sounds or palpable pressure is obtained due to hypotension, vasoconstriction, hypothermia, or dysrhythmias. Second, these devices provide information needed to make initial decisions by determining an approximate mean or systolic blood pressure. Third, these instruments automatically repeat the measurement, therefore allowing greater productivity of personnel during an emergency. They thus fulfill a useful function in the initial management of the patient in shock prior to the insertion of a indwelling arterial catheter.

Table 2.2. Noninvasive Blood Pressure Studies: Correlation with Intraarterial (Direct) Measurements

			Direct-Indirect Systolic Pressure[a]		
Reference	Technique	Age Range and Conditions	Average Difference ± S.D.	Range	Correlation Coefficient
Cohn[32]	Auscultation/ palpation	Severely hypotensive adults	High peripheral resistance: 64 mmHg Low peripheral resistance: 6.5 mmHg	10–164 mmHg −20–+64 mmHg	
Elseed et al[43]	Auscultation Palpation Manual Doppler	Normotensive 1–11 years	6.8 ± 5.7 mmHg* 11.4 ± 8.2 mmHg 5.7 ± 6.3 mmHg 23% of readings >5 mmHg	−10–+24 mmHg 10–30 mmHg	 r = .74*
Reder et al[110]	Manual Doppler (Pedisphyg) Arteriosonde Doppler	1 day–9 years	97% of indirect readings within ± 3 mmHg of direct 10.7 mmHg, 40% of readings >10 torr difference		r = .99 r = .83
Dweck et al[41]	Arteriosonde Doppler	Premature and term newborns (<4 days old)	P_s: 3 mmHg P_d: −5 mmHg		r = .75 r = .80
McLaughlin et al[89]	Manual Doppler	Premature and term newborns (<5 days old) P_s = 10–80 mmHg	P_s: 96% of indirect readings within ± 3 mmHg of direct	0–10 mmHg	
Gordon et al[61]	Manual Doppler	Premature newborns	P_s: −0.6 ± 3.4 mmHg P_d: −1.33 ± 2.6 mmHg		r = .98
Hernandez et al[68]	Manual Doppler	Normotensive 4 weeks–14 years	P_s: 5.0 mmHg 77% of patients >5 mmHg error during at least one reading		P_d: r = .75

Segall et al[132]	Auscultation Auscultation Manual Doppler Manual Doppler	Normotensive adults	P_s: −1.9 ± 3.0 mmHg P_d: 0.2 ± 3.5 mmHg P_s: 0.1 ± 2.2 mmHg P_d: −0.3 ± 2.1 mmHg		r = .97 r = .96 r = .99 r = .98
Black et al[16]	Manual Doppler	Infants	P_s: 2.5 ± 2.0 mmHg P_d: 3.3 ± 2.4 mmHg		
Ramsey[107]	Oscillometry	14 adults 3 children (7–73 paired readings per patient)	P_m: −2.3 ± 4.2 mmHg	−7.7–+5.6 mmHg	r = .98
Yelderman and Ream[151]	Oscillometry	Adults	P_m: −1.4 ± 6.2 mmHg	−7.2–+9.2 mmHg	r = .87
Kimble et al[81]	Oscillometry	Premature and term newborns	P_m: 0.2 ± 3.8 mmHg		r = .85
Friesen and Lichtor[51]	Oscillometry	1 day–22 weeks	P_s: 15% of readings >10 mmHg error P_d: 21% of readings >10 mmHg error		r = .96 r = .94
Colan[23]	Oscillometry	1 day–48 months	P_s: 6% of readings >10 mmHg error P_d: 3% of readings >10 mmHg error		r = .98 r = .94
Bruner[27]	Oscillometry				P_s: r = .59 P_m: r = .66

* Author's recalculation.
P_s = Systolic blood pressure
P_d = Diastolic blood pressure
P_m = Mean blood pressure

Echocardiography

During the past two decades, the use of ultrasonic waves to analyze the beating heart has increased our knowledge of cardiac structure and function tremendously. This noninvasive technique presently allows rapid and repeatable bedside evaluation of the size and motion of all cardiac structures and their interrelationships without pain or obvious biological risk. Echocardiography has become the standard for the appraisal of atrioventricular valve motion and function and systolic time intervals. Its major use in pediatric cardiology is the evaluation of abnormal intracardiac relationships found in congenital malformations, and is particularly useful in the study of the critically ill newborn who may consequently undergo a more efficient cardiac catheterization. The major uses of echocardiography in the pediatric ICU are (1) measurements of LV volume and function, (2) analysis of LV regional wall motion abnormalities, (3) determination of stroke volume and cardiac output, (4) estimation of LV filling pressure, (5) recognition of right-to-left intracardiac shunts, (6) detection of pericardial fluid, and (7) estimation of pulmonary artery pressure.

M-mode echocardiography

M-mode ("motion") echocardiography (MME) is the study of cardiac structures moving in one plane, toward and away from the transducer, with time. Sound waves are generated at a very high frequency (2.5 to 5.0 million cycles per second, or MHz) by a piezoelectric crystal which compresses and expands when activated by an electrical signal, thus transforming electrical into mechanical energy. An advancing sound wave which strikes an interface of two different densities, such as that between the septal wall and ventricular cavity, will be reflected back to the transducer if the angle of incidence is approximately 90 degrees to the surface of the interface. The transducer produces a wavefront during 1/1000 second and receives reflected wavefronts during 999/1000 second, transforming mechanical energy back into electrical energy. The length of time required for the round trip is measured, and since the average velocity of sound through human tissue is known, the distance between the transducer and the reflective interface is easily calculated and recorded. Other sound waves pass to deeper structures, require a longer time to return their reflected waves to the transducer, and are recorded "below" the more superficial structures. When the recording device applies time to the x-axis, an M-mode tracing of all structures intercepted by the beam is produced. The structures easily viewed in children with normal intracardiac anatomy are (1) all four cardiac valves, (2) the LV, right ventricle (RV), and left atrial cavities, (3) the RV anterior wall, LV posterior wall, and intraventricular septum, and (4) the pericardium (Fig. 2.2).

However, several factors prevent MME from providing a complete anatomic evaluation. The advancing sound wavefront must be nearly perpendicular to the interface, so that the angle of incidence approximates the angle of reflection. The majority of waves will then return to the transducer instead of scattering. This requirement is usually satisfied by changing the angle the transducer makes to the chest, and therefore to the heart. A more serious problem is caused by the absorption of nearly all sound waves by air located anywhere between the chest wall and epicardium: pneumomediastinum, pneumothorax, or pneumopericardium.

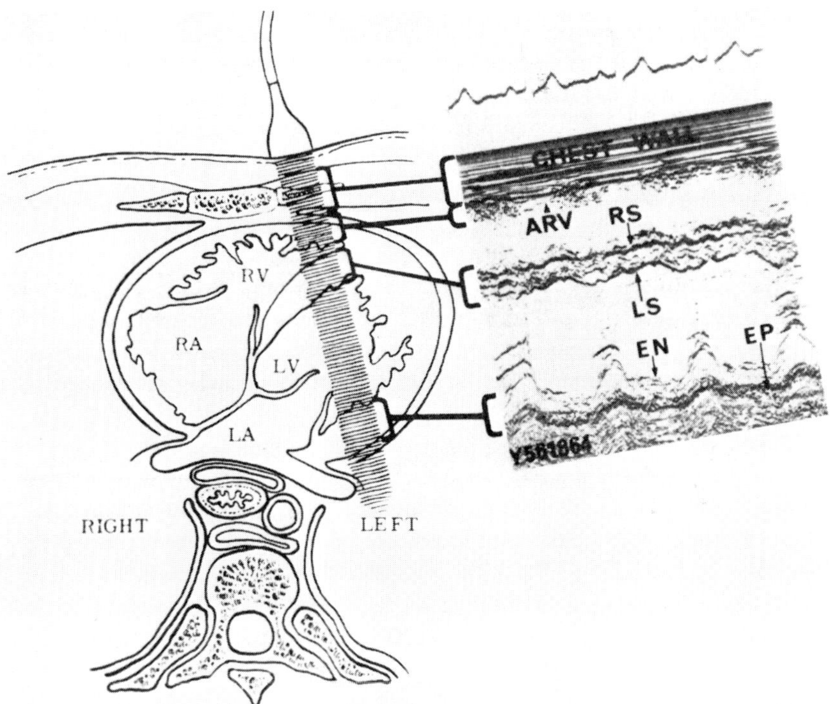

Fig. 2.2. Diagram and echocardiogram showing how echocardiography can obtain an "ice-pick", one-dimensional view of the heart through the right and left ventricles. ARV, anterior right ventricular wall; RS, right septum; LS, left septum; EN, posterior left ventricular endocardium; EP, posterior left ventricular epicardium; RA, right atrium; RV, right ventricle; LV, left ventricle; LA, left atrium. (Feigenbaum H 1981 Echocardiographic evaluation of cardiac chambers. In: Echocardiography, 3rd edn. Lea & Febiger, Philadelphia.)

This may be overcome by moving the transducer to a different intercostal space or to the subxiphoid or suprasternal position. Such changes of angle and position are commonly necessary in the ICU patient. M-mode measurements of chamber size and function using the subxiphoid view are generally comparable to those obtained from the standard left parasternal position.[131]

The most important limitation of MME is its singular "ice-pick" view of the heart which permits visualization of only a small part of any chamber at one time. The structures listed above may be viewed in turn by changing the transducer's orientation to the chest. The technician must scrupulously adhere to recognized standards of transducer position and angle to ensure that the true minor axis of the LV and the proper left atrial dimension are recorded. The interpreter must likewise adhere to established guidelines to accurately and reproducibly measure cardiac distances and timing intervals.[118]

Two-dimensional echocardiography

The development of two-dimensional echocardiography (2DE) was a major advance in overcoming the limitations of MME. Instead of emitting an "ice-pick" of sound waves, the 2DE transducer emits a wedge-shaped, 30 to 90 degree plane of sound waves with the apex of the wedge located at the transducer. The motion of structures is recorded at 30 frames per second as movement toward and away from the transducer as well as in one dimension perpendicular to this. Different transducer orientations show different structures. The four-chamber views (Fig. 2.3) show the two atria and ventricles, both atrioventricular valves, and the interatrial and interventricular septa. The long axis view (Fig. 2.4) shows the left atrium, LV, RV outflow tract, mitral, aortic, and pulmonic valves, pulmonic and aortic roots, and the interventricular septum. The short axis views (Fig. 2.5) show the LV, papillary muscles, aortic and pulmonic valves and their great vessel roots, tricuspid valve, interatrial and interventricular septa, and the proximal right and left coronary arteries. The entire left ventricular cavity can thus be viewed, and the true minor axis, major axis, and cavity area can be readily measured.

Echocardiographic estimation of LV size, function, and regional wall motion

A great need existed for a portable, accurate, reproducible, and easily repeated measurement of LV contractile performance and size, including linear cavity distances and volumes. For years, these measurements could be determined only by high-quality contrast left ventriculography during cardiac catheterization. For this, contrast material is injected directly into the ventricle while filming fluoroscopic images of sequential stages of the cardiac cycle at a rapid rate, usually 60 frames per second. Although angiography continues to be the standard, several sources of systematic error exist.[123,150] LV volumes may be overestimated by failing to detect a sharp endocardial edge, by not accounting for the space occupied by the papillary muscles and trabeculae carneae within the LV body, by rotation of the heart during the cardiac cycle, and by magnification of the portion of the heart located near the periphery of the screen. Also, one must assume that the LV is a rotationally symmetrical ellipsoid: the projection on the plane of the major axis is an ellipsoid. Standard measurement techniques use either the major and minor axes, or major axis and area, in one or two views, to determine the ventricular volume. A factor is applied to correct for magnification errors, and the resulting value is inserted into a regression equation (established by measuring the volume displaced by a dog ventricular cast) to correct the echo volume to a "true" volume. Finally, the presence of contrast material in the LV may depress contractility and increase LV volumes.

Angiography and other techniques may be used to measure the LV end-diastolic and end-systolic volumes (LVEDV and LVESV). Their difference, the stroke volume (SV), is the amount of blood ejected from the heart during each cardiac cycle. The ratio of SV/EDV is the ejection fraction (EF), a potent index of LV contractility. For adult males, LVEDV established by contrast angiography is normally 70 $\pm$ 20 ml/m^2 (mean $\pm$ SD), and EF is 0.67 $\pm$ 0.08.[79] For infants less than 2 years old, LVEDV normally is 42 $\pm$ 10 ml/m^2, and EF is 0.68 $\pm$ 0.05. For children older than two years, LVEDV is 73 $\pm$ 11 ml/m^2, while EF is 0.63 $\pm$ 0.05. However, these pediatric normal values were established by studying only 19 children less than 2 years of age, and 66 percent of all children in the study received "light" nitrous oxide and/or halothane anesthesia during the catheterization, which may have unknowingly altered the normal volumes through a reduction in myocardial contractility.[63]

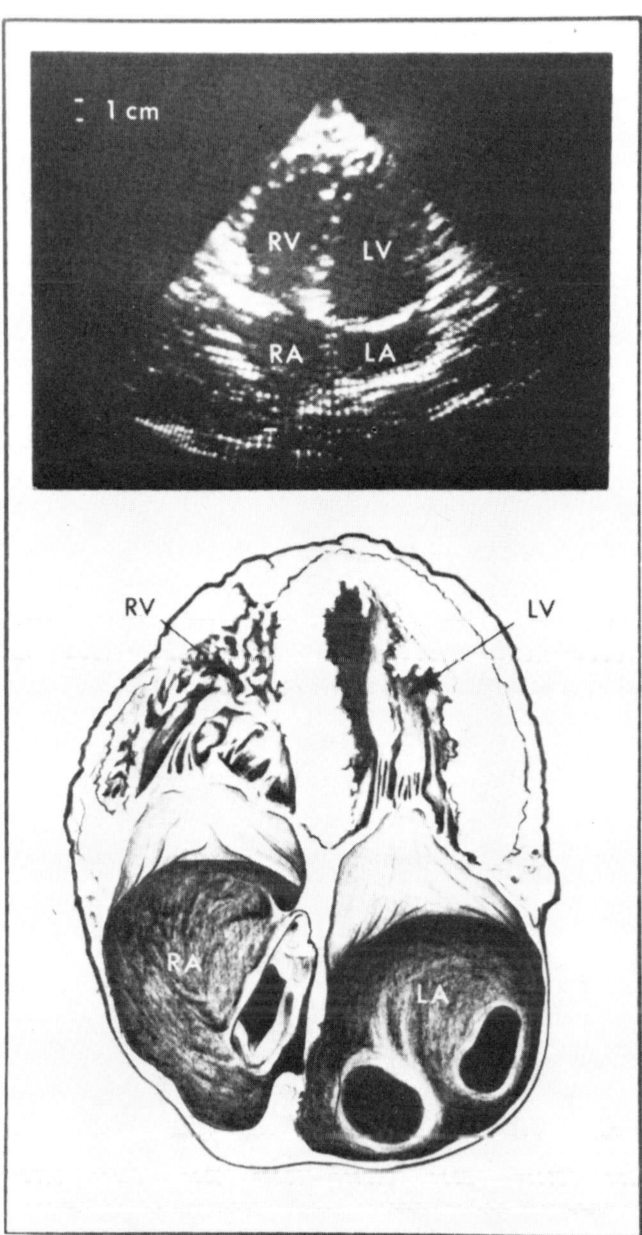

Fig. 2.3. Two-dimensional echocardiogram and anatomic specimen of an apical four-chamber examination of the heart. Abbreviations as in Fig. 2.2. (Feigenbaum H 1981 Echocardiographic evaluation of cardiac chambers. In: Echocardiography, 3rd edn. Lea & Febiger, Philadelphia, and Rogers EW, Feigenbaum H, and Weyman AE 1979 Echocardiography for quantitation of cardiac chambers. In: Yu PN and Goodwin JF (ed) Progress in Cardiology, vol. 8. Lea & Febiger, Philadelphia.)

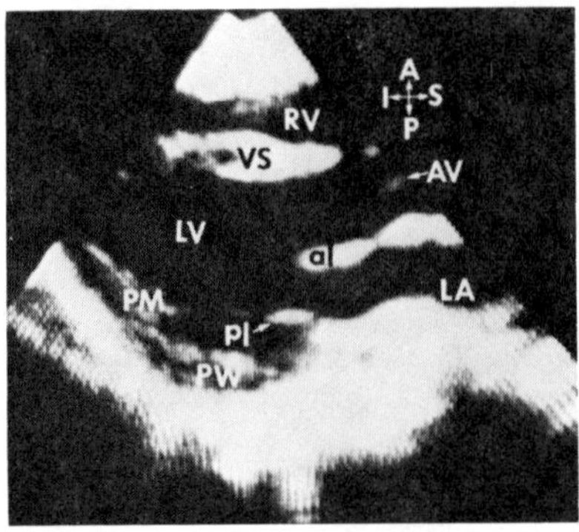

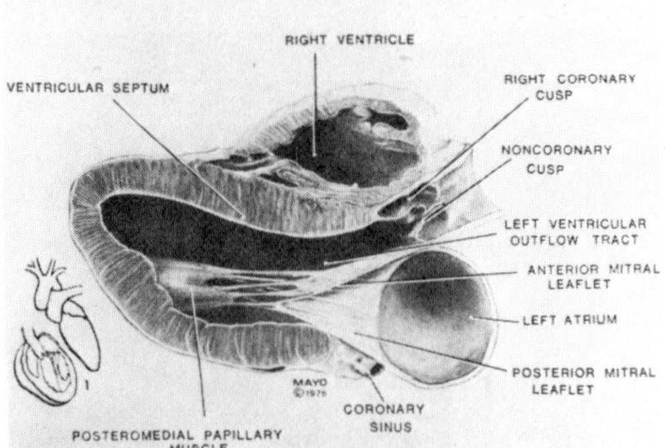

Fig. 2.4. (A) Long-axis view of LV, with apex located to left and aortic valve located to right of image. A and P, anterior and posterior; I and S, inferior and superior; AV, aortic valve; VS, ventricular septum; al and pl, anterior and posterior mitral valve leaflets; PM papillary muscle; PW, posterior wall; other abbreviations as in Fig. 2.2. (B) Drawing of same section. (Tajik AJ, Seward JB, Hagler DJ, Mair DD, and Lie JT 1978 Two-dimensional real-time ultrasonic imaging of the heart and great vessels: Technique, image orientation, structure, identification, and validation. Mayo Clinic Proceedings 53:271.)

With the advent of MME, LV cavity size could be measured noninvasively. Since the LV cavity normally assumes the approximate shape of a prolate ellipse (Fig. 2.6), the plane of the minor axis lies at the mid-point between the two ends of the major axis and perpendicular to it. The intersection of this plane with the LV cavity inscribes a circle. The internal diameter of that circle at diastole and systole ($LVID_d$ and $LVID_s$) can be measured. Left ventricular chamber size is a linear function of body surface area.[59] $LVID_d$ is so reproducible that a change greater than 5 percent reflects a true change in the ventricular size.[103] Furthermore, this test is more specific for LV cavity enlargement than chest radiography, since cardiomegaly defined by CXR may be due instead to pericardial effusion, RV

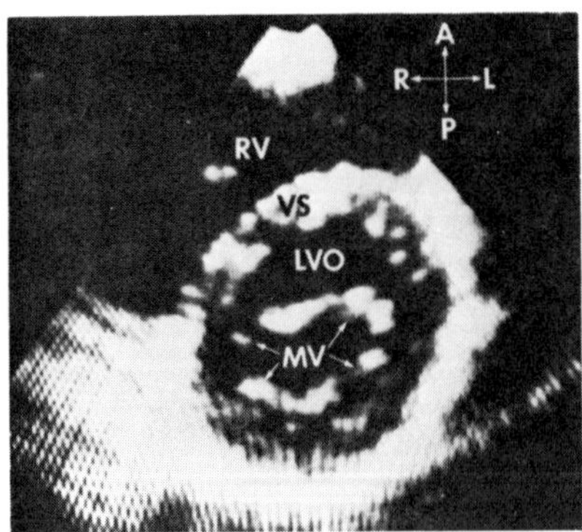

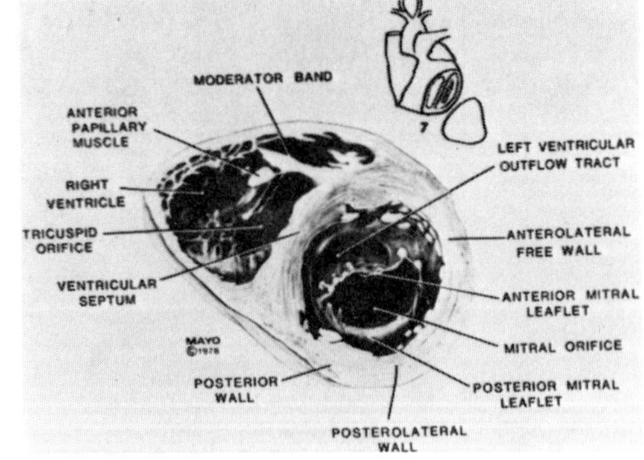

Fig. 2.5. (A) Short-axis view at level of mitral valve leaflets. LV is posterior and appears circular; RV is anterior and appears triangular. LVO, LV outflow tract; MV, mitral valve anterior and posterior leaflets; other abbreviations as in Figs. 2.2 and 2.4. (B) Drawing of same section. (Tajik AJ, Seward JB, Hagler DJ, Mair DD, and Lie JT 1978 Two-dimensional real-time ultrasonic imaging of the heart and great vessels: Technique, image orientation, structure, identification, and validation. Mayo Clinic Proceedings 53:271.)

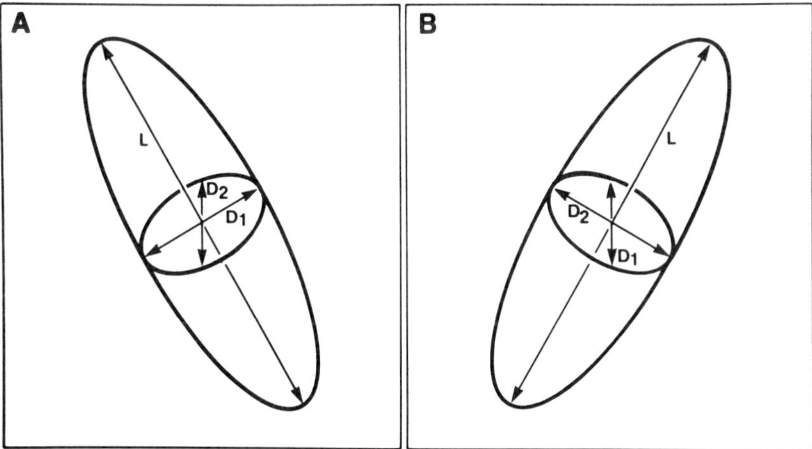

Fig. 2.6. (A & B) Two views of a prolate ellipse and its three axes. L, long axis; D_1 and D_2, minor axes. (Feigenbaum H 1981 Echocardiographic evaluation of cardiac chambers. In: Echocardiography, 3rd edn. Lea & Febiger, Philadelphia, and Rogers EW, Feigenbaum H, Weyman AE 1979 Echocardiography for quantitation of cardiac chambers. In: Yu PN, Goodwin J (ed) Progress in Cardiology, Vol. 8. Lea & Febiger, Philadelphia.)

dilatation, or ventricular hypertrophy. Initial studies demonstrated a good correlation between $LVID_d$ determinations by MME and by angiography.[14,49] In fact, children with *normal LV size* had a very good correlation (r = .91) by these techniques. However, those children with LV enlargement, an abnormally oriented ventricular septum, or previous RV surgery had a poor correlation for $LVID_d$.[14]

Besides measuring LV size, MME can be used to estimate LV function. The fractional shortening of the left ventricle,

$$\%SF = \frac{100 \times (LVID_d - LVID_s)}{LVID_d}$$

measures the extent of LV contraction along the minor axis. Fractions below 28 percent represent reduced contractility, and values below 20 percent indicate severe depression of the contractile state. This is the echocardiographic test of contractility most commonly used. The mean velocity of circumferential fiber shortening is the ratio of LV fractional shortening to ejection time: VCF = percent SF/ET. This test measures the rate of contraction of the minor axis. Normal values range between 1.02 and 1.94 circ./sec.[44] LV posterior and septal wall motion can also be quantified.

Formulas have been developed to correlate linear MME LV dimensions with volumes and ejection fractions obtained by angiography. The key assumptions are (1) LV contraction is symmetric without asynergy, (2) LV is a sphere, not an ellipse, and (3) the true minor axis can be accurately identified. These assumptions are often wrong. Although LV contractility may be uniform in normal hearts, grossly asymmetrical contraction is present in about 60 percent of patients with myocardial infarction,[84] and in an undetermined fraction of critically ill children without apparent myocardial ischemia. If the LV cavity is assumed to approximate a sphere, the linear dimensions might be cubed to estimate a volume. Although a few investigators were able to find a reasonably good correlation between ejection fraction based on M-mode measurements and left ventriculography,[137] many other laboratories were unable to satisfactorily correlate MME and angiographic measurements of cardiac volumes, stroke volume, EF, or cardiac output in adults with symmetric or asymmetric contractility[48,84,109,122] or in children.[96,126] In fact, percent SF and mean velocity of circumferential fiber shortening were inaccurately estimated in children with LV enlargement when compared with angiography.[14] The prevailing evidence in children thus suggests that MME measurements can be used to accurately determine the linear minor axis systolic and diastolic dimensions in children with normal LV size only, and cannot accurately determine LV volume or EF.

Since MME allows imaging of only a limited portion of the LV at any instant, it cannot be used to adequately assess the motion of all its walls. An area of regional dysfunction can be overlooked, simply because the region is not present in the area scanned by the transducer beam. The development of 2DE gave noninvasive measurements of LV regional wall motion new credibility, since areas of asynergy invisible to the MME beam could now be measured more accurately.[65] LV volume measurements also became more reliable with 2DE. Using a four-chamber image, the LV endocardial surface may be traced and the area obtained by planimetry. The length of the LV major axis is measured, and a regression equation applied to calculate LV volume (Fig. 2.7).

The validity of volume measurements by 2DE was tested both in spherical balloons containing a known, variable volume of saline, and in formalin-fixed canine hearts.[42] A close linear correlation ($r = 0.99$) was found between the volume determined directly and by 2DE for both models. Further, the true volumes and EF of a beating canine heart correlated closely with their 2DE estimates ($r = .97$ and .92, respectively). Direct and 2DE measurements of volume determined instantaneously throughout the cardiac cycle correlated very closely. The 2DE volumes underestimated true volume at any point during the cardiac cycle by less than 7 percent in this model. Other studies of adults with radiopaque myocardial markers implanted around the LV demonstrated excellent correlations for LVEDV and EF between 2DE and fluoroscopic determinations.[123] Studies of children with congenital heart disease showed a good correlation ($r \geq .85$) between measurements from several 2DE views and angiographic determinations of LVEDV, LVESV, SV and EF.[96,126] Likewise, RV size by 2DE has been shown to correlate closely with autopsy casts.[19,48]

Investigators have tested these correlations in adults using a variety of formulas to describe the left ventricular shape as an ellipse, a truncated ellipse, a truncated cone, or a hemisphere-cylinder. Correlation coefficients differ markedly between laboratories when the same formula is used, and in the same laboratory when different formulas are used. Some formulas yield a high correlation, while others yield an unacceptably low, nonpredictive value. Therefore, regression analysis of institutional 2DE and angiographic data should be performed in each laboratory before using 2DE alone to predict the true LV volume.

Correlations have not been established for left ventricular volumes of unusual shapes, such as left ventricular septal convexity associated with increased positive end-expiratory pressure.[75] Accuracy is wholly dependent upon a high-quality echocardiogram showing the entire chamber with a sharp endocardial surface. In ad-

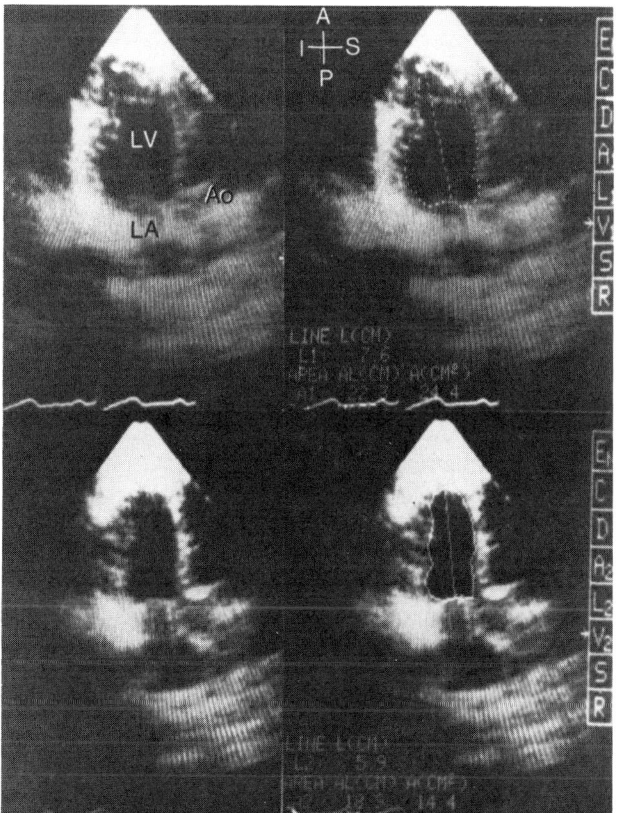

Fig. 2.7. Modified four-chamber view to visualize the entire LV cavity. Upper frames: end-diastole; lower frames: end-systole. Right frames show light-pen tracing of endocardial surface and LV major axis used to compute LV volume. Abbreviations as in Figs. 2.2 and 2.4. (Silverman NH, Ports TA, Snider AR, Schiller NB, Carlsson E, Heilbron DC 1980 Determination of left ventricular volume in children: Echocardiographic and angiographic comparisons. Circulation 62:548–557, by permission of the American Heart Association, Inc.)

dition, intraobserver and interobserver variability may be important. One experienced group determined these variables and recommended that changes of at least 15 percent for LVEDV, 25 percent for LVESV, and 10 percent for EF (representing the 95 percent confidence limits) should be demonstrated before concluding that an observed change is real.[33,62] This use of 2DE may be valuable for critically ill children, since angiography entails the hazards of excessive time, patient transport, scheduling difficulties, expense, ectopic beats induced by catheter manipulation, and alteration of the hemodynamic state by contrast dye.[122] Two-dimensional echocardiography allows repeated analysis of unlimited cardiac cycles at relatively low expense and without hazards.

Echocardiographic estimations of cardiac output and stroke volume

Stroke volume has been estimated from MME measurements of aortic valve motion, including separation between aortic valve cusps, systolic ejection time, and posterior aortic root excursion during ejection.[35] Stroke volume has also been calculated from the mitral valve echos using the maximum separation of the anterior and posterior mitral valve leaflets, maximum slope of mitral valve opening, heart rate, and the PR interval.[34] A good correlation of stroke volume was found between mitral valve echos and Fick, or thermodilution, techniques ($r = .90$).[45] Mitral and aortic valve echocardiographic techniques depend on the presence of a structurally normal, competent valve.

Echocardiographic estimation of LV filling pressure

Total blood volume is often estimated from LVEDV (see the section *Intravascular volume determinations*). As an index of preload, LVEDV is a major determinant of cardiac output. In turn, LVEDV is a function of (1) alterations in venous return caused by changes in body posture, (2) conditions which lower peripheral vascular resistance, such as exercise, hypoxia, and anemia, (3) altered distribution of blood between the intrathoracic and extrathoracic compartments, as determined by body position, intrathoracic pressure, intrapericardial pressure, and venous tone, and (4) atrial contribution to ventricular filling. Since these factors all influence the diastolic stretching of the myocardium, they affect LVEDV.[21]

LVEDV measurements have historically been difficult to obtain in the ICU. Until bedside radionuclide angiography became available for this purpose, alternate methods were sought. Estimation of the LV end-diastolic pressure (LVEDP) by mean pulmonary artery wedge pressure (PAWP) measurements became a standard technique. However, the assumption that end-diastolic volume and end-diastolic pressure are directly related is flawed. In particular, the left ventricular compliance (dv/dp) relationship is curvilinear, with progressively smaller volume increments causing progressively higher filling pressures.[58,64] Furthermore, LV diastolic compliance is reduced by myocardial ischemia, positive end-expiratory pressure, RV overload, hemorrhagic and septic shock, dopamine, and isoproteronol. In contrast, heart failure, volume overload, cardiomyopathy, and nitroprusside increase the diastolic compliance.[125] Since several of these factors may be present in any patient, the assumption of constant ventricular compliance is potentially seriously wrong. PAWP may change due to a change in LV compliance alone, not due to an alteration of LVEDV. For example, no relationship between PAWP and LVEDV was found in adults with cardiac disease or sepsis, possibly due to a shift in compliance in these states.[31]

Despite the demonstrated inability to construct a Frank-Starling curve (plotting LVEDP versus stroke volume index) when LV compliance is altered, measuring PAWP may be useful when its value is greatly increased. Also, if an intravenous infusion of a small aliquot causes a large increase in PAWP, LV compliance may be assumed to be low. Further, PAWP estimates the intravascular hydrostatic pressure of the Starling equation. Clinicians therefore need an accurate, noninvasive method of estimating LVEDP or PAWP. Qualitative and quantitative analysis of mitral valve motion by MME has yielded conflicting conclusions. At first, premature mitral valve closure was believed to represent an abnormally elevated LVEDP.[44,92] Other investigators found that the mitral valve may close later, not earlier, than normal in the presence of increased LVEDP.[87] In another line of investigation, an excellent correlation was noted between the ratio of two easily measured mitral valve diastolic time intervals and PAWP in adults.[7,8] However,

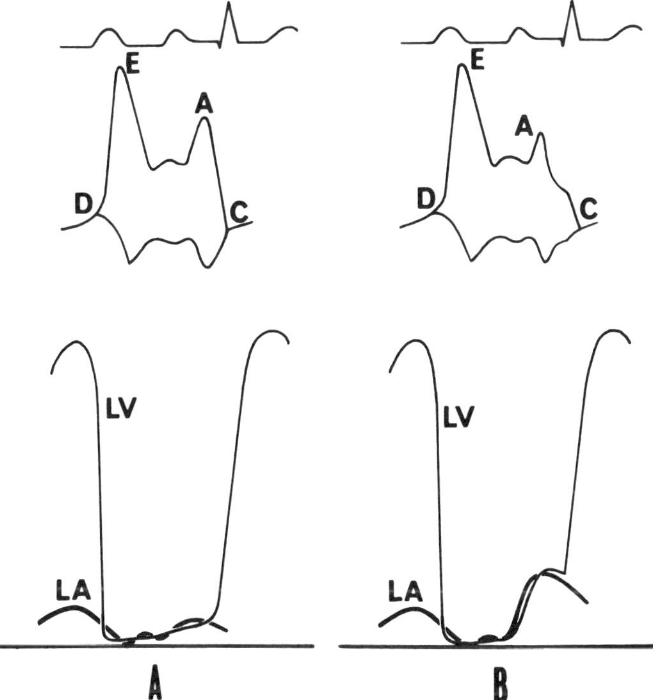

Fig. 2.8. Diagrams showing mitral valve echogram and LA and LV pressures in the presence of normal (left) and increased (right) LVEDP with a prominent "B-bump." (Feigenbaum H 1981 Hemodynamic information derived from echocardiography. In: Echocardiography, 3rd edn. Lea & Febiger, Philadelphia.)

these studies require independent confirmation, since in the author's experience, it does not apply to children (unpublished data).

Elevated LVEDP is sometimes associated with an abnormal echogram of anterior mital valve leaflet closure. Closure normally occurs with a smooth, uninterrupted, posterior motion of the anterior leaflet until it coapts with the posterior leaflet at the onset of systole (Fig. 2.8). When LVEDP is increased, this posterior motion is interrupted by a plateau which occurs at the instant the LVEDP and left atrial pressures equalize, with a momentary cessation of flow prior to ventricular systole. This plateau, generally present when LVEDP exceeds 20 mmHg, may be the most reliable echocardiographic sign of increased LVEDP.[5,46,99] However, no one has yet conclusively demonstrated a predictive correlation between echocardiographic mitral valve motion and LVEDP.[8,87] Since a reduction of LV compliance in the critically ill patient may increase PAWP without altering LVEDV, noninvasive, accurate estimation of LVEDV should be more useful than LVEDP in determining intravascular volume.

Contrast echocardiography

Echocardiography is useful in the detection of right-to-left intracardiac shunts. Saline or blood, once shaken in a syringe, contain invisible, brightly echodense microcavitations which are normally trapped completely in the pulmonary microcirculation and do not pass into the left heart. By noting whether these dots appear in the left atrium, left ventricle, or aorta, a right-to-left shunt at the level of the atria, ventricles, or great vessels, respectively, will be defined. In the postoperative open-heart surgery patient with persistant cyanosis, echocardiography can define whether hypoxemia is due to residual right-to-left intracardiac shunting or to pulmonary disease.[15,40,140]

As a research tool, cardiac output may be estimated using contrast 2DE. Following the injection of solution, the intensity of light eminating from the microcavitations is measured by focusing a simple photometer on the screen image of the RV cavity. The appearance and disappearance (decay) of these bright dots from the RV, and their change in luminescence with time, yields a curve identical to that of indocyanine green or thermal dilution. This densitometric dilution technique depends on the injection of a constant amount of bubbles in each injectate. The area under the curve produced by this technique compares favorably to that produced by indocyanine green ($r = .77 - 0.96$) between 1.7 and 7.07 L/min flow.[18,37] Refinements of standardization and improved reproducibility have been achieved using new contrast agents, such as CO_2, pressurized blood, and CO_2-releasing sugars. Currently, the technique lacks adequate calibration to determine absolute values of cardiac output.[38] Nevertheless, it may still be useful in determining relative changes in cardiac output in critically ill patients. Of course, a right-to-left atrial shunt through a patent foramen ovale would reduce its accuracy.

Detection of pericardial effusions

Pericardial effusions are easily identified by M-mode echocardiography as an enlargement of the potential pericardial space betwen the normally apposed visceral and parietal layers. Although the size of the effusion may be evident by echocardiography, its hemodynamic effects are generally not. This technique may define whether a pericardial effusion (and presumed cardiac tamponade), ventricular dysfunction, or hypovolemia is the cause of reduced cardiac output following open-heart surgery. Postpericardiotomy syndrome and pericarditis are also accurately identified.

Noninvasive assessment of pulmonary artery pressure

Both M-mode and Doppler ultrasonography have been used to detect the presence of pulmonary hypertension.[80] Several investigators have attempted to correlate MME RV (pulmonary valve) systolic time intervals with phasic or mean pulmonary artery pressures. The ratio of RV preejection period (PEP) to RV ejection time (ET) was initially reported to predict pulmonary artery hypertension in children with left-to-right shunts[69,111,130] and infants with pulmonary hypertension due to noncardiac disease.[66,112,113] However, a thorough evaluation of this technique by Silverman et al[127] in infants and children with ventricular septal defects showed a poor correlation with pulmonary artery diastolic or mean pressures or pulmonary vascular resistance. Neither a flat diastolic slope nor mid-systolic pulmonary valve closure universally reflects pulmonary hypertension.[45]

Using pulsed Doppler technique to sample the RV outflow tract, Kitabatake et al[83] noted that adults with pulmonary hypertension had decreased time-to-peak flow during RV systole ($r = -.88$, $p < .0001$). This interesting finding requires confirmation by other laboratories.

Although left ventricular systolic time intervals (particularly PEP/ET) are one of the oldest quantitative, noninvasive tests used to the evaluate LV performance, these have not enjoyed the widespread popularity of other echocardiographic and nuclear function studies because of the need for high-fidelity equipment and meticulous attention to detail. These intervals provide no anatomic information, and their pathophysiologic basis is more complex than other tests. Several good reviews are available on this subject.[86,147]

Radionuclide Imaging

Radioisotope evaluation[152] of the circulation includes (1) analysis of ventricular function by labeling the blood pool within a chamber,[138] (2) detection and quantitation of intracardiac shunts,[72] (3) identification of ischemic or infarcted myocardium,[105] (4) measurement of intravascular volume, and (5) functional metabolic imaging with positron emission tomography (PET). Of these, left ventricular function (especially beat-by-beat) analysis has the greatest utility in the pediatric ICU, and will be discussed in relatively great detail.

First-pass technique[12,60,104]

Radioisotope angiography was initially performed in a manner similar to contrast ventriculography. Following the injection of a bolus of radiolabeled substance into a peripheral or central vein, a scintillation camera is placed over the anterior chest wall to record the pattern of blood flow during the first pass of the agent through sequential chambers of the heart. Since the number of radioactive counts is evenly distributed within the blood pool of a cardiac chamber, the number of counts measured at any instant is directly proportional to the chamber volume at that moment. Unlike contrast ventriculography or echocardiography, no assumptions regarding ventricular shape or uniformity of wall contraction are needed, and any such abnormalities do not reduce the accuracy of these measurements. Potassium perchlorate (6 mg/kg) is administered orally to block thyroid uptake of radionuclide. In vivo red blood cell labeling is performed using IV stannous pyrophosphate followed 15 to 20 minutes later by the administration of technetium 99m pertechnetate (^{99m}Tc). For adults, the radiation exposure is approximately 1.50 mrad, or 4 percent of the whole body radiation required for cardiac catheterization with angiography.[135] The dose used in children also compares favorably with contrast angiography.[100] Counts are measured at least 20 times per second. One drawback, the amount of statistical variation in the counts, may be overcome by summing several cardiac cycles and statistically "smoothing" the data.[121]

The ejection fraction calculated by this technique has a high correlation with LV contrast angiography ($r = .95$) across a broad range of normal and abnormal values. Interobserver and intraobserver variability showed no statistically significant difference between two data pairs in one study, although the actual differences ranged from 2 to 9 percent.[94,153] Hemodynamic stability is required for less than 1 minute to collect the data as the bolus passes through the heart. Studies may therefore be repeated frequently, although multiple injections of tracer are needed to obtain serial measurements or multiple views.

Multiple-gated acquisition blood pool imaging

Multiple-gated acquisition (MUGA) blood pool imaging technique avoids these difficulties.[13,135,153] Stannous pyrophosphate is again injected in order to prepare the patient's red blood cells for subsequent in vivo labeling with ^{99m}Tc pertechnetate, and the radiolabel is allowed to reach equilibrium in the vascular space. An electronic circuit activates (gates) the scintillation camera during selected time periods of the cardiac cycle relative to the R wave. Since insufficient counts are detected during one cardiac cycle to yield an adequate image for quality viewing and analysis, several hundred beats are ECG-synchronized and "overlapped" by a computer according to the R wave. A computer-driven cursor can be placed on the image in the region of interest, and the regional activity calculated at each instant to produce a time-activity curve. These summations yield high-count density images with good spatial resolution. MUGA scans can be used to obtain (1) quantitative hemodynamic data, especially EF, SV, and cardiac output (HR $\times$ SV); (2) multiple cardiac projections after a single injection of tracer; (3) serial studies before and after therapeutic interventions up to 4 hours following an injection; and (4) analysis of regional wall motion disorders (hypokinesia, akinesia, dyskinesia) by viewing the reproduced image at different sequential points during the cardiac cycle as an endless-loop cine. Hemodynamic stability is required during the period of data collection: 20 to 25 frames per second may be obtained to characterize a complete cardiac cycle in approximately 2 minutes,[90] although most studies are performed within 8 minutes. These counts must be adjusted for background activity eminating from overlapping or underlapping blood-containing structures such as the left atrium, aorta, and the lungs.

An excellent correlation for LVEF was found between MUGA scans and contrast ventriculography.[29] A point-by-point comparison of these two techniques showed a high correlation coefficient ($r = .96$) at all time intervals within one cardiac cycle. Interobserver variation was less than 2 percent. In addition, LVEF determined by two MUGA studies of the same patient 1 hour apart varied only 5.7 ± 4.8 percent ($\pm$SD) of EF value.[104] Normal adult values for LVEF by MUGA scan are $.62 \pm 0.7$ ($\pm$SD). RV volumes and ejection fraction have also been determined by first-pass and gated equilibrium techniques, with low intraobserver and interobserver error and a high degree of correlation with invasive studies. In-house normal values are essential for the proper interpretation of these studies.

The MUGA scan has several disadvantages. An expensive camera, computer, and a specialized technician are required. The equipment is portable, although not compact. This technique has found its greatest utility in the study of stable patients who could be moved to the diagnostic nuclear cardiology suite, although equipment can be moved if necessary.

Nuclear cardiac probe

A highly promising new tool in radionuclide cardiac imaging is the nuclear cardiac probe,[144–146] dubbed the "nuclear stethoscope" (Fig. 2.9). This device is particularly well-suited for monitoring, rather than diagnostic, purposes. It is relatively inexpensive ($25,000 to $32,000), portable, and provides a continuous beat-by-beat analysis of LV function. The device consists of a ECG-gated, thallium-activated, sodium iodide gamma scintillation crystal mounted on an arm and precisely

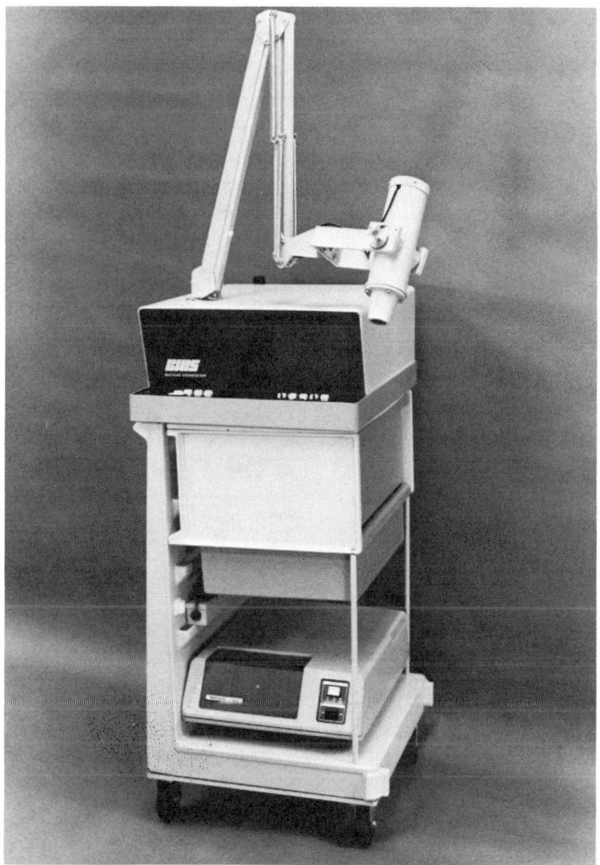

Fig. 2.9. The cardiac nuclear probe. (Courtesy of Bios, Inc.)

positioned over the chest at the bedside. The crystal of the probe is much thicker, and therefore much more sensitive to the same level of radioactive counts produced by the heart. An LV-time activity curve is produced instead of an LV cavity image. Spatial resolution is sacrificed for improved temporal resolution and greater sensitivity. Strategies were developed to allow an integrated microprocessor and technician to "recognize" the LV by its characteristic time-activity curve, since the shape of the chamber was no longer visualized (Fig. 2.10). Due to increased sensitivity, a curve could now be generated *for each beat*, instead of relying on the summation of several hundred beats to represent the average beat. Global LV function is therefore monitored on a beat-to-beat basis. First pass studies are also possible. The detector head senses all counts indiscriminantly within a 7 cm^2 area located 2 cm inside the chest. This area must lie completely within the LV cavity. An adapter can be obtained to reduce the field size for smaller subjects.

Validation studies of EF in adults have shown a remarkably good correlation (r = .92) between first-pass nuclear angiography and nuclear probe values, regardless of the presence of low EF or regional wall abnormalities. Reproducibility was excellent (r = .94) when a repeat study was performed, including removing and

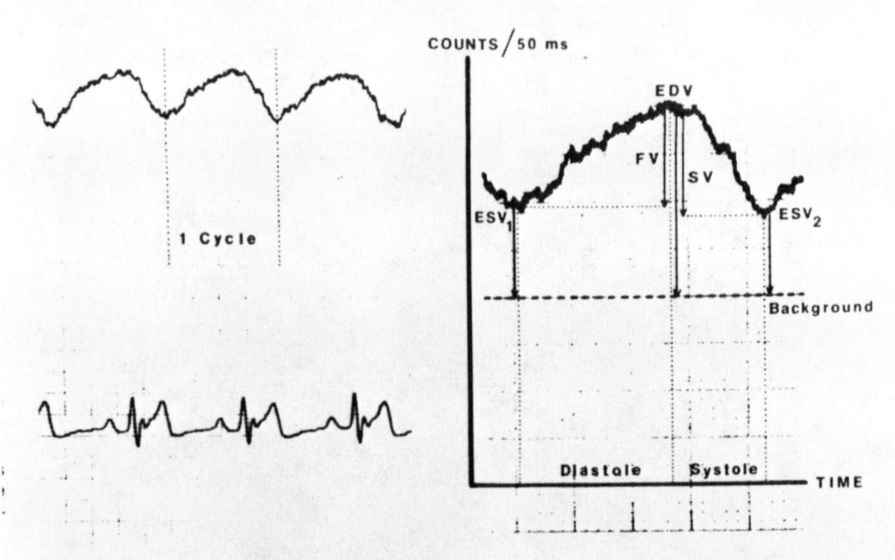

Fig. 2.10. (A) Beat-to-beat left ventricular time-activity curve obtained with the cardiac probe. (B) One cardiac cycle with definition of some left ventricular variables. EDV, end-diastolic volume; ESV_1, end-systolic volume of the previous beat; ESV_2, end-systolic volume of the same beat; FV, filling volume; SV, stroke volume. (Camargo EE, Harrison KS, Wagner HN, Bourbuignon MH, Reid PR, Alderson PO, Baxter RH 1980 Noninvasive beat-to-beat monitoring of left ventricular function by a nonimaging nuclear detector during premature ventricular contractions. American Journal of Cardiology 45:1219.)

repositioning the camera without the use of external chest markings. Interobserver and intraobserver error was extremely low, and beat-to-beat variability during a stable period was less than 6 percent EF units.[11] The nuclear probe is also an effective screening device in identifying adults with abnormal LV performance.[134] In infants and children with congenital cardiac malformations, EF obtained using the nuclear probe correlated well ($r = .93$, $p < .001$) with MUGA or angiography in children with over 5 years of age, although less well in children below 5 years of age ($r = .72$, $p < .02$).[129] The accuracy of EF measurements obtained with this technique is heavily dependent upon the computer software used.

An exciting improvement in this area is the development of a miniature detector which can be strapped to the chest to continuously measure LV function.[70] One such detector is made of cadmium telluride, measures 3.5 cm in diameter, 2 cm long, weighs 6 ounces, and is mounted on foam rubber adapters. A single dose of ^{99m}Tc-labeled red blood cells allows LV function monitoring for at least 12 hours, and possibly up to between 18 and 24 hours. Multiple injections would be safe and feasible for additional periods. LVEF obtained with this module correlated reasonably well in adults with MUGA technique ($r = .76$). Although this device is presently an experimental prototype, it offers great promise in the bedside assessment of global LV function in critically ill patients.

Radionuclide detection of intracardiac shunts

The first-pass technique may also be used for detection and quantitation of intracardiac shunts. Left-to-right shunts may be visualized by inspecting all cardiac chambers for early recirculation during the first pass of ^{99m}Tc. Detection of small shunts requires computer analysis of the radioactive counts over the right lung during the recirculation phase. Tiny shunts (QP:QS < 1.2:1) are not recognized by this method and rely on contrast angiography for diagnosis.[3,53,91] Right-to-left shunts may be identified by detecting counts over the carotid artery before they appear over the pulmonary artery, lungs, and left ventricle. False-positive right-to-left shunts of small magnitude (up to 5 percent) may be found in children with no shunt identified by standard Fick technique. Otherwise, quantitative analysis appears to be accurate.[102]

These techniques may be used for the bedside evaluation of residual shunts in patients following open-heart surgery. Both residual left-to-right shunts, which cause congestive heart failure, and right-to-left shunts, which cause cyanosis, may be recognized and quantified in lieu of cardiac catheterization. LV and RV contractility and size may also be assessed. However, qualitative analysis of postoperative right-to-left intracardiac shunting is commonly performed instead using 2DE, to avoid the use of cumbersome equipment, non-cardiology personnel (depending on the institution), and exposure to radiation.[15,40,140]

Myocardial imaging

Noninvasive radionuclide imaging of regions of myocardial ischemia, infarction, or scar has blossomed in the past 10 years.[28] Two general classes of radiopharmaceutical agents are useful: those which lodge in the cardiac microvasculature during their initial passage[82] and soluble agents which rapidly enter the intracellular space. This latter group consists of inert gases (krypton and xenon) and potassium analogues (thallium, cesium, rubidium) which distribute in the same intracellular space as potassium. Although myocardial distribution of inert gases depends only on regional blood flow, tissue concentration of the potassium analogues depends on both regional blood flow and active membrane transport using the Na-K ATPase enzyme system.[20,23] Thus, impairment of active membrane function by hypoxia in the presence of normal myocardial perfusion may result in the reduced uptake of such agents[2,85] and appear as a "cold spot."

The clinical uses of myocardial perfusion imaging with potassium analogues, particularly thallium 201, include (1) diagnosis and sizing of acute myocardial infarction and (2) diagnosis of coronary artery disease on the basis of perfusion defects which appear during resting studies or following exercise. Filling defects may be found in areas of transient ischemia, acute necrosis, severe ischemia adjacent to regions of acute necrosis, or scar due to old myocardial infarction. In the patient with suspected ischemic heart disease, the scan may be normal at rest, yet have a focal defect of tracer uptake during or immediately following exercise. The sensitivity and specificity for detecting myocardial ischemia by exercise thallium imaging is in the range of 85 to 90 percent, compared with 65 to 70 percent for exercise electrocardiography.[105]

A different group of labeled substances concentrate in zones of ischemic or infarcted myocardium and display "hot spots" due to relatively nonspecific biochemical reactions with constituents of damaged myocardial cells.[148] Such radiopharmaceuticals include ^{99m}Tc-stannous pyrophosphate and other ^{99m}Tc-labeled phosphates and diphosphonates. A second group of agents concentrate in infarcted myocardium by forming an immune complex of various myocardial constituents with their radiolabeled antibodies, such as antibodies to myosin and myoglobin.

A third group of agents concentrates in the acutely infarcted tissue by labeling the inflammatory infiltrate present. Examples include an in vivo method for labeling leukocytes with ^{67}Ga-citrate and in vitro labeling[28] of leukocytes with ^{111}In.

These techniques are mentioned to show the current direction of research concerning noninvasive imaging of damaged myocardium. Fortunately, this is a rare problem in the acutely ill infant or child, although a patient with cardiomyopathy, RV hypertrophy, tumor, Kawasaki disease, anomalous left coronary artery, or other coronary artery malformations may benefit from such techniques.

Intravascular volume determinations[98,149]

Whether they are the cause or effect of circulatory failure, abnormalities of intravascular volume are of keen interest to the pediatric intensivist. The red cell and plasma volumes can be determined simultaneously using readily distinguished isotopes, then summed to yield the total blood volume. Alternatively, but less accurately, total blood volume may be estimated by measuring the red cell volume and venous hematocrit, then applying a factor to the venous hematocrit to calculate the approximate body venous hematocrit. This factor is altered by shock, anemia, or edema. Red cell volume is measured directly using one of several labels of autologous or homologous red cells: (1) ^{51}Cr, accurate within 2 percent, with a very long half-life which makes repeat measurements difficult,[74] (2) ^{99m}Tc-pertechnate, with a short half-life ($T_{1/2}$ 6.1 hours) but which requires great care in the volumetric addition of red cells to a stannous chloride and pertechnate solution, and (3) ^{11}C-carbon monoxide, which requires an on-site cyclotron due its very short half-life of 21 minutes (See the section *Metabolic imaging techniques* (*PET scans*)). These techniques all require equilibration of the labeled red blood cells in the vascular space for up to 20 minutes, during which the patient should be in a steady state without intravascular volume additions or losses. Elution of ^{51}Cr is negligible during this time period, although the other agents may have a significant elution.

The direct measurement of plasma volume is usually performed with radioiodinated albumin (^{125}I or ^{131}I). Although this technique is accurate, its potential thyroid toxicity requires pharmacologic blocking with potassium iodide for 2 days before injection and 2 weeks thereafter.[74] However, protein may be lost from the circulatory space at a variable rate depending on the disease state. Therefore, following an injection, the "true" value must be obtained by extrapolation back to the time of injection. Also, repeat measurements require repeat injections. For these two reasons, measuring the red cell volume, with subsequent estimation of total blood volume, is simpler and less hazardous, although potentially less accurate, than measuring both red cell and plasma volumes.

Blood volume measurement in children requires specialized equipment and technical assistance, making round-the-clock availability difficult. A steady state is particularly difficult to guarantee. Because of these problems, changes in total blood volume are often estimated from changes in LVEDV, as measured by 2DE or a radionuclide technique.

Metabolic imaging techniques (PET scans)[120,128]

Tissue integrity and viability can be assessed following the injection of a positron-emitting radiopharmaceutical tracer which labels the counterparts of a normal constituent of a biological system. Such tracers include (1) blood pool labeling agents (^{11}C-carbon monoxide, ^{15}O-carbon monoxide), (2) indicators of blood flow (^{13}N-ammonia, ^{68}Ga microspheres, ^{81}Rb, ^{82}Rb), and (3) indicators of metabolism (^{11}C-palmitate, ^{13}N-amino acids). Virtually any physiologic substance involved in metabolism can be labeled and used as a tracer, which theoretically allows almost any physiological process to be imaged and quantified. For example, radiolabeled fatty acids such as ^{11}C-palmitate should be taken up by normal myocardium and used as its primary metabolic fuel. Hypoxic or ischemic injury therefore results in reduced myocardial uptake of this agent. Radiolabeled ammonia studies show regional myocardial perfusion defects similar to the potassium analogue tests.[143] Tomographic slices are reconstructed by computer from images detected by a bank of 48 scintillation detectors surrounding the patient. Although structural resolution is inferior to computerized tomography, PET images quantitate regional biochemical events in three dimensions.[128] Since some potentially useful isotopes are extremely short-lived (less than 20 minutes), an on-site cyclotron must be available for the synthesis of ^{13}N-ammonia and $^{81}Rb^{+}$. However, $^{82}Rb^{+}$ can be obtained using a portable generator. Due to its extremely short half-life (75 seconds), sequential images can be obtained at intervals as short as 5 minutes.[10] PET might eventually permit the study of all three major segments of myocardial performance: regional blood flow, mechanical function, and myocardial metabolism. Conceivably, this new method may establish the metabolic link between flow and mechanical function. However, it should be emphasized that this technique is available in only a few medical centers, requires specialized physicians and technicians, and extremely expensive, nonportable equipment. Its usefulness in the serial evaluation of children with myocardial disease is presently untested.

Doppler Cardiac Output

Doppler ultrasonography has become a useful, accurate method of determining systemic blood flow (cardiac output) in children. The Doppler effect is a change in the observed (apparent) frequency of a wave from its true frequency due to motion of the source or target. For cardiac evaluation, source sound waves are produced by a stationary transducer and strike a moving target (blood cells, cardiac valve, or vessel wall). Ordinarily, many frequency shifts are recorded when evaluating (interrogating) the many velocities within a blood stream, since viscous drag of the blood nearest the vessel wall reduces its velocity compared with the central stream. Each frequency shift represents a single velocity. Fast Fourier transform spectral analysis is used to separate these velocities and their distribution during the period of a cardiac cycle. As currently displayed (Fig. 2.11), the grey scale is proportional to the number of red blood cells (RBC) moving at a given velocity, so that the darkest line at any instant represents the most frequently occurring (modal) velocity present.[9,141] By the Doppler equation,

$$\text{Blood flow velocity} = \frac{(F_1 - F_0)\ (\text{velocity of sound in blood})}{(2\ F_0)\ (\cos\ \theta)}$$

where velocity of sound in blood = 1580 m/sec, F_0 = transmitted frequency, F_1 = reflected frequency, the numerator is divided by 2 because sound travels from and to the transducer, and θ is the angle of incidence between the sound wave and the direction of blood flow. Cosine θ may be assumed to equal one ($\pm$6 percent)

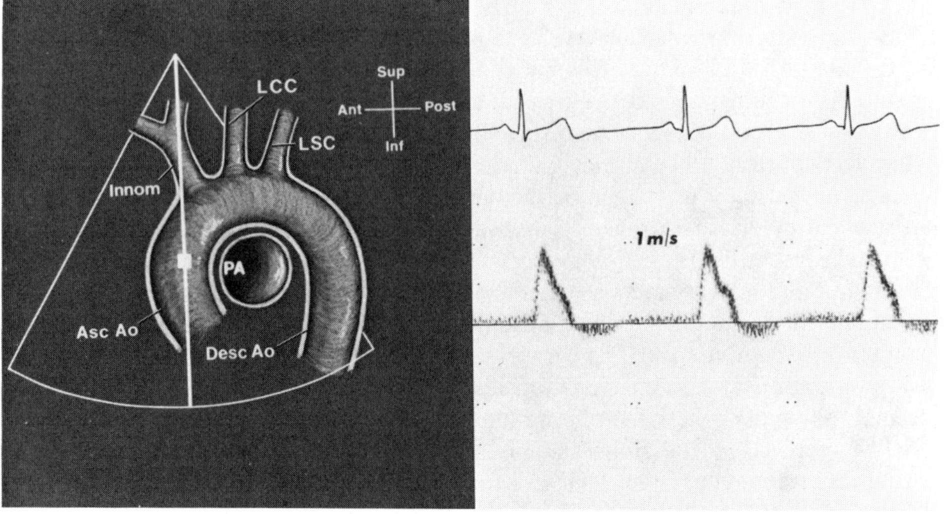

Fig. 2.11. Pulsed Doppler and two-dimensional ultrasonographic evaluation of ascending aortic blood flow from the suprasternal notch. Upper frame: diagram of aortic arch; lower frame: Doppler velocity recording. The mean velocity is obtained by dividing the area under the curves by the length of time recorded, using several cardiac cycles. (Courtesy of Irex Corporation, a Johnson and Johnson Company.)

for angles between −20 and +20 degrees. An ideal (0 degree) angle may be achieved by directing the beam from the suprasternal notch into the ascending aorta.[24] This contrasts with the ideal 90 degree angle needed for standard imaging echocardiography. In a sense, Doppler and 2D ultrasonography are complementary, since 2DE demonstrates the anatomic aspects of the cardiac walls and valves without providing information about functional aspects of blood moving within a cavity, whereas Doppler provides only a functional description of blood movement within a chamber, but no anatomic definition. Two types of Doppler ultrasound technique are currently in use: continuous wave (CW) and pulsed Doppler (PD). Continuous wave Doppler uses two transducers, one which transmits and one which receives sound energy. No visual selection of an area of the heart or great vessels by imaging echocardiography is possible. Using continuous wave Doppler, the velocities of *all* RBCs in the path of flow are detected and recorded. When interrogating the ascending aorta from the suprasternal notch, the maximum frequency shift is assumed to arise from blood flow in the central aortic stream. However, the RBCs lying near the vessel wall move more slowly due to viscous friction. These lower velocities are ignored when calculating flow. Instead, a flat velocity profile is assumed to be present, wherein all RBCs move at approximately the same speed at any instant in time. If the velocity profile is not flat, aortic flow will be overestimated by CW technique. The mean velocity during the cardiac cycle is obtained by planimetry of the area under the velocity-time curve and dividing by systolic and diastolic times. Confounding signals which may arise from the innominate and pulmonary arteries must be eliminated by repositioning the transducer during acquisition of data.[73]

Pulsed Doppler allows a single transducer to both send and receive bursts of signals. Range-gating is therefore permitted, whereby the transducer listens to the returning wave only during a selected period of time (sample volume) corresponding to a particular distance from the transducer, instead of listening continuously. PD may be incorporated with 2DE, so that the linear aortic dimension may be determined. Assuming the aortic cross-section to be circular, the aortic cross-sectional area equals r^2, or $d^2/4$. Since flow (Q) is the product of velocity and area,[4]

$$(Q) = \text{mean aortic velocity} \times \text{aortic cross-sectional area} \times 60$$

Several technical problems may reduce the accuracy of PD or CW ultrasonography. With PD, high velocities arising from flows deep within the chest of some adults cannot be measured and require CW Doppler. PD may seem at first to be more accurate than CW since the sample volume may be placed "precisely" by 2DE. However, the azimuthal plane (in front of or behind the plane of the 2DE beam) is never defined. Although the sample volume may appear to be placed properly, it might actually be placed in the wrong stream. Furthermore, significant underestimation of flow occurs if a beam aimed partly outside the aortic wall using either CW or PD.[24] Deviation of the incident beam by more than 20 degrees from the axis of blood flow also underestimates cardiac output.[141] Further, cross-sectional aortic area and velocity cannot be measured simultaneously at the identical level of the aorta using CW. When using PD, the flow is usually sampled in the proximal ascending aorta (where the flow profile is assumed to be flat) at its central portion, where the maximum aortic flow velocity (frequency shift) is recorded.[73] When using CW, the transducer must be aimed without the benefit of imaging. Since the aortic velocity is assumed to be highest at the narrowest aortic diameter, the CW transducer is aimed blindly at the portion of the aorta which yields the highest aortic systolic velocity (and highest pitched signal), while the echo transducer is later used to measure the narrowest aortic diameter. Finally, the internal diameter of the ascending aorta must be measured accurately and therefore must be visualized completely. This is not always possible. The aortic area increases approximately 15 percent during systole and may be a further source of error.[24] For ease of calculation and to avoid arguments concerning accuracy, serial determinations of the peak systolic velocity may be used in lieu of cardiac output computations for the purposes of tracking a given patient's progress.

Validation studies of cardiac output using these techniques have been performed on dogs and humans. Using pulsed Doppler and 2D ultrasonic beams aimed at the aorta of open-chest dogs, an excellent correlation for cardiac output was noted between thermodilution and PD techniques ($r = .96$)[50] and between PD and flowmeter measurements during right heart extracorporeal bypass ($r = .98$ between .75 and 5 L/min cardiac output).[47] Reproducibility studies in adults have shown a 6 to 9 percent coefficient of variation.[57] Intraobserver and interobserver variability were less than 5 percent.[139] In adults, CW Doppler cardiac output differed by .21 percent ± 8.6 percent (S.D.) from thermodilution values.[73] In one study, only 15 percent of adult ICU patients could not be adequately studied due to the presence of subcutaneous air, spinal abnormality, or very tight skin in the post-operative period.[73]

In infants and children, a good correlation was noted between Fick and Doppler determinations from the suprasternal notch approach (Doppler = 1.07 × Fick −

4.5; r = .98).[4] Because of the occasional technical difficulty in obtaining an accurate suprasternal notch cross-section of the ascending aorta, cardiac output has been determined by measuring flow through the mitral valve orifice by placing the PD sample volume in the LV inflow region. θ was nearly zero degrees, an important factor. The mitral valve orifice area was obtained by planimetry. An excellent correlation was obtained between cardiac output measured by mitral valve PD analysis and by right heart bypass using a calibrated roller pump (r = .97). Moreover, the mitral valve technique allows determination of pulmonary blood flow in patients with left-to-right shunts originating beyond the atrial level.[47,95] The main pulmonary artery may also be interrogated for determination of pulmonary blood flow, which equal systemic blood flow in the absence of any intracardiac shunts.

These Doppler techniques therefore offer much promise in the noninvasive, accurate assessment of beat-to-beat changes in cardiac output and stroke volume, as well as changes over longer periods of time. The technique requires patience and skill to achieve reliable tracings, and the equipment costs approximately $6000 for CW and much more for a PD/2DE system.

Myocardial Enzyme Analysis[133]

Although acute myocardial infarction (AMI) is rare in children, its diagnosis may be aided by the presence of abnormally elevated myocardial enzyme levels. Serum glutamic oxaloacetic transferase (SGOT), creatinine phosphokinase (CPK) and lactate dehydrogenase (LDH) are released from myocardial cells into the serum, and reach peak concentrations at characteristic times following infarction. The diagnostic usefulness of these tests is therefore improved by their serial analysis. SGOT levels generally offer no additional value over CPK and LDH levels. Increased total CPK levels are sensitive but not specific for AMI.[52] Increased LDH levels provide good sensitivity, specificity, and therefore good predictability of AMI, which is enhanced by combining it with CPK measurements.[17,52]

Isoenzyme analysis may be helpful in patients whose history, ECG, and serial total enzyme levels are nondiagnostic for AMI. CPK isoenzymes are separable due to differences in their electrical charge or immunochemical properties. The greatest concentration of CPK-MB is found in myocardial tissue, with less present in skeletal muscle. CPK-MB activity is below 2 percent in healthy adults.[88] The major clinical use of CPK-MB isoenzyme analysis is the detection of AMI within 24 hours of admission, since it reaches its peak level between 12 and 18 hours. Although this is the most sensitive test available for the detection of AMI (100 percent), it lacks specificity, and may also be increased in patients with acute or chronic myocardial disease, myocarditis, pericarditis, cardiac surgery, or trauma, or a host of rare problems.

Abnormal LDH isoenzymes have also been a popular marker for AMI. Of the five LDH isoenzymes, LDH_1 is the myocardial fraction, but LDH_2 always predominates in healthy subjects. Within 2 days following AMI, 80 percent of patients will have an increase in LDH_1 above LDH_2, or "flip." Although not as sensitive as CPK-MB, it is remarkably specific. The combination of these tests in adults complaining of chest pain is a powerful tool for the diagnosis of AMI. The presence of increased CPK-MB and LDH flipped pattern in the first 48 hours after suspected AMI yields a positive predicted value of virtually 100 percent.[52]

Transcutaneous Oxygen Tension Monitoring of Blood Pressure

Peabody et al.[101] have studied the correlation between mean aortic pressure and the energy required to maintain a constant (44°C) electrode temperature of a standard transcutaneous PO_2 electrode. Of 18 premature and term infants, 15 demonstrated a good correlation between these measurements (r = .91 between 29 and 72 mmHg). Factors affecting the correlation adversely were the presence of a previous cutdown in the extremity used and increased skin thickness. The response to changes in blood pressure were prompt and the difference between paired measurements using the two techniques in any infant was less than 4 percent. Although this technique appears simple, and may be useful, independent validation studies are needed. A separate recording system is required.

Computer Axial Tomography

Two types of computed tomographic scanning are currently used to image cardiovascular structures.[25] Dynamic scanning addresses the rapid changes in cardiac function and blood flow by repeating scans rapidly at the same body level. When an iodinated contrast medium is injected, a "poor man's angiogram" is produced. A second scanning protocol takes serial, 5 to 10 mm thick, single scans at adjacent levels to encompass the entire heart and great vessels. An intravenous infusion of contrast medium over 5 to 10 minutes is usually needed to identify the chamber lumen. Some scanners have computer software which stack adjacent individual slices to recreate images along any longitudinal plane. The radiation dose is considerably less than that required for conventional cineangiography. At present, this technique has been useful in identifying patients with an aortic aneurysm, LV or left atrial thrombus, pulmonary embolus, cardiac neoplasm, and pericardial diseases such as an effusion, cyst, calcification, or congential defect. In adults, this technique has proved useful in the noninvasive assessment of coronary artery bypass graft patency[26] and may help determine the extent of a myocardial infarction.[39]

The dynamic spatial reconstructor (DSR) is a major improvement in computed tomography.[114] This multiple x-ray source scanner images the entire heart in a fraction of a second and repeats the scan many times each second. This electronically pulsed scan achieves its image at high speed without the blurring ordinarily caused by cardiac contraction, breathing, or the movement of bowel or blood. It was designed to make simultaneous measurements of myocardial structure and function, instead of making isolated measurements of each. Ventricular wall thickness and chamber volumes may be measured. Cardiac output may be determined using indicator dilution technique to analyze the instantaneous concentration of contrast medium within a carotid artery. This technique may eventually allow quantitative analysis of coronary artery lumen diameters viewed in cross-section. Using the computer to stack serial slices in different planes, the technician can show cut-away views to look inside the chambers. Although a prototype scanner exists only at the Mayo Clinic, this technology may eventually be a quantum leap in the evaluation of myocardial structure and function.

Cardiac Output by Gas Exchange Analysis

Several techniques are available for the noninvasive assessment of cardiac output by analysis of instantaneous gas concentrations and oxygen and carbon dioxide consumptions.[55,56,71] These techniques have several disadvantages. They require

(1) a cooperative subject or a steady state, (2) a long, slow exhalation, (3) accurate gas analysis to determine gas concentrations and tidal volumes, and (4) an on-line computer. Cardiac output estimates made from thermodilution and respiratory gas exchange measurements during a rebreathing maneuver demonstrated reasonably good correlation during normal cardiac output states, but very poor correlation in adults with hemorrhagic shock.[71] In general, other noninvasive techniques are more widely available, more accurate, and less expensive.

Roentgendensitometry Cardiac Output[119]

Although indicator dilution technique using indocyanine green remains the standard for quantitation of cardiac output, other substances have proved useful. Thermodilution has become a widely accepted technique due to the ready application of computer analysis to indicator curves and the harmlessness of the biological indicator. Several other indicator substances have also been used: ^{99m}Tc-labeled red blood cells, x-ray contrast medium (roentgendensitometry), microbubbles by echocardiography, and respiratory gas analysis. With the roentgendensitometric method, indicator dilution technique is used with radiographic contrast medium serving as the indicator. Contrast injected through a central vein moves sequentially through the cardiac chambers. As it moves, it interrupts an x-ray or gamma-ray beam aimed through the heart to a plate under the patient's back containing a sensor system of six solid state crystals. Each crystal is connected to a separate pen recorder, causing simultaneous transcriptions of six contrast dilution curves. The radiation beam passes through one or more cardiac chambers and inscribes a complex curve with multiple deflections, each proportional to the attenuation of the photon beam by contrast material as it moves through several cardiac chambers located in the path of the beam. Statistical moment analysis yields a value which may be correlated with cardiac output by thermodilution. Unfortunately, this correlation is poor ($r = -.63$). This technique has also been advocated by its inventors for the detection of intracardiac shunts[36] and pulmonary circulation times, but has not yet become popular.

Magnetic Resonance Imaging[77]

Like PET scanning, nuclear magnetic resonance imaging (MRI) is in its infancy. The technique is based on the ability to induce and monitor resonance of the magnetic moment of nuclei in the presence of large (static) and weak (varying) magnetic fields. The property of tissues composing a lesion is its fingerprint. Lipid, calcified tissue, and connective tissue are readily identifiable in the iliac and carotid arteries. Imaging of the coronary arteries is not yet possible.

SUMMARY

Cardiologists, radiologists, and intensivists have expended a tremendous effort creating and validating noninvasive tests of cardiac performance. As summarized in Table 2.1, several techniques may be used to measure each variable. The author recommends that a clinician interested in the noninvasive measurement of circulatory performance begin by recognizing the facilities available in all divisions of his institution, especially cardiology, radiology, and nuclear medicine. Because of the variable correlation between a noninvasive test and the standard at different institutions, in-house validation studies should be performed in children for each technique. It is hoped that the establishment of protocols for each test will allow smoother operation at the busy bedside of a very ill child. If a major test category is desired but no type of technique available, the intensivist should review the pros and cons of each technique within that category. He could poll all personnel who might have a strong interest in establishing one particular technique, since most techniques require a great start-up effort in each institution.

As demonstrated by the range of techniques available, noninvasive measurements of circulatory function have become very important in the evaluation of hemodynamically stable adults who can be transported to a study facility within the institution. In time, performance of many of these tests will be commonplace at the bedside of critically ill adults, and eventually in critically ill children.

ACKNOWLEDGEMENTS

The advice of Robert Hirsch, Ph.D. (statistics) and William Follansbee, M.D. (nuclear cardiology) is greatly appreciated.

REFERENCES

1. Adams FH, Emmanouilides GC 1983 Heart Disease in Infants, Children and Adolescents, 3rd edn. Williams & Wilkins, Baltimore
2. Adolph R, Romhilt D, Nishiyama H, Sodd V, Blue J and Gabel M 1976 Use of positive and negative imaging agents to visualize myocardial ischemia. Circulation 54(Supplement II): 220 (abstract)
3. Alderson PO, Jost RG, Strauss AW, Boonvisut S, Markham J 1975 Radionuclide angiography: Improved diagnosis and quantitation of left to right shunts using area-ratio techniques in children. Circulation 51: 1136
4. Alverson DC, Eldridge M, Dillon T, Yabek SM, Berman W 1982 Noninvasive pulsed Doppler determination of cardiac output in neonates and children. Journal of Pediatrics 101: 46
5. Ambrose JA, Teichholz LE, Meller J, Weintraub W, Pichard AD, Smith H, Martinze EE, Herman MV 1979 The influence of left ventricular late diastolic filling on the A wave of the left ventricular pressure trace. Circulation 60: 510
6. Apple HP 1980 Automatic noninvasive blood pressure monitors: What is available. In: Gravenstein JS (ed) Essential noninvasive monitoring in anesthesia. Grune & Stratton, New York
7. Askenazi J, Koenigsberg DI, Ribner HS, Plucinski D, Silverman IM, Lesch M 1983 Prospective study comparing different echocardiographic measurements of pulmonary capillary wedge pressure in patients with organic heart disease other than mitral stenosis. Journal of the American College of Cardiology 2: 919
8. Askenazi J, Koenigsberg DI, Ziegler JH, Lesch M 1981 Echocardiographic estimates of pulmonary artery wedge pressure. New England Journal of Medicine 305: 1566
9. Baker DW 1980 Application of pulsed Doppler techniques. Radiologic Clinics of North America 18: 79
10. Beller GA, Hoop B, Parker JA, Smith TW 1975 Sequential myocardial imaging with rubidium-82, an ultrashort lived radionuclide. Circulation 51, 52(Supplement II): 110 (abstract)
11. Berger HJ, Davies RA, Batsford WP, Hoffer PB, Gottschalk A, Zaret BJ 1981 Beat-to-beat left ventricular performance assessed from the equilibrium cardiac pool using a computerized nuclear probe. Circulation 63: 133
12. Berger HJ, Zaret BJ 1981 Nuclear Cardiology, part II. New England Journal of Medicine 305: 855
13. Berman DS, Maddahi J, Garcia EV, Freeman MR, Shak PK 1981 Assessment of left and right ventricular function with multiple gated equilibrium cardiac blood pool scintigraphy. In: Berman DS and Mason DT (eds) Clinical Nuclear Cardiology. Grune & Stratton, New York

14. Bhatt DR, Isabel-Jones JB, Villoria GJ, Nakazawa M, Yabek SM, Marks RA, Jarmakani JM 1978 Accuracy of echocardiography in assessing LV dimensions and volume. Circulation 57: 699
15. Bjorkhem G, Lundstrom NR 1979 Echocardiographic studies of children operated on for congenital heart disease: evaluation in the immediate postoperative period. European Journal of Cardiology 10: 429
16. Black IF, Kotrapu N, Massie H 1972 Application of Doppler ultrasound of blood pressure measurement in small infants. Journal of Pediatrics 81: 932
17. Blomberg DJ, Kimber WD, Burke MD 1975 Creative kinase isoenzymes: predictive value in the early diagnosis of acute myocardial infarction. American Journal of Medicine 59: 464
18. Bommer W, Neef J, Neumann A, Weinert L, Lee G, Mason DT, DeMaria AN 1978 Indicator-dilution curves obtained by photometric analysis of two-dimension echo-contrast studies. American Journal of Cardiology 41: 370 (abstract)
19. Bommer W, Weinert L, Neumann A, Neef J, Mason DT, DeMaria A 1979 Determination of right atrial and right ventricular size by two-dimensional echocardiography. Circulation 60: 91
20. Bonte FJ, Parkey RW, Stokely EM, Lewis SE, Horwitz LD, Curry GC 1973 Radionuclide determination of myocardial blood flow. Seminars in Nuclear Medicine 3: 153
21. Braunwald E 1980 Contraction of the normal heart. In: Heart Disease. WB Saunders, Philadelphia
22. Braunwald E 1980 The physical examination. In: Heart Disease. WB Saunders, Philadelphia
23. Britten JS, Blank M 1968 Thallium activation of the Na^+K^+ activated ATPase of rabbit-kidney. Biochemical Biophysiology Acta 159: 160
24. Brubakk AO, Gisvold SE 1982 Pulsed Doppler ultrasound for measuring blood flow in the human aorta. In: Hatle L and Angelsen B (eds) Doppler Ultrasound in Cardiology: Physical Principles and Clinical Applications. Lea & Febiger, Philadelphia
25. Brundage BH 1983 Computed tomography: a new view of cardiovascular disease. Primary Cardiology, July: 57
26. Brundage BH, Lipton MJ, Herfkens RJ, Berninger WH, Redington RW, Chatterjee K, Carlsson E 1980 Detection of patent coronary bypass grafts by computed tomography. Circulation 61: 826
27. Bruner JM, Krenis LJ, Kunsman JM, Sherman AP 1981 Comparison of direct and indirect methods of measuring arterial blood pressure—Parts I, II, and III. Medical Instrumentation 14: 182, 15: 11, 97
28. Buja LM, Parkey RW, Bonte FJ, Willerson JT 1979 Pathophysiology of "cold spot" and "hot spot" myocardial imaging agents used to detect ischemia or infarction. In: Willerson JT (ed) Nuclear Cardiology. FA Davis, Philadelphia
29. Burow RD, Strauss HW, Singleton R, Pond M, Rehn T, Bailey IK, Griffith LC, Nickoloff E, Pitt B 1977 Analysis of left ventricular function from multiple gated acquisition cardiac blood pool imaging. Circulation 56: 1024
30. Caffey JP 1978 Pediatric X-Ray Diagnosis, 7th edn. Year Book, Chicago
31. Calvin JE, Driedger AA, Sibbald WJ 1981 Does the pulmonary capillary wedge predict left ventricular preload in critically ill patients? Critical Care Medicine 9: 437
32. Cohn JN 1967 Blood pressure measurement in shock. Journal of American Medical Association 199: 118
33. Colan SD, Fujii A, Borrow KM, MacPherson D, Sanders SP 1983 Noninvasive determination of systolic, diastolic and end-systolic blood pressure in neonates, infants, and young children: comparison with central aortic pressure measurements. American Journal of Cardiology 52: 867
34. Corya BC, Rasmussen S 1981 Assessing left ventricular function with intervention echocardiography. Journal of Cardiovascular Medicine 6:574
35. Corya BC, Rasmussen S, Phillips JF, Black MJ 1981 Forward stroke volume calculated from aortic valve echograms in normal subjects and patients with mitral regurgitation secondary to left ventricular dysfunction. American Journal of Cardiology 47: 1215
36. DelGuercio LRM, Engler PE, Maluso PJ, Wagner RS, Davachi R, Cohn JD 1976 Shunts detected by roentgen densitometry. Circulation 53, 54(Supplement II): 111 (abstract)
37. DeMaria AN, Bommer W, Riggs K, Dajee A, Miller L, Mason DT 1980 In vivo correlation of cardiac output and densitometric dilution curves obtained by contrast 2D echocardiography. Circulation 62(Supplement II): 101 (abstract)
38. DeMaria AN, Bommer W, Takeda P, Mason DT, Kwan OL, Rasor J 1983 Value of limitations of contrast echocardiography in cardiac disease. In: Fowler NO (ed) Noninvasive Diagnostic Methods. FA Davis, Philadelphia
39. Dougherty PW, Lipton MJ, Berninger WH, Skioldebrand CG, Carlsson E, Redington RW 1981 The detection and quantification of myocardial infarction in vivo using transmission computed tomography. Circulation 63: 597
40. Duff DF, Gutgesell HP 1977 The use of saline or blood for ultrasonic detection of a right-to-left shunt in the early postoperative patient. American Heart Journal 94:402

41. Dweck HS, Reynolds DW, Cassady G 1974 Indirect blood pressure measurement in newborns. American Journal of Diseases in Children 127: 492
42. Eaton LW, Maughan WL, Shoukas AA, Weiss JL 1979 Accurate volume determination in the isolated ejecting canine left ventricle by two-dimensional echocardiography. Circulation 60:320
43. Elseed AM, Shinebourne EA, Joseph MC 1973 Assessment of techniques for measurement of blood pressure in infants and children. Archives of Disease in Childhood 48: 932
44. Feigenbaum H 1981 Echocardiographic evaluation of cardiac chambers. In: Echocardiography, 3rd edn. Lea & Febiger, Philadelphia
45. Feigenbaum H 1981 Hemodynamic information derived from echocardiography. In: Echocardiography, 3rd edn. Lea & Febiger, Philadelphia
46. Feingenbaum H, Dillon JC, Haine CL, and Chang S 1970 Effect of elevated atrial component of left ventricular pressure on mitral valve closure. American Journal of Cardiology 25: 95 (abstract)
47. Fisher DC, Sahn DJ, Friedman MJ, Larson D, Valdes-Cruz LM, Horowitz S, Goldberg SJ, Allen HD 1983 The effect of variations on pulsed Doppler sampling site on calculation of cardiac output: An experimental study in open-chest dogs. Circulation 67: 370
48. Folland ED, Parisi AF, Moynihan PF, Jones DR, Feldman CL, Tow DE 1979 Assessment of left ventricular ejection fraction and volumes by real-time, two-dimensional echocardiography. Circulation 60: 760
49. Fortuin NJ, Sherman ME, Hood WP, Craige E 1971 Determination of left ventricular volumes by ultrasound. Circulation 44: 575
50. Friedman MJ, Salin DJ, Larson D, Flint A 1980 2D echo-range gated Doppler measurements of cardiac output and stroke volume in open chest dogs. Circulation 62(Supplement III): 101 (abstract)
51. Friesen RH, Lichtor JL 1981 Indirect measurement of blood pressure in neonates and infants utilizing an automatic noninvasive oscillometric monitor. Anesthesia and Analgesia 60: 742
52. Galen RS 1975 The enzyme diagnosis of myocardial infarction. Human Pathology 6: 141
53. Gates GF, Orme HW, Pore EK 1974 Cardiac shunt assessment in children with macroaggregated albumin technicium-99m. Radiology 112: 649
54. Geddes LA, Chaffee V, Whistler SJ, Bourland JD, Tacker WA 1977 Indirect mean blood pressure of the anesthetized pony. American Journal of Veterinary Research 38. 2055
55. Geisler FH, Farrell EJ, Siegel JH 1978 A new noninvasive method for the simultaneous determination of CO, VA/QC disparity, and the magnitude of peripheral perfusion, suitable for use in the critically ill patient. Journal of Trauma 18: 751
56. Gilbert R, Auchincloss JH 1970 Comparison of single-breath and indicator-dilution measurement of cardiac output. Journal of Applied Physiology 29: 119
57. Gisvold SE, Brubakk AO 1982 Measurement of instantaneous blood-velocity in the human aorta using pulsed Doppler ultrasound. Cardiovascular Research 16: 26
58. Glanz SA, Parmley WW 1978 Factors which affect the diastolic pressure-volume curve. Circulation Research 42: 171
59. Goldberg SJ, Allen HD, Sahn DJ 1975 Pediatric and Adolescent Echocardiography. Year Book, Chicago
60. Gordon DG, Ashburn WL, Slutsky RA 1981 Assessment of ventricular function by first-pass radionuclide angiography. In: Berman DS and Mason DT (eds) Clinical Nuclear Cardiology. Grune & Stratton, New York
61. Gordon LS, Johnson PE, Penido JR, Printup CA, Dietrick WR, Buggs H 1974 Systolic and diastolic blood pressure measurements by transcutaneous Doppler ultrasound in premature infants in critical care nurseries and at closed-heart surgery. Anesthesia and Analgesia 53: 914
62. Gordon EP, Schnittger I, Fitzgerald PJ, Williams P, Popp RL 1983 Reproducibility of left ventricular volumes by two-dimensional echocardiography. Journal of the American College of Cardiology 2: 506
63. Graham TP, Jarmakani JM, Canent RV, Morrow MN 1971 Left heart volume estimation in infancy and childhood. Reevaluation of methodology and normal values. Circulation 43: 895
64. Grossman W, McLaurin LP 1976 Diastolic properties of the left ventricle. Annals of Internal Medicine 84: 316
65. Haendchen RV, Wyatt HL, Maurer G, Zwehl W, Bear M, Meerbaum S, Corday E 1983 Quantitation of regional cardiac function by two-dimensional echocardiography. Circulation 67: 1234
66. Halliday H, Hirschfeld S, Riggs T, Liebman J, Fanaroff A, Bormuth C 1977 Respiratory distress syndrome: echocardiographic assessment of cardiovascular function and pulmonary vascular resistance. Pediatrics 60: 444
67. Hearst JW 1982 The Heart, 5th edn. McGraw-Hill, New York
68. Hernandez A, Boldring D, Hartmann AF 1971 Measurement of blood pressure in infants and children by the Doppler ultrasonic technique. Pediatrics 48: 788

69. Hirschfeld S, Meyer R, Schwartz DC, Korfhagen J, Kaplan S 1975 Echocardiographic assessment of pulmonary artery pressure and pulmonary vascular resistance. Circulation 52: 642
70. Hoffer PB, Berger HJ, Steidley J, Brendel AF, Gottschalk A, Zaret BL 1981 A miniature cadmium telluride detector module for continuous monitoring of left ventricular function. Radiology 138: 477
71. Homer LD, Denysyk B 1975 Estimation of cardiac output by analysis of respiratory gas exchange. Journal of Applied Physiology 39: 159
72. Howman-Giles RB, Gilday DL, Mason DT, Berman DS 1981 Nuclear cardiology in pediatrics: Evaluation of intracardiac shunts and additional congenital disorders. In: Berman DS and Mason DT (eds) Clinical Nuclear Cardiology. Grune & Stratton, New York
73. Huntsman LL, Stewart DK, Barnes SR, Franklin SB, Colocousis JS, Hessel EA 1983 Noninvasive Doppler determination of cardiac output in man: Clinical validation. Circulation 67: 593
74. International Committees for Standardization in Hematology 1973 Standard techniques for the measurement of red cell and plasma volume. British Journal of Haematology 25: 795
75. Jardin F, Farcot JC, Boisante L, Curien N, Margairaz A, Bourdarias JP 1981 Influence of positive end-expiratory pressure on left ventricular performance. New England Journal of Medicine 304: 387
76. Joly HR, Weil MH 1969 Temperature of the toe as an indication of the severity of shock. Circulation 39: 131
77. Kaufman L, Crooks L, Sheldon PI, Hricak H, Herfkens R, Bank W 1983 The potential impact of nuclear magnetic resonance imaging on cardiovascular diagnosis. Circulation 67: 251
78. Keith JD, Rowe RD, Vlad P 1978 Heart Disease in Infancy and Childhood, 3rd edn. MacMillan, New York
79. Kennedy JW, Baxley WA, Figley MM, Dodge HT, Blackmon JR 1966 Quantitative angiocardiography. The normal left ventricle in man. Circulation 34: 272
80. Kerber RE, Martins JB, Barnes R, Manuel WJ, Maximov M 1979 Effects of acute hemodynamic alterations on pulmonic valve motion. Experimental and clinical echocardiographic studies. Circulation 60: 1074
81. Kimble KJ, Darnall RA, Yelderman M, Ariagno RL, Ream AK 1981 An automated oscillometric technique for reestimating mean arterial pressure in critically ill newborns. Anesthesiology 54: 423
82. Kirk GA, Adams R, Jansen C, Judkins MP 1977 Particulate myocardial perfusion scintigraphy. Its clinical usefulness in evaluating coronary artery disease. Seminars in Nuclear Medicine 7: 67
83. Kitabatake A, Inoue M, Asao M, Masayama T, Tanouchi J, Morita T, Mishima M, Uematsu M, Shimazu T, Hori M, Abe H 1983 Noninvasive evaluation of pulmonary hypertension by a pulsed Doppler technique. Circulation 68: 302
84. Kronik G, Slany J, Mösslacher H 1979 Comparative value of eight M-mode echocardiographic formulas determining left ventricular stroke volume: a correlative study with thermodilution and left ventricular single-plane cineangiography. Circulation 60: 1308
85. Levenson NI, Adolph RJ, Romhilt DW, Gabel M, Sodd V, August LS 1975 Effects of myocardial hypoxia and ischemia on myocardial scintigraphy. American Journal of Cardiology 35: 251
86. Lewis RP 1983 The use of systolic time intervals for evaluation of left ventricular function. In: Fowler NO (ed) Noninvasive Diagnostic Methods in Cardiology. FA Davis, Philadelphia
87. Lewis JR, Parker JO, Burggral GW 1978 Mitral valve motion and changes in left ventricular end-diastolic pressure: a correlative study of the PR-AC interval. American Journal of Cardiology 42: 383
88. Lott JA, Stang JM 1980 Serum enzymes and isoenzymes in the diagnosis and differential diagnosis of myocardial ischemia and necrosis. Clinical Chemistry 26: 1241
89. McLaughlin GW, Kirby RR, Kemmerer WT, deLemos RA 1971 Indirect measurement of blood pressure in infants utilizing Doppler ultrasound. Journal of Pediatrics 79: 300
90. Maddahi J, Berman DS, Silverberg R, Charuzi Y, Buchbinder N, Gray R, Waxman A, Vas R, Shak PK, Swan HJC, Forrester J 1978 Validation of a 2-minute technique for multiple gated scintigraphic assessment of left ventricular ejection fraction and regional wall motion. Journal of Nuclear Medicine 19: 669
91. Maltz DL, Treves S 1973 Quantitative radionuclide angiography: determination of Qp:Qs in children. Circulation 47: 1049
92. Mann T, McLaurin L, Grossman W, Craig E 1975 Assessing the hemodynamic severity of acute aortic regurgitation due to infective endocarditis. New England Journal of Medicine 293: 108
93. Maresh MM, Washburn AH 1938 Size of the hearts of normal children: II. Roentgen ray studies. American Journal of Diseases in Children 56: 33
94. Marshall RC, Berger HJ, Costin JC, Freedman GS, Wolberg J, Cohen LS, Gottschalk A, Zaret

BL 1977 Assessment of cardiac performance with quantitative radionuclide angiocardiography. Circulation 56: 820

95. Meijboom EJ, Valdes-Cruz LM, Horowitz S, Sahn DJ, Larson DF, Young KA, Lima CO, Goldberg SJ 1983 A two-dimensional Doppler echocardiographic method for calculation of pulmonary and systemic blood flow in a canine model with a variable-sized left-to-right extracardiac shunt. Circulation 68: 437
96. Mercier JC, DiSessa TG, Jarmakani JM, Nakanishi T, Hiraishi S, Isabel-Jones J, Friedman WF 1982 Two-dimensional echocardiographic assessment of left-ventricular volumes and ejection fraction in children. Circulation 65: 962
97. Moss AJ, Adams FH 1965 Auscultatory and intraarterial pressure: a comparison in children with special reference to cuff width. Journal of Pediatrics 66: 1094
98. Najean Y, Cacchione R 1977 Blood volume in health and disease. Clinics in Hematology 6: 543
99. Nimura Y, Matsumoto M, Shimada H, Nagata S, Oyama S, Takahashi Y, Abe H, Kitabatake A, Matsuo H 1971 Unusual configuration of ultrasound cardiogram of mitral valve observed in some cases with myocardial disease of unknown cause. Medical Ultrasonics 9: 108
100. Parker JA, Treves S 1977 Radionuclide detection, localization, and quantitation of intracardiac shunts and shunts between great arteries. Progress in cardiovascular disease 20: 121
101. Peabody JL, Willis MM, Gregory GA, Severinghaus JW 1979 Reliability of skin TcPO2 electrode heating power as a continuous noninvasive monitor of mean arterial pressure in sick newborns. Birth Defects: Original Article Series, 15: 127
102. Peter CA, Armstrong BE, Jones RH 1981 Radionuclide quantitation of right-to-left intracardiac shunts in children. Circulation 64: 572
103. Pietro DA, Voelkel AG, Ray BJ, Parisi AF 1981 Reproducibility of echocardiography. A study evaluating the variability of serial echocardiographic measurements. Chest 79: 29
104. Pitt B, Strauss HW 1977 Evaluation of ventricular function by radioisotopic technics. New England Journal of Medicine 296: 1097
105. Pitt B, Strauss HW 1979 Clinical application of myocardial imaging with Thallium-201. In: Willerson JT (ed) Nuclear Cardiology. FA Davis, Philadelphia
106. Posey JA, Geddes LA, Williams H, Moore AG 1969 The meaning of the point of maximum oscillations in cuff pressure in the indirect measurement of blood pressure. Cardiovascular Research Center Bulletin 8: 15
107. Ramsey M 1979 Noninvasive automatic determination of mean arterial pressure. Medical and Biological Engineering and Computing 17: 11
108. Ramsey M 1980 Noninvasive blood pressure monitoring methods and validation. In: Gravenstein JS (ed) Essential Noninvasive Monitoring in Anesthesia. Grune & Stratton, New York
109. Rasmussen S, Corya BC, Phillips JF, Black MJ 1982 Unreliability of M-mode left ventricular dimensions for calculating stroke volume and cardiac output in patients without heart disease. Chest 81: 614
110. Reder RF, Dimich I, Cohen ML, Steinfeld L 1978 Evaluating indirect blood pressure of three systems in infants and children. Pediatrics 62: 326
111. Riggs T, Hirschfeld S, Borkat G, Knoke J, Liebman J 1978 Assessment of the pulmonary vascular bed by echocardiographic right ventricular systolic time intervals. Circulation 57: 939
112. Riggs T, Hirschfeld S, Bormuth C, Fanaroff A, Liebman J 1977 Neonatal circulatory changes on echocardiography. Pediatrics 59: 338
113. Riggs T, Hirschfeld S, Fanaroff A, Liebman J, Fletcher B, Meyer R, Bormuth C 1977 Persistence of fetal circulation syndrome: an echocardiographic study. Journal of Pediatrics 91: 626
114. Ritman EL 1983 The dynamic spatial reconstructor. Modern Problems in Paediatrics 22: 38
115. Roberts NK, Gelbland H 1977 Cardiac Arrythmias in the Neonate, Infant and Child. Appleton-Century-Crofts, New York
116. Roy RC, Morgan L, Beamer D 1983 Factitiously low blood pressure from the DinamappTM Anesthesiology 59: 258
117. Rudolph AM 1974 Congenital Diseases of the Heart. Year Book, Chicago
118. Sahn DJ, DeMaria A, Kisslo J 1978 Recommendations regarding quantitation in M-mode echocardiography: results of a survey of echocardiographic measurements. Circulation 58: 1072
119. SanFilippo JA, Cohn J, Gupte P, Barbata J, Feldman M, DelGuercio LRM 1981 Invasive cardiopulmonary monitoring. Surgery 90: 313
120. Schelbert HR, Phelps ME, Kuhl DE 1981 Positron emission tomography of the heart: A new method for the noninvasive assessment of regional myocardial blood flow, function, and metabolism. In: Berman DS and Mason DT (eds) Clinical Nuclear Cardiology. Grune & Stratton, New York
121. Schelbert HR, Verba JW, Johnson AD, Brock GW, Alazraki NP, Rose FJ, Ashburn WL 1975

Nontraumatic determination of left ventricular ejection fraction by radionuclide angiocardiography. Circulation 51: 902
122. Schiller NB, Acquatella H, Ports TA, Drew D, Georke J, Ringertz H, Silverman NH, Brundage B, Botvinick EH, Boswell R, Carlsson E, Parmley WW 1979 Left ventricular volume from paired biplane two-dimensional echocardiography. Circulation 60: 547
123. Schnittger I, Fitzgerald PJ, Daughters GT, Ingels NB, Kantrowitz NE, Schwarzkopf A, Mead CW, Popp RL 1982 Limitations of comparing left ventricular volumes by two dimensional echocardiography, myocardial markers, and cineangiography. American Journal of Cardiology 50: 512
124. Showman A, Betts EK 1981 Hazard of automatic noninvasive blood pressure monitoring. Anesthesiology 55: 717
125. Sibbald WJ, Calvin JE, Driedger AA 1982 Right and left ventricular preload and diastolic ventricular compliance: implications in critically ill patients. In: Shoemaker WC and Thompson WL (eds) Critical Care: State of the art, Vol. 3. Society of Critical Care Medicine, Fullerton, CA
126. Silverman NH, Ports TA, Snider AR, Schiller NB, Carlsson E, Heilbron DC 1980 Determination of left ventricular volume in children: Echocardiographic and angiographic comparisons. Circulation 62: 548
127. Silverman NE, Snider AR, Rudolph AM 1980 Evaluation of pulmonary hypertension by M-mode echocardiography in children with ventricular septal defect. Circulation 61: 1125
128. Sobel BE, Ter-Pogossian MM, Geltman EM 1981 Positron-emission tomography in cardiac evaluation. Hospital Practice 16: 93
129. Spicer R, Rabinovitch M, Rosenthal A, Pitt B 1984 Measurement of left ventricular ejection fraction in pediatric patients utilizing the nuclear stethoscope. American Journal of Cardiology 53: 211
130. Spooner EW, Perry BL, Stern AM, Sigmann J 1978 Estimation of pulmonary/systemic resistance ratios from echocardiographic systolic time intervals in young patients with congenital or acquired heart disease. American Journal of Cardiology 42: 810
131. Starling MR, Crawford MH, O'Rourke RA, Groves BM, Amon KW 1980 Accuracy of subxiphoid echocardiography for assessing left ventricular size and performance. Circulation 61: 367
132. Stegall HF, Kardon MB, Kemmerer WT 1968 Indirect measurement of arterial blood pressure by Doppler ultrasonic sphygmomanometry. Journal of Applied Physiology 25: 793
133. Stein EA, Kaplan LA 1983 Serum enzymes, isoenzymes, myoglobin, and contractile proteins in acute myocardial infarction. In: Fowler NO (ed) Noninvasive Diagnostic Methods in Cardiology, FA Davis, Philadelphia
134. Strashun A, Horowitz SF, Goldsmith SJ, Teichholz LE, Dicker A, Miceli K, Gorlin R 1981 Noninvasive detection of left ventricular dysfunction with a portable electrocardiographic gated scintillation probe device. American Journal of Cardiology 47: 610
135. Strauss HW, Zaret BL, Hurley PJ, Natarajan TK, Pitt B 1971 A scintiphotographic method for measuring left ventricular ejection fraction in man without cardiac catheterization. American Journal of Cardiology 28: 575
136. Sy WP 1981 Ulnar nerve palsy possibly related to use of automatically cycled blood pressure cuff, Anesthesia and Analgesia 60: 687
137. Teichholz LE, Cohen MV, Sonnenblick EH, Gorlin R 1974 Study of left ventricular geometry and function by B-scan ultrasonography in patients with and without asynergy. New England Journal of Medicine 291: 1220
138. Twieg D, Parkey RW, Willerson JT 1979 Scintigraphic evaluation of left ventricular function. In: Willerson JT (ed) Nuclear Cardiology, FA Davis Philadelphia
139. Valdes-Cruz LM, Horowitz S, Mesel E, Salin DJ, Fisher DC, Larson D, Goldberg SJ, Allen HD 1983 A pulsed Doppler echocardiographic method for calculation of pulmonary and systemic flow: accuracy in a canine model with ventricular septal defect. Circulation 68: 597
140. Valdes-Cruz LM, Pieroni DR, Roland JA, Shematch JP 1977 Recognition of residual postoperative shunts by contrast echocardiographic techniques. Circulation 55: 148
141. Valdes-Cruz LM, Sahn DJ 1982 Two-dimensional echo Doppler for noninvasive quantitation of cardiac flow: a status report. Modern Concepts for Cardiovascular Disease 51: 123
142. VanderArk CR, Ballontyne F, Reynolds EW 1973 Electrolytes and the electrocardiogram. In: Fisch C (ed) Complex Electrocardiography I. FA Davis, Philadelphia
143. Walsh WF, Fill HR, Harper PV 1977 Nitrogen-13-labeled ammonia for myocardial imaging. Seminars in Nuclear Medicine 7: 59
144. Wagner HN 1982 The nuclear cardiac probe. Hospital Practice 17: 163
145. Wagner HN, Rigo P, Baxter RH, Alderson PO, Douglass KH, Housholder DF 1979 Monitoring ventricular function at rest and during exercise with a noninvasive nuclear detector. American Journal of Cardiology 43: 975

146. Wagner HN, Wake R, Nickoloff E, Natarajan TK 1976 The nuclear stethoscope: a simple device for generation of left ventricular volume curves. American Journal of Cardiology 38: 747
147. Weissler AM 1977 Systolic-time intervals. New England Journal of Medicine 296: 321
148. Willerson JT, Parkey RW, Buja LM, Bonte FJ 1979 Technicium^{99M} stannous pyrophosphate "hot spot" imaging to detect acute myocardial infarcts. In: Willerson JT (ed) Nuclear Cardiology. FA Davis, Philadelphia
149. Wright RR, Tono M, Pollycove M 1975 Blood volume. Seminars in Nuclear Medicine 5: 63
150. Yang SS, Bentivoglio LG, Maranhao V, Goldberg H 1978 From Cardiac Catheterization Data to Hemodynamic Parameters, 2nd edn. FA Davis, Philadelphia
151. Yelderman M, Ream AK 1979 Indirect measurement of mean blood pressure in the anesthetized patient. Anesthesiology 50: 253
152. Zaret BL 1979 Key references: Cardiovascular nuclear medicine. Circulation 60: 210
153. Zaret BL, Strauss HW, Hurley PJ, Natarajan TK, Pitt B 1971 A noninvasive scintiphotographic method for detecting regional ventricular dysfunction in man. New Journal of Medicine 284: 1165
154. Zuberbuhler JR 1981 The cardiac physical examination. In: Clinical Diagnosis in Paediatric Cardiology. Churchill Livingstone, Edinburgh

3

Invasive Assessment of the Failing Circulation

David B. Swedlow
David E. Cohen

The purpose of the pediatric intensive care unit is to restore health in a child with failing vital organ systems. For the circulation, this means restoring a normal balance between supply and demand of substrate to the body. The function of the heart is to pump substrate-rich blood to the periphery, while the function of the remainder of the cardiovascular system is to distribute the substrate in a manner appropriate to supply the body's needs.

Invasive monitoring allows the clinician to evaluate the circulation, to recognize potential and actual problems, and to adjust the circulation with rapid feedback. Invasive monitoring provides objective data to be used in conjunction with clinical assessment. The circulation can be evaluated for preload, afterload, contractility, and substrate delivery and utilization using objective and numerical data that allow a more precise quantification than is available with noninvasive means. Continuous invasive monitoring facilitates the recognition of potential problems before they become major catastrophes. For example, a situation in which central filling pressure and blood pressure are both falling in the context of a postoperative patient strongly suggests hypovolemia, whereas a falling blood pressure and rising filling pressure suggest congestive or restrictive heart failure. A fall in mixed venous $P_{\bar{v}}O_2$ suggests an alteration in the balance between peripheral substrate supply and demand before the patient has suffered irreversible tissue hypoxia.[21,80,125] Invasive monitoring facilitates adjustment and "fine tuning" of the circulation. A clinician may use small volume infusions and measure the changing blood pressure and/or cardiac output with immediate feedback.[138]

When is invasive monitoring more appropriate than noninvasive monitoring? This question requires evaluation of the relative advantages of invasive versus noninvasive monitoring. The details of this evaluation depend on the type of invasive monitoring being considered, the need for the data, and the risk to the child. A common use of invasive monitoring involves the measurement of blood pressure, blood gases, or electrolytes on a continuous or frequent intermittent basis. When sudden and dramatic swings in blood pressure, gas exchange, or fluid and electrolytes are anticipated, the clinician should consider a monitoring system that allows convenient and perhaps continuous access to the circulation or convenient access to the subject's vascular tree. Continuous monitoring allows the clinician, anticipating sudden catastrophic swings in vital signs, to set minimum and maximum alarm limits. Certain measures are not currently available noninvasively. Cardiac output is an example of a measure for which there are no noninvasive methods that are considered sufficiently accurate and reliable. In other cases, there are noninvasive measurements available, but they are not judged sufficiently accurate or reliable. Measurement of arterial blood gas tensions is one such example. Transcutaneous blood gas electrodes are available commercially, but do not always produce reliable data during periods of hemodynamic instability.

There are several disadvantages of invasive versus noninvasive monitoring. Insertion of an invasive device involves some pain for the noncomatose child. Infection is a risk because the invasive device must pass through the integument.[6,141] There is the obvious risk of bleeding as the catheter device is inserted into the vessel and the less obvious risk of bleeding upon accidental disconnection of a device in continuity with the vascular space. Some invasive monitors may cause physical damage to structures within the body, such as pulmonary artery rupture or thrombosis.[8,94,96,127] Receiving increasing attention is the cost associated with capital outlay and supplies as well as the hidden cost of increased nursing personnel required to maintain the patency and sterility of invasive devices.[32]

When considering invasive monitoring, the clinician first needs to determine that cardiopulmonary instability exists and that invasive monitoring exists that addresses the instability. Second, he must determine that the usual noninvasive means to assess the circulation are inadequate or unreliable in terms of accuracy, precision, or continuity. Third, the clinician must weigh the risk/benefit ratio involved with each invasive monitoring decision. If the need for data plus the danger of not having the data outweighs the risk to the patient and cost associated with the invasive monitor, then the risk/benefit analysis favors invasive monitoring. The clinician must then select the most appropriate invasive monitor and insert it in a safe and effective manner.

In this chapter we will consider technical issues common to all invasive monitoring including insertion techniques, complications, catheter materials, and protocols for their use. We will then discuss physiologic variables that are measurable by invasive monitoring, beginning with the most commonly monitored variable and progressing to the least commonly monitored variable. For each variable we will discuss physiologic considerations surrounding that variable, the technology of measurement concerned with that variable, and any specific problems that may arise. Whenever appropriate, we will first discuss intermittent methods and then move to continuous or indirect measurements.

TECHNICAL ISSUES RELATING TO CATHETERIZATION

Arterial Catheter Insertion Sites

The majority of invasive monitoring requires the insertion of a catheter through the integument and into the vascular space of the child. Part of the decision process for choosing an invasive monitor in a child revolves around the technical considerations of size, location, ease of securing the catheter, risk of infection, and other complications relating to the site.

In the arterial tree, one of the major considerations for site determination is the verification of collateral circulation. Many arteries have limited anastomotic pathways to provide circulation in the event of a partial or complete occlusion of the primary vessel. For example, the fingers are supplied by the superficial and deep palmar arches. This anastomotic network is supplied by the radial and ulnar arteries. In many individuals, the palmar arches are supplied by only one functional artery with no collateral available.[28,135] Documentation of adequate collateral circulation can be performed by using the modified Allen's test.[3,117] In this maneuver, one compresses both the radial and ulnar arteries at the wrist with firm pressure, while simultaneously squeezing the subject's hand in an attempt to empty the soft tissues of blood. While maintaining the pressure on the radial artery, one releases the pressure on the ulnar artery and looks for the appearance of a capillary flush on the palmar surface of the hand within 7 seconds. If the palmar flush does not occur soon after release, the clinician should assume that the collateral circulation to the palmar arch via the ulnar artery is inadequate to supply nutrient flow to the hand in the event that the radial artery is occluded. He should seek an alternative site for catheterization.[15] The palmar flush technique can be used in any size patient including an infant or newborn. In a small child, it may be easier to perform a modified Allen's test using a finger plethysmograph wrapped around the soft tissue pad of the thumb or first finger when testing for ulnar collateral flow or the fifth finger when testing for radial collateral flow.[19] The plethysmographic wave form is displayed on an oscilloscope. Both arteries are compressed while the clinician observes the disappearance of the plethysmographic wave form. Each individual artery can be tested for patency by releasing the pressure over that artery and watching the reappearance of the plethysmographic wave form indicating adequate flow to the monitored digit. However the modified Allen's test is done, its performance is important in order to insure that partial or complete obstruction of the catheterized vessel will not result in damaging ischemia to the hand.[38,70,82,143]

Radial artery

The radial artery is probably the most common site chosen for systemic arterial pressure monitoring via invasive monitors.[133] The radial artery courses near the superficial tissues of the wrist so that catheters can be secured to the volar aspect of the wrist. In a high percentage of patients, there is adequate collateral flow from the ulnar artery. The wrist is taped in an extended position on an arm board with adequate padding under the joint of the wrist. The hand and fingers are taped facing upward and the site is prepped and draped. The reader will find a discussion of insertion techniques below.

Ulnar artery

The ulnar artery runs along the medial aspect of the forearm becoming relatively superficial about 1 cm proximal to the wrist. The ulnar forms one half of the usual supply of the palmar arches.[28,135] Before the clinician cannulates the ulnar artery, he should check the patency of the radial artery using the modified Allen's test. The ulnar artery is less commonly used than the radial because it lies deeper than the radial artery and because it is more difficult to cannulate. Nevertheless, when one cannot palpate the radial artery but has documented its presence via the modified Allen's test, the ulnar artery represents an acceptable choice for catheterization.[66,77]

Brachial artery

Moving proximally in the arterial tree one next considers the brachial artery in the antecubital fossa. This artery has long been the favorite of radiographers and cardiologists but may present a significant risk of median nerve damage in the intensive care situation.[93] There is no formal test for adequate collateral circulation for the brachial artery. An additional problem with the brachial artery is that it is very difficult to secure a catheter across the elbow joint, which tends to flex unless it is splinted in an extended posture by uncomfortable and bulky arm boards.

Axillary artery

At first glance, the axillary artery might seem to be an unusual vessel to choose for arterial catheterization because of its awkward location deep within the soft tissues of the upper arm. However, the axillary artery has a rich collateral circulation supplying the rest of the arm in the event that it becomes blocked.[136] The axillary artery is frequently approached via cutdown but may be palpated and approached percutaneously using the standard Seldinger technique.[4,35] With a vessel close to the central circulation, one needs to be very careful about flushing small clots or air bubbles retrograde in the arterial tree to the subclavian arteries where small emboli may travel via the carotid circulation to the brain.[76] When the usual peripheral vessels are unavailable due to previous use or thrombosis, the axillary artery represents an excellent choice for catheterization in the intensive care unit environment.

Subclavian artery

Still more proximal in the arterial tree is the subclavian artery. The subclavian artery is rarely chosen as a site for elective catheterization due to the very high risk of embolization into the cerebral and coronary circulations. However, during emergency resuscitations, a subclavian vein catheterization attempt may inadvertently yield a subclavian artery. Extreme caution must be exercised in maintaining patency of the vessel and in insuring that no clots or air bubbles are flushed into the catheter.

Aorta

Most proximal in the arterial tree is the aorta. The aorta is rarely used for monitoring outside of the neonatal period because of the high risk of embolization to the brain and coronaries. In the neonate however, aortic catheterization via the umbilical artery represents a major route of arterial access. Two umbilical arteries are located in the umbilicus, at locations 4 o'clock and 8 o'clock. The larger and patulous single umbilical vein typically is located at the 12 o'clock position. The umbilical arteries are relatively thick walled vessels which easily go into spasm in response to mechanical trauma. Once the lumen of the umbilical artery is identified, a 3.5 French or 5.0 French end-hole catheter can be inserted and threaded into the central circulation. The goal of umbilical artery catheterization is to reach the central aorta and to place the tip of the catheter either in the descending thoracic aorta or in the abdominal aorta below the origins of the renal and mesenteric arteries. While the aorta is the simplest and most convenient systemic artery to cannulate in the newborn, its prolonged use has major complications associated with it. The most worrisome are necrotizing enterocolitis; thrombosis, blanching, and cyanosis of the lower extremities; and paraplegia.[5,10,71,83,134] The catheter tip should be placed such that it does not traumatize the takeoff of the hepatic, splenic, superior or inferior mesenteric, or renal arteries. Since the aortic catheter in newborns is frequently used for infusion of hypertonic solutions and vasoactive drugs, one should attempt to minimize the likelihood that these potentially damaging agents will find their way directly into major splanchnic viscera. The high position appears to be associated with a lower *number* of *observed* complications than the low position, but the *severity* of complications tends to be greater with high catheters than low catheters.[83] Complications that occur with the high position appear to be related to the infusion of hypertonic or vasoactive drugs into major abdominal vessels with possible occlusion or compromise to the mesenteric vessels and resulting damage to the gut. With the low position, complications tend to be embolic phenomena resulting in either partial or total ischemia of a segmental patch of skin or muscle tissue. The complication rate is relatively low with both approaches, and the difficulty of obtaining arterial vascular access in the newborn makes the umbilical artery a popular vessel in this select population.

Femoral artery

More distal in the arterial tree, one comes to the femoral arteries. In years past, the femoral artery was a favorite site for arterial catheterization because it was easily accessible and easily catheterized.[42] However, experience with pediatric femoral artery catheterization has revealed that this approach carries with it a significant risk of vascular damage to the involved leg.[9,18,88] We prefer to avoid the femoral artery for prolonged catheterization when alternative sites are available. However, during resuscitation or extreme hypotension when no other major vessels are palpable, the femoral artery may represent the only viable choice for gaining access to the arterial system. In the event that the clinician chooses to use the femoral artery for invasive monitoring, the usual mode of access is via the percutaneous Seldinger technique. The structures in the femoral triangle include the femoral nerve, which is most lateral, the femoral artery, the femoral vein, an empty space, and finally the lymphatics, the most medial structure in the femoral triangle. Because the femoral triangle is in the midst of a major body crease, it is often difficult to secure the catheter in such a way that flexure of the hips does not cause kinking and dysfunction of the catheter.

Temporal artery

The temporal artery is an easily palpated vessel, fairly distal in the circulation, located in the superficial tissues of the scalp anterior and superior to the pinna of the ear. It is easily identified in the newborn. Although this vessel seems ideally located for cannulation, there is a major complication associated with it that has virtually eliminated its use in most neonatal centers. There is a major risk of embolization into the internal cerebral circulation from retrograde flushing of small thrombotic material or air from the tip of the catheter. It can travel down into the external carotid artery and into the common carotid circuit from whence the embolus may travel into the cerebral circuit. There have been several case reports of devastating cerebral infarcts attendant to the use of superficial temporal arteries for systemic blood pressure monitoring.[102,126] For this reason most neonatal centers have abandoned the use of this technique.

Dorsalis pedis and posterior tibial arteries

Moving more distal in the circulation one comes to the dorsalis pedis and posterior tibial arteries, the two major arteries supplying the foot. As in the hand, the tissues in the foot are supplied by a superficial and deep arch which in turn is supplied by contributions from the relatively superficial dorsalis pedis artery and the more deeply lying posterior tibial artery. Because of this anastomotic channel, the performance of a modified Allen's test in a manner similar to that employed by the radial and ulnar arteries in the wrist are to be greatly encouraged. A modified Allen's test may be performed in the foot, either by manually squeezing the tissues of the foot while compressing the vessels and watching for a capillary flush upon release of one of the vessels or alternatively by using a plethysmograph on either the great toe or the fifth toe while releasing the opposite vessel. Although there are no published standards for a normal Allen's test in the foot, common sense suggests that a capillary flush appearing within 7 seconds is probably acceptable evidence for adequate collateral circulation in the foot. The dorsalis pedis artery runs fairly superficial in the dorsal aspect of the foot between the second and third metatarsal. It is relatively straight at this point in its course and is easily transfixed with a catheter using a percutaneous Seldinger or catheter-over-the-needle approach. The relatively flat surface of the dorsal aspect of the foot makes securing a catheter in this position simple.[68,144] The posterior tibial artery is more difficult to cannulate.[128,129] This artery winds its way around and goes deep to the medial malleolus. It is in close proximity to the posterior tibial nerve. The difficult location of this vessel and its proximity to a major nerve makes cannulation of this vessel considerably more risky and therefore less commonly used in the pediatric population than other vessels.

Access to the Central Venous Circulation

Access to the central venous circulation provides many challenges to the pediatric critical care physician. Access to the central circulation allows measurement of filling pressures and facilitates adjustment of cardiac performance in the child whose circulation is failing. Many drugs are either hypertonic, hypotonic, sclerotic, or damaging to peripheral tissues and should be infused only into a deep vein with a relatively high flow.

Internal jugular vein

One of the classic sites for gaining access to the central venous circulation is the internal jugular vein. There have been a number of approaches to this vein described in the literature,[30,109] In all approaches, the operator attempts to identify the jugular vein and fix its position by manipulation of the shoulders, head and neck. Typically, the operator places a small shoulder roll under the patient's shoulders in an attempt to extend the neck on the body. If the operator is attempting to cannulate the right internal jugular vein, he turns the patient's head to the left thus stretching the right internal jugular vein and fixing it in position. With the head rotated to the left, the operator can identify the landmarks in the following manner: first palpating the sternal notch and then the tip of the mastoid process, the operator draws a line between these two structures and divides that line in half. This central point marks the location of the carotid artery. Approximately 1 cm lateral and caudad to this point is the usual entry site for the middle jugular vein approach. The user first inserts his needle into the skin, directing the needle caudad and toward the ipsilateral nipple. The needle is advanced while gentle aspiration on the syringe is maintained. Upon entry into the vein, the operator will be rewarded by a flash of blood. At this point, a through-the-needle or catheter-over-the-needle approach may be used. The various approaches to the internal jugular vein have advantages and disadvantages which balance the relative ease and success rate against the complication rate and risk of hitting other structures such as carotid artery, subclavian artery or brachial plexus. In general, preference for one approach over another tends to be dictated by local customs and prejudice modulated by experience. The reader is referred to reviews by Rosen[109] and Sanford[119] on this subject for further information and a discussion of complications.

External jugular vein

The external jugular vein provides an alternative to the internal jugular vein. The external jugular vein courses superficially in the anterior cervical triangle from a generally anterior to a generally posterior position. In situations of hypovolemia, it is often difficult or impossible to identify this vessel. However with patients who have adequate central blood volume, this vessel is generally easy to identify. It lies superficially and is easily entered percutaneously. Once the vessel is identified, the typical approach to the external jugular vein is with a "J" wire. Using this technique, a soft braided wire with a preformed "J" at one end is inserted through the introducer needle and threaded centrally past the clavicle into the central circulation. The introducer needle is removed and a monitoring catheter is threaded over the guide wire into the central circulation. The major problem with this technique is unpredictable results.The success rate of this technique varies between 25 and 70 percent.[16,89] The major problem involves threading the "J" wire past the clavical into the thorax. Inexperienced operators will often waste precious time persisting with this technique instead of going to the more traditional and secure internal jugular vein approach. The theoretical advantage of the external jugular vein is that it does not offer the same risk of carotid puncture or subclavian puncture as does the internal jugular vein. However, since the external jugular vein is a relatively low flow system when compared to the internal jugular vein, the risk of thrombosis may be higher. The unreliable results that one obtains with this system make it less than an ideal site of entry. If the operator chooses to use the external jugular vein and wishes to confirm the location of the catheter for monitoring purposes, a chest X-ray is necessary, since in a large number of cases, the catheter winds its way out of the thorax into the vessels of the arm rather than being centrally located.

Subclavian vein

The subclavian vein offers one of the most secure and simple methods of providing access to the central circulation currently available. Favored by the surgeon, it represents an ideal site for long term cannulation of the central circulation due to the relative ease of securing the catheter by fixation to the skin on the large and broad surface of the chest.[53,65,74,98,111] In this approach, the subclavian vein is approached with an introducer needle by "walking" the tip of the needle under the clavicle until one identifies the vein by aspirating blood. The user then inserts a guide wire followed by a monitoring catheter. The major complications of the subclavian vein approach are subclavian artery puncture or plural membrane laceration and pneumothorax.[65] The operator should always obtain a chest radiograph following insertion of a subclavian catheter.

Basilic and cephalic veins

Moving distal in the venous circulation, one comes to the basilic and cephalic veins in the antecubital fossa of the arm.[110,137] These vessels are often difficult to cannulate in small children, but in larger children are accessible using either the catheter-over-needle or Seldinger technique. The vessels are identified as they course superficially in the antecubital fossa and entered with a needle or catheter. A long catheter is then threaded retrograde toward the heart in an attempt to enter the central circulation. The major problem aside from technical difficulty of insertion and threading with these approaches is the fact that a large length of potentially thrombogenic catheter material is in a low flow vessel. This situation predisposes to thrombosis and thrombophlebitis of the brachial and cephalic veins.

Femoral vein

The last major site of access to the central circulation is the femoral vein.[112] This is frequently the site of choice for entry during a resuscitation and following major trauma to the upper extremities, head, or neck area. The femoral vein is medial to the femoral arterial pulse in the femoral triangle. Having gained access to the femoral vein, the operator can thread a catheter into the central circulation traversing the inferior vena cava. A major acute problem associated with femoral venous catheterization is perforation of vessel walls and retroperitoneal bleeding that is very difficult to diagnose and recognize.

Validating the location of the catheter

No matter how the operator enters the venous circulation, he must validate the location of the catheter before using the catheter as a monitor of central venous pressures. There are four major methods of validating the location of the catheter in the right atrium: (1) pressure wave form analysis and display, (2) electrocardiographic validation, (3) radiographic imaging techniques, and (4) Doppler contrast echocardiography.

Pressure wave form analysis and display With this technique, the operator makes use of the fact that venous pressure wave forms are different in the periphery compared to the central intrathoracic circulation. Figure 3.1 demonstrates a typical progression of wave form morphology as the catheter traverses the peripheral venous circulation across the diaphragm into the thoracic circulation, then through

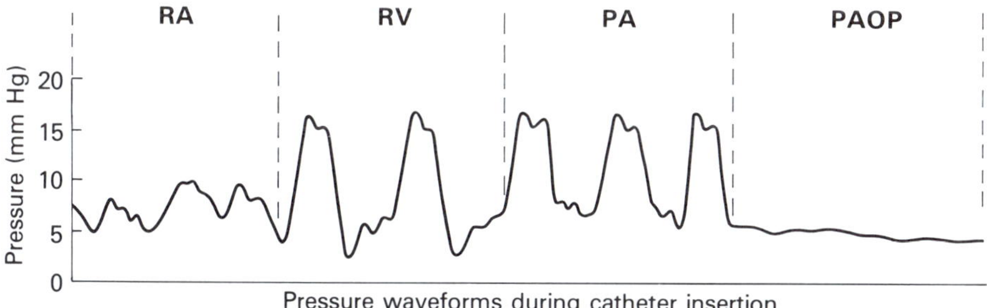

Fig. 3.1. Change in pressure waveform morphology as pulmonary artery catheter is inserted from peripheral vein through the chambers of the heart into the pulmonary artery.

Note the sudden rise in diastolic pressure as the catheter advances from right ventricle to pulmonary artery. As the catheter occludes the pulmonary artery, one sees the characteristic phase-delayed, amplitude-dampened estimate of LAP in the trace of the pulmonary artery occluded pressure. (See text for abbreviation definitions.)

the tricuspid valve into the right ventricle, and finally out the pulmonary artery outflow track and into the pulmonary artery itself. The central venous pressure wave form becomes more negative during inspiration, as opposed to an abdominal venous pressure tracing in which the pressure tends to become more positive during inspiration. In certain cases, one may be able to identify the classic "a" and "v" waves of the right atrium. The right ventricle pressure wave form is that of a relatively large box-like square wave with a typical end diastolic rise that makes identification of the right ventricle simple. As the catheter traverses the right ventricle and the pulmonary valve, the wave form changes from a relatively square ventricular tracing with an end diastolic pressure rise that is usually quite low, to the more typical arterial tracing of the pulmonary artery. The pulmonary artery systolic pressure tends to be the same as the right ventricular systolic pressure unless there is pulmonary outflow obstruction. The diastolic pressure suddenly rises from a relatively low end diastolic pressure of the right ventricle to the higher diastolic pressure of the pulmonary artery. In Raphaely's series of 68 consecutive pulmonary artery catheterizations in 49 children,[104,105] he was able to identify the progress of the tip of the pulmonary artery catheter as it traversed the central circulation by pressure display alone in approximately 33 percent of the cases recorded.

Electrocardiography One method that is available to the clinician at the bedside but not commonly employed is electrocardiography. The operator fills the catheter with a conductive solution, typically saline, and attaches it via a metal hub to the chest lead of an electrocardiogram. While monitoring the chest lead of the ECG, the operator advances the catheter. As the catheter traverses the right atrium, the operator notes a large and biphasic "P" wave. The point at which the P wave is maximal in amplitude and nearly equal in positive and negative direction is generally assumed to be the midpoint of the right atrium.[78,108] This can be confirmed later by chest radiograph.

Radiography By far radiography is the most common means of validation of catheter location. In the simplest case, the location of the central venous pressure (CVP) catheter may be verified by simple chest x-ray noting the position at the tip of the catheter. When inserting a pulmonary artery catheter, the operator may choose to use continuous fluoroscopy with image intensification to reduce the exposure to the patient and operating personnel. In this technique, the patient needs to be placed on a radiolucent table. Under direct fluoroscopic visualization, the operator threads the catheter through the central circulation into the right ventricle and finally out the pulmonary artery outflow tract into the pulmonary artery. This makes visualization very simple and provides confirmation of catheter position but has the major disadvantage that fluoroscopy equipment, personnel and exposure is required in order to place the catheter. Because the CVP port in a pulmonary catheter may be too far or too close to the distal pulmonary artery port and thus not lie in the right atrium, the pediatric operator is advised to check the location of the central venous pressure port by injecting contrast material through the CVP port while the fluoroscopy is running or by taking an x-ray. In our experience, nearly 25 percent of standard sized catheter CVP ports fail to locate in the right atrium using the femoral approach.

Echocardiography In echocardiography, the echo transducer is placed over the precordium and directed toward the cardiac chambers. The catheter will create echo shadows as it interrupts the Doppler beam. In this manner, the location of the tip of the catheter can be verified.

Percutaneous and Surgical Cutdown Approaches

The clinician may use a variety of techniques for gaining access to the arterial and venous circulation. Chief among these are the Seldinger technique, the catheter-over-the-needle-technique and the sheath technique, and the catheter-through-the-needle technique.

Seldinger technique

In the Seldinger technique, first described in 1953, a narrow bore needle is inserted through the skin and used to identify the lumen of the target vessel.[122] Once blood has flashed back through the lumen of the finder needle, the operator inserts a fine gauge braided wire through the lumen of the needle into the vein or artery. The needle is held in place while the guide wire is threaded into the vessel. Once the wire is securely in the vessel, the introducer needle is removed over the wire keeping the wire in place within the vessel. The monitoring catheter is then threaded over the guide wire through the skin and into the target vessel, using the guide wire as a tracking system to gain secure entrance into the vessel. Once the catheter itself is inserted and threaded into the target vessel, the guide wire is pulled back through the monitoring catheter and discarded. The technique is easy to master and allows access to very small vessels since only one needle insertion is required to identify the vessel.

Catheter-over-the-needle technique

In the catheter-over-the-needle technique the needle and catheter are inserted as a unit through the skin with the needle protruding distal to the tip of the catheter by a small margin. As the needle enters the target vessel, the flashback of blood identifies the event of entry. At this point, the needle and catheter unit are inserted together, and the catheter is slid over the needle into the lumen of the target vessel.

The introducer needle is then withdrawn from the catheter leaving the catheter in place in the target vessel. This technique is commonly used for radial artery and dorsalis pedis artery catheterization. The major advantage of this technique is that the equipment is very simple. The major disadvantage is that as the catheter is inserted into the target vessel over the introducer needle, the catheter may displace the target vessel from the introducer finder needle and distort the landmarks.

A variant of the catheter-over-the-needle approach is the sheath technique. In this method, a sheath is inserted over a needle (or in the modified Seldinger approach over a guide wire) and the final monitoring catheter is inserted through the indwelling sheath. The sheath catheter may be left in place serving as an alternate source of infusion if there is a side hole assembly.

Catheter-through-the-needle technique

An older technique used in the approach to the antecubital fossa is the catheter-through-the-needle technique. A relatively large bore needle is inserted into a superficial venous vessel. With the needle in place, a catheter is inserted through the bore of the needle and threaded into the target vessel to the central circulation. After the catheter is inserted into the target vessel, the finder needle is withdrawn over the indwelling catheter.

Surgical cutdown

When percutaneous methods fail or the operator is unable to use them because he cannot identify the vessel by palpation or location, a surgical cutdown may be required. After prepping and draping the field in a sterile manner, a small incision is made in the skin and the vessel is identified. Ligatures or stay sutures may be threaded around the target vessel to assist the operator in holding the vessel in place. An arteriotomy or venotomy is then made through which a monitoring catheter is inserted. The operator may choose to ligate the vessel proximal and distal to the entry site in an attempt to control bleeding or may elect not to ligate the vessel and thus allow recannulization of the vessel after removal of the monitoring catheter. In either case, the monitoring catheter is brought out through the surgical wound or through an ancillary stab wound and the primary wound is closed. The surgical cutdown has the dramatic advantage of allowing access to the circulation in the most profound of low flow states, but can only be conducted when adequate surgical technical experience and skill are available.

Complications

There are many complications attendant to venous and arterial catheterization, including thrombosis of the target vessel, platelet consumption and thrombocytopenia, bacterial infection, accidental disconnection, traumatic rupture, and knotting of the catheter.

Thrombosis of the target vessel

This is one of the more common complications. Direct trauma to the intima of the target vessel may trigger the clotting cascade and result in the formation of a thrombus surrounding the monitoring catheter, which may progress to partial or total occlusion of the vessel.[13,14,33] In most cases with adequate collateral circulation, there is little physiologic consequence to this kind of thrombotic occlusion.[13,44] However, when the vessel is centrally located or is an end artery, then thrombosis may prove disastrous.[18] An arterial thrombectomy may be required in order to restore circulation to the affected limb. Bedford[12,13] has studied the incidence and occurrence of arterial thrombosis as it relates to site of insertion and catheter construction for radial artery catheters. He found that straight Teflon nontapered catheters of low external diameter had the lowest incidence of thrombotic occlusion. Furthermore, he found that the incidence of occlusion appears to rise as the duration of catheterization increases. Arterial cannulation of less than 3 days duration was not associated with significant arterial thrombosis, whereas catheterization of greater than 3 days duration was associated with significant thrombosis.

Platelet consumption and thrombocytopenia

An infrequently recognized but commonly occurring complication associated with indwelling venous catheters is platelet consumption and resulting thrombocytopenia.[106] In this situation, polyvinyl chloride catheters, such as pulmonary artery Swan-Ganz catheters that are left in place for several days, may accelerate platelet consumption by two- or threefold. Richman demonstrated a markedly decreased survival time of radiolabeled platelets in rabbits in whom a 7 French pulmonary artery catheter was inserted. In these animals, the decreased rate of platelet survival was associated with uptake of isotope in the spleen and liver suggesting that the reticuloendothelial system is involved with the removal of the damaged platelets. In patients in whom pulmonary artery catheters were used for prolonged periods of time, thrombocytopenia was directly proportional to the duration of catheterization.[115,132] When pulmonary catheters were removed, the platelet counts rose dramatically on the second day after removal and remained stable thereafter. No other etiology was noted to explain the thrombocytopenia.

Bacterial infection

The incidence of bacterial colonization and overt infection increases with the duration of catheterization.[43] Raphaely[104,105] demonstrated that the overall incidence of catheter related sepsis in children was 17 percent in association with pulmonary artery Swan-Ganz catheters in place for a wide variety of indications.

Accidental disconnection

Accidental disconnection may result in severe and life threatening hemorrhage. Though the hemorrhage associated with arterial cannula disconnections is often dramatic and highly visible, the disconnection associated with the lower pressure venous circuit may be equally devastating and may go unnoticed for a sufficiently long period of time that the child may suffer a significant loss of blood. Continuous and alarmed pressure monitoring of all arterial and central venous pressure catheters is necessary to delete this preventable event.

Traumatic rupture

Traumatic rupture of a vessel either by the guide wire or the catheter itself may occur as it traverses peripheral vessels toward the central circulation. In the umbilical artery of the newborn, perforation of the posterior wall of the aorta may occur if the umbilical artery catheter is forced against resistance. This may go initially unrecognized but may result in catastrophic retroperitoneal hemorrhage, shock, and death. A catheter inserted into the central venous circulation may perforate the thin walled right atrium and even on occasion the thicker walled right ventricle causing either bleeding into the mediastinum or pericardium depending on the location of the perforation.

Knotting of the catheter

A pulmonary artery or central venous pressure catheter may be threaded into the central circulation with such zeal and disregard for landmarks that the catheter may wind itself into a knot within the chambers of the heart and present a serious problem of extraction.[45,75] Sophisticated catheter techniques exist that enable these knotted catheters to be removed without the need for surgical exploration of the thorax and cardiac cavities.[40] Occasionally however, surgical removal is necessary.

Catheter Materials

There are a variety of catheter materials that have profound implications for the performance of the catheter within the central circulation. The most commonly used material is polyvinyl chloride (PVC). This is a very workable and easily manufactured material that can be extruded in multilumen configurations. It is the typical catheter material of pulmonary artery catheters. The major problem with PVC is that it is highly thrombogenic in comparison with other materials and thus accelerates platelet consumption and thrombus formation on the catheter surface.[99,115] Adult experience has suggested that within a mean of 104 minutes after insertion of polyvinyl chloride catheters into the central circulation, serious clot formation had occurred on the surface of the catheter.[63] Because of this finding, many pediatric centers have ceased to use polyvinyl chloride catheters in patients with right to left shunts at the cardiac level fearing embolization to the systemic circulation.

Newer catheter materials such as polyurethane, Teflon, and silicone have markedly improved thrombogenic properties when compared to polyvinyl chloride but have their own problems. Polyurethane is easily workable but does not lend itself to multilumen extrusion. Teflon is very stiff and extremely difficult to bond to other plastic materials requiring complex fittings to attach to intravenous hubs. Because of its stiffness, Teflon represents a poor choice for prolonged central venous catheterization due to the concern over cardiac chamber perforation. Silicone material is extremely nonthrombogenic and very flexible causing little trauma to vessels. The major problem with silicone is that it is so flexible that it is very difficult to guide, having no intrinsic stiffness of its own. It may require a stylet for proper placement. The stiffness of the stylet introduces problems of perforation once again. Newer techniques of heparin bonding to catheter materials may offer a significant reduction in thrombogenicity.[64]

Protocols for Care of Catheters

Each institution should establish protocols for the care of indwelling vascular catheters. These protocols must address certain issues common to all catheterizations, such as dressing changes, heparin flushing, accidental disconnection, and bacterial colonization. In many institutions, dressings are changed on a daily basis in an attempt to keep down bacterial colonization at the entry site. Continuous heparin infusions with flow-limiting devices are used in most pediatric centers in an attempt to keep the catheters patent for long periods of time. Luer-locked connectors make accidental disconnection of interlocking devices less likely. It is our practice to perform daily or every other day line cultures with blood samples drawn through the catheter in critically ill children. Although there is no guarantee that the organisms cultured from the line itself will be the same organism causing bacterial sepsis, the clinician is well advised to cover those organisms that have grown from the line cultures until peripheral blood culture results are available.

MEASUREMENT OF PRIMARY CIRCULATION VARIABLES

Systemic Arterial Blood Pressure

Of all the primary variables that a clinician may wish to monitor invasively, systemic arterial blood pressure represents the key variable in a critically ill child. If the patient has an inadequate blood pressure to supply substrate across the resistant vessels of the body, the tissue will die. Extreme life threatening alterations of physiology typically manifest themselves with sudden and often catastrophic changes in blood pressure. This dependence on blood pressure monitoring might come as a parodox to the physiologically minded physician who tends to focus on flow to the periphery rather than the absolute driving pressure. However, if the pressure is inadequate, there will be no flow. Variations in the relationship between flow and pressure constitute a major problem for the physician. The vascular tree serves as the compliance and resistance vessels for the distribution of the stroke volume. As the pulsatile flow empties into the distensible aorta, aortic pressure rises. This increase in central vascular pressure relative to peripheral vascular pressure will result in a bulk movement of blood down the vascular tree. Along with this flow, there will be a pressure wave that is propagated along the vascular tree. Components of the wave form tend to propagate at different velocities, resulting in distortion of the pressure wave form as it propagates.[56,72,95] There may be reflected or standing waves that are set up as previous pressure waves reflect back from the periphery into the major circulation. The net result of these technical phenomena is that the pressure wave form is distorted as it propagates and that the systolic and diastolic pressures are both higher and lower respectively, the further distal they are measured in the vascular tree.[68] Unlike systole and diastole which are affected by this process of amplification, the mean blood pressure is typically unaffected.

The technology available for blood pressure monitoring consists of vascular catheters, pressure tubing and connectors, transducers, amplifiers, and display devices. The technical system begins with a vascular catheter which allows continuous access to the circulation. Catheters used in children should be relatively nonthrombogenic and of a sufficiently narrow gauge so that they will fit into the small pediatric vessel without occluding the lumen of that vessel. A variety of catheter and needle device kits are available from various manufacturers. The precise selection of which device to use represents a combination of local custom and design characteristics.

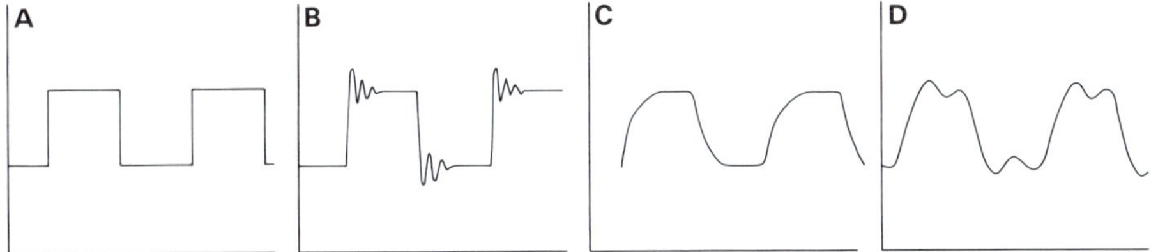

Fig. 3.2. Resonance and damping. (A) A square wave input signal is shown. (B) Resonance occurs as there is overshoot and undershoot at the characteristic resonant frequency of the system. (C) Excessive damping is shown as energy is dissipated in the system due to viscous loss. (D) The usual mixture of both resonance and damping seen in most real systems is shown.

The catheter must be connected in some manner to the monitor and measurement device. This connection introduces numerous artifactual problems associated with damping and resonance phenomena.[123] All physical systems subjected to oscillation exhibit the characteristics of resonance and damping. Much as a bell when struck with a clapper will resonate at a characteristic natural frequency, so too, will a column of fluid within a pressure catheter tend to oscillate or resonate at a characteristic natural frequency.[113] This tendency of physical systems to vibrate at a natural frequency is known as *resonance*. In addition to having a natural frequency of oscillation, the concept of resonance also carries with it the tendency of a physical system to amplify oscillations supplied to it that are close to the natural frequency. Figure 3.2 shows a tracing taken from a pressure tubing to which has been applied a single square wave pressure input. In panel A, the pressure is suddenly raised, held at the new level for a period of time, and then suddenly dropped back to the resting baseline. Figure 3.2A shows the actual input signal as applied to the pressure tubing. Figure 3.2B demonstrates the phenomena of resonance. The upstroke of the pressure wave causes an overshoot. The system tends to oscillate around the new set point at a frequency determined by its resonant frequency. These oscillations tend to dampen until a new steady state is reached. In a similar fashion, when the input signal suddenly returns to baseline, the recorded pressure will undershoot and resonate until the signal dampens at the new baseline value. This phenomenon, when translated to the periodic oscillation caused by the pressure generated by each heart beat, will cause an artifactual increase in the systolic pressure measured by the system and at the same time cause an artifactual decrease in the diastolic pressure. The opposite of resonance is *damping*. As fluid oscillates back and forth in the pressure tubing, viscous forces between the fluid column and the wall of the catheter tend to dissipate the kinetic energy of the moving column of fluid. As the column of fluid vibrates back and forth, more energy is dissipated. The amplitude of the oscillations gradually die out. If these viscous forces are large or if there are compressible media in the fluid such as air bubbles, much of the kinetic energy of the oscillation may be absorbed or dissipated by this phenomenon and the wave form may be distorted, as is seen in Figure 3.2C. In this case the system is said to be dampened. The systolic pressure will be lower than that originally applied to the system and the diastolic pressure will be higher. Usually, the phenomena of resonance and damping occur together (Fig. 3.2D). Although the systolic and diastolic pressures are adversely affected, the mean blood pressure measurement is rarely affected. Therefore, in situations in which excessive resonance or damping are present, the clinician should monitor mean blood pressure—a measurement relatively insensitive to these artifacts.

The physical characteristics of the plumbing system that tend to influence its resonant frequency behavior and damping are the overall length of the catheter, the thickness, the stiffness and rigidity of the tubing wall and the lumenal diameter of the pressure tubing.[113,116] Systems that are short in overall length (less than 4 feet), are of narrow bore, and have a very stiff wall material exhibit little or no significant ringing or damping artifact at heart rates typically encountered in children. Conversely, long, wide bore, and flexible tubing tends to introduce significant artifacts of ringing or damping which may seriously distort the pressure wave form and adversely affect the accuracy of the systolic and diastolic pressure reading. An alternative to using pressure tubing is mounting the pressure transducer directly on the catheter itself. This improves the fidelity of the recording system, but requires small and rugged transducers.

An integral component of the monitoring system is the pressure transducer. A transducer is a device which converts one form of energy to another. In the case of blood pressure monitoring, a transducer converts potential energy (pressure) into electrical energy, which is then input to an amplifier and analyzed for output readings. Transducers can be divided into two general categories: the wheatstone bridge and the solid state piezo-electric crystal. In the wheatstone bridge, four elements are arranged in a diamond-shaped pattern bridged in the middle by a current or voltage measuring device.[27] One of the four elements behaves in a variable fashion depending on the pressure or deformation applied to it by some sliding membrane. In the classic configuration, the active elements are resistors. The fourth element is usually a strain gauge whose resistance varies in a predictable fashion with the amount of stretch applied to it. The four elements are mounted in such a way that as the diaphragm of the pressure transducer is made to move by the applied pressure transmitted by the pressure tubing, the strain gauge is either stretched or compressed. This change in length causes the strain gauge to change its resistance, which results in an unbalancing of the wheatstone bridge. This unbalancing generates a voltage drop and current flow. It is this voltage drop or current flow that is actually measured and displayed by blood pressure monitors.

In the second major form of pressure monitoring technology, a piezo-electric crystal is exposed to a pressure which causes it to deform. This deformation alters the crystal structure of the piezo-electric device in such a manner that it generates a very small voltage. This voltage is then amplified by the monitor and displayed. The major advantage of piezo-electric crystals is that they are less prone to drift and are more rugged in construction than the strain gauge device. In addition, they can be made quite small for use in direct catheter-mounted applications.

A common problem in the application of invasive monitoring in the critically ill child is the confusion caused by the observation that the invasively monitored blood pressure is not always identical to the noninvasively cuff-measured blood pressure.[59] There is a tendency to assume that one of the two methods is in error. Of course, one can never be certain which method is the offending culprit. More often than not, neither method is in error, but rather, the two pressures are indeed not equal. There are several reasons for the observed differences between cuff-measured and invasive catheter-measured systemic arterial pressures. Some are

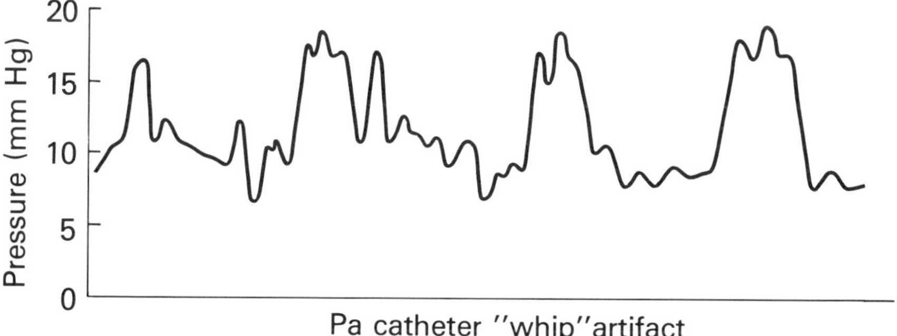

Fig. 3.3. Catheter whip occurs when a free floating catheter is flung about a vessel or cardiac chamber. Inertial forces create artifactual pressure "spikes" in the waveform.

artifactual and some are real. Artifacts include differences caused by resonance and damping phenomena, catheter whip effect, and hydrostatic differences between the site of measurement and the pressure transducer.

Resonance and damping problems have already been discussed. They are not always easily recognized or corrected, although careful attention to plumbing and connections can greatly minimize their effect.

Catheter whip phenomenon refers to the artifact caused by the forceful "flinging" of the tip of an intravascular catheter within a vascular chamber. As the catheter is whipped about, the inertia of the blood or fluid column within the catheter lumen causes an artifactual pressure to be transmitted through the tubing to the transducer.[60] Catheter whip is most commonly seen in pulmonary artery catheters lying within the ventricular cavity, but it can also be seen with small arterial catheters lying within a large vessel such as the aorta or femoral artery. Catheter whip may be easily recognized from the characteristic pressure tracing on the oscilloscope such as shown in Figure 3.3. It tends to occur in conditions of a hyperdynamic circulation. Very little can be done to correct catheter whip except repositioning the catheter.

Hydrostatic pressure differences are responsible for the majority of *artifactual* differences between invasive and noninvasive blood pressure measurements. The cuff measures ambient systolic pressure in the underlying artery *at the site of the cuff*. Transducers measure pressure in the vessel *with reference to an arbitrarily defined* "zero" point. If the "zero" point for the transducer is at the level of the site of the catheter, say the radial artery, and the patient is sitting up with the arm dependent, than there will be an artifact of hydrostatic pressure introduced between the cuff and the transducer equal to the vertical distance (converted to appropriate units) between the cuff site and the transducer "zero" point. The hydrostatic artifact can be eliminated simply by selecting a "zero" reference site that is level with the site of the cuff-measured pressure.

Even when artifactual errors have been accounted for, there are still differences observed between cuff- and direct-pressure measurements. These differences are real and often meaningful in a clinical sense. The cuff pressure measures the pressure exerted on the lateral walls of the vessel tending to open the vessel. It is an "ambient" or static pressure, devoid of aspects relating to blood flow or velocity.

Direct measurements of intravascular pressure are influenced by a kinetic component of blood flow in addition to the ambient or static pressure. The usual vascular catheter employed in clinical use is an end-hole catheter. As such, it presents a column of nonmoving fluid within the catheter lumen facing the oncoming and moving blood in the vessel. At the interface between the moving blood in the vessel and the nonmoving fluid in the catheter, the blood must be stopped. Since the blood has mass (m), and a velocity (v), it possesses kinetic energy equal to $1/2\ mv^2$ that must be converted to potential energy as the blood column is stopped at the catheter-blood interface. One form of potential energy is pressure. In fact, the total pressure measured by an end-hole catheter placed within a moving column of blood is the sum of the static and dynamic pressure components. In contrast, the cuff technique only measures the static pressure. Therefore, under normal conditions, the direct pressure measured with an end-hole catheter within the vessel will always be higher than the simultaneously measured cuff pressure. The more hyperdynamic the circulation, the higher will be the blood velocity in the vessel, and the larger will be the dynamic component of the invasively measured pressure. Under normal conditions, this difference—which is real and not artifactual—accounts for a difference between cuff and direct pressure of approximately 8 to 16 mmHg.[34,48] Under conditions of a hyperdynamic circulation, such as may occur during sympathetic stimulation or peripheral vasodilation, the observed difference between cuff and direct pressures may exceed 25 to 30 mmHg. The difference is real, and it is meaningful in terms of assessing the state of the circulation.

Filling Pressures

Second to systemic arterial blood pressure, the most common pressure that is invasively monitored in critically ill children is the central circulation filling pressure. The usual sites of filling pressure measurement are the central venous pressure (CVP), the right atrial pressure (RAP) and the left atrial pressure (LAP). The rationale for measuring filling pressures is to estimate preload for the heart.

Preload is the resting fiber length immediately prior to ventricular contraction. In the ideal situation, one would like to measure resting fiber length directly or at least the ventricular chamber volume at end-diastole. At present, however, there is no practical way to obtain either of these measurements. If it is assumed that the ventricular compliance is known and is constant, then one can simply measure absolute intraventricular end-diastolic pressure and from this measurement calculate ventricular volume. From this, one can calculate resting fiber length. Of course, the actual filling pressures that distend the ventricle are the transmural pressures—the pressure within the cavity minus the pleural pressure.

There is a long history of estimating preload from filling pressures using the assumption of a known and constant ventricular compliance. The original Starling relationship demonstrates the phenomenon in which useful cardiac work increases as preload, or resting fiber length, increases.[130] This concept was extended by Sarnoff to the relationship between filling pressure (RAP or CVP) and stroke volume or cardiac output (Fig. 3.4).[120]

One problem faced by the clinician wishing to manipulate the circulation is which filling pressure to measure, the right sided CVP, or RAP, or the left sided LAP.

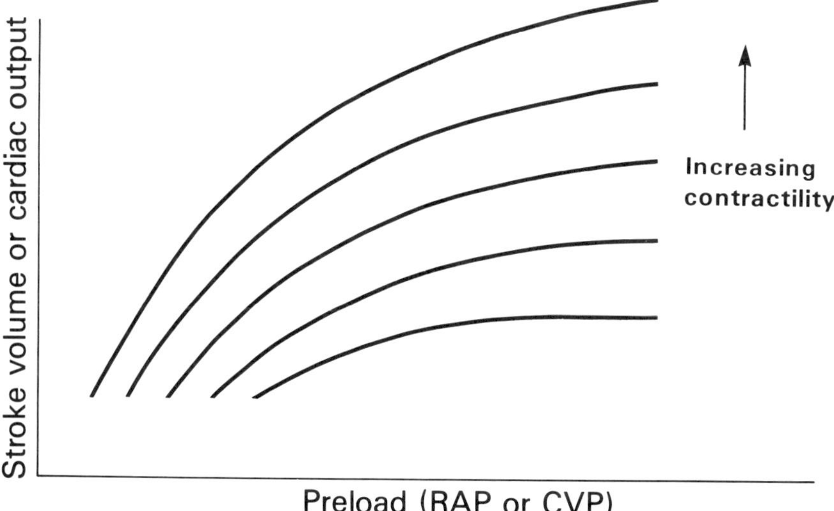

Fig. 3.4. The ventricular function relationship showing a rise in stroke volume or cardiac output as the estimate of preload—right atrial pressure (RAP) or central venous pressure (CVP) in this case—is increased. There is a family of ventricular function curves, each one depicting a different state of myocardial contractility.

One way to resolve this question is to determine which ventricle is predominately responsible for the circulatory dysfunction. Ideally, both left and right filling pressures should give the same estimates of preload. Such is not always the case. In some clinical situations, left and right ventricle functions are disparate. The most obvious example of this situation is in isolated left coronary artery occlusive disease with isolated left ventricular dysfunction due to coronary ischemia.[49] Of course, this is very unusual in the pediatric population unless one is dealing with anomalous coronary arteries or Kawasaki's disease. More common conditions in children in which left and right sided filling pressures may not be equal are sepsis, burns, and major trauma. Even here, the right and left pressures are usually close in value and can generally be assessed by measurement of the CVP alone. In conditions of volume overload or hypovolemia, the two sides of the heart are almost always equally effected and one need not pursue left sided filling pressures in the usual cases.

There are several common sources of error in interpretation of right and left sided filling pressures which the clinician should keep in mind. The most significant problem is that the filling pressures do not in fact measure classic preload, that is, resting fiber length. Each filling pressure measurement is several steps removed from the corresponding measure of preload. For example, the CVP is a reflection of the mean RAP, which is a reflection of right ventricular end diastolic pressure. The latter—if ventricular compliance is known and constant—is affected by right ventricular end-diastolic volume, which bears a loose relationship (depending on geometry) to the preload itself, the resting fiber length of right ventricular muscle fibers. The user must recognize, however, that the weak link in the above chain is that the ventricular compliance is, in fact, neither known nor constant over time.[2,25] Over the span of minutes and perhaps hours, if myocardial ischemia and edema does not intervene, the ventricular compliance probably does stay relatively constant, so that acute changes in filling pressures probably do reflect acute changes in preload. From day to day or patient to patient, however, compliance of the ventricle may change dramatically as myocardial ischemia and edema waxes and wanes.[54] For this reason, trusting absolute values for filling pressures is usually fraught with disappointment, although moment-to-moment changes in filling pressure are probably appropriate to follow. Much as the CVP only indirectly assesses right sided preload, the pulmonary artery occluded pressure (PAOP) or pulmonary capillary wedge pressure (PCWP) also indirectly assesses left sided preload, with the additional approximation that PAOP or PCWP only approximates the mean LAP. Despite the above problems of uncertain and changing ventricular compliance, many clinicians are comfortable assessing cardiac function using estimates of filling pressures.

Filling pressure measurements are not without technical problems of their own. Aside from artifactual problems similar to those discussed above under systemic arterial pressure, there is the effect of positive end-expiratory pressure (PEEP). PEEP affects the raw measured values of filling pressure, whether right or left sided, by partial transmission of an elevated airway pressure to the intrathoracic vascular structures.[39] For example, in a child with severe adult respiratory distress syndrome (ARDS) being treated with 20 cm H_2O PEEP and mechanical ventilation, the peak inflating pressure may be as high as 50 to 60 cm H_2O. This may result in a mean airway pressure of approximately 30 cm H_2O. The compliance of the lung and chest may be such that one-half of this mean airway pressure, or 15 cm H_2O, is transmitted to the pleural space surrounding the atria and ventricles. If we were following the raw CVP and the measurement was 17 cm H_2O, we might be led to the conclusion that the preload was high, and that the patient might be helped by diuretic therapy. If, on the other hand, we took into account the elevated mean pleural pressure of 15 cm H_2O, then the conclusion would be quite different. In this case, the net transmural distending pressure contributing to ventricular preload is really the raw measured value of 17 cm H_2O minus the mean pleural pressure of 15 cm H_2O or only 2 cm H_2O. These data lead to the conclusion that a volume challenge is in order, rather than diuretic therapy. The net effect of positive transmitted airway pressure is to decrease the effective transmural distending pressure contributing to preload.

There are several means of estimating the mean pleural pressure opposing intravascular distending pressure.[1] One is to measure the pressure in the pleural space directly with a fluid filled catheter or a transducer tipped catheter.[37,87] This requires a surgical incision, or thoracostomy, to place the catheter, a risky procedure in conditions of severe lung disease with stiff lungs and hypoxia. In addition, the fluid filled catheter may develop an air-fluid interface in the pleural space if there is a small pneumothorax.[1] This air-fluid interface will result in surface tension forces, which rival the magnitude of the measured intrapleural pressure. Thus, the intrapleural catheter is not a commonly used method.

An alternative to direct intrapleural pressure measurement is to estimate the pleural pressure by taking advantage of the fact that the esophagus is a tubular structure lying within the mediastinum, in close physical contact with the pleural space. The assumption is that pressure in the pleural space will be transmitted to the esophagus and can thus be measured within the esophagus by means of an air-filled balloon lying within the esophagus.[1,61] Care must be taken not to overdistend the balloon so that the muscular esophagus is not stimulated to peristaltic activity. In general, this technique of estimating pleural pressure by measuring intraesophageal pressure works well. Esophageal balloons are available commercially in sizes ranging from 8 French to 14 French as parts of a triple lumen sump-type nasogastric tube. There is a large experience with their use in estimating pleural pressure in the pediatric population.[11] Care must be taken to position the balloon properly. The manufacturer recommends that the balloon be positioned at or near the midline inferior to the carina in the distal third of the thoracic esophagus, in close proximity to the heart.[92] One problem with this approach is that the cardiac mass may lie on top of the esophagus in this position and falsely elevate the measured esophageal pressure by direct compression of the measuring balloon.

In addition to the decrease in effective filling pressure, elevated pleural pressures have at least two other effects on the circulation. One effect is that an elevated intrathoracic pressure will tend to impede venous return to the heart and thereby decrease preload.[26,55,100] If PEEP is high enough, the pressure transmitted to the pleural space from the airway will act to compress the vascular structures and thereby decrease the volume of the ventricle at the end of diastole. Such a decrease in end-diastolic volume will result in a shortening of resting fiber length and thus, a diminution of preload. A second effect is that afterload on the left ventricle is decreased by a reduction of ventricular cavity size.[22] Afterload is the ventricular wall tension during contraction. The major determinants of the wall tension during contraction are the impedance to ventricular ejection, or the aortic pressure, and the ventricular cavity size. Anything that decreases the size of the ventricular cavity, such as extracardiac compression by an elevated intrathoracic pressure, will decrease effective ventricular afterload, and usually improve ventricular function. Thus, it is important to consider the pleural pressure in conditions when high mean airway pressures are being used.

The first consideration after deciding to measure filling pressure is how best to obtain access to the central circulation and which side should be the target. Right sided filling pressures are usually measured via the CVP or RAP. A catheter may be placed through large veins in the neck, the arm, or the groin and threaded into the central circulation.

Obtaining access to the left side of the heart is far more complicated. In the noncardiothoracic surgery patient, the only practical means by which left sided filling pressures may be measured is via PAOP or PCWP.[73] The theory behind the use of PAOP is quite simple. If the catheter lies within the pulmonary artery and a balloon is inflated at the tip of the catheter, then the tip will be carried along with the blood flow through the vessel as the catheter is advanced until it impinges on a vessel smaller than the diameter of the balloon, at which time it is said to be "wedged." Distal to the balloon is a column of blood within the remaining pulmonary artery; this extends into and through the associated pulmonary capillary network and pulmonary venous network and leads all the way to the left atrium. Under usual conditions, the PAOP measured in this way will be an accurate reflection of mean left atrial pressure, and hence can be used to estimate left sided filling pressures in much the same way that LAP may be used if measured directly with a left atrial catheter. Since continuous inflation of the balloon might lead to pulmonary ischemia and infarction in the lung supplied by the occluded vessel, the balloon can only be inflated intermittently when estimates of left sided filling pressure are desired. In practice, the catheter tip is usually left in a main branch of the pulmonary artery with the balloon deflated. In most situations, the pulmonary artery diastolic pressure (PADP) is very closely related to the PAOP.[73] One can thus use the PADP as a continuous assessment of left sided pressures.

There are many complications reported with the use of pulmonary artery catheters, including dysrhythmias on insertion, catheter knotting within the ventricular or atrial cavity, damage to cardiac valves, thrombus formation on the surface of the catheter, cardiac perforation and tamponade, infection, pulmonary artery rupture, pulmonary infarcts, and others.[8,94,96,127] In children, an additional problem occurs not commonly seen in adults. That is, that the time required to place the catheter in a very small child may be very long. In Raphaely's series, despite the use of image intensification fluoroscopy to facilitate catheter placement in most of the catheterizations, the average time from skin entry to validation of catheter tip location was 45 minutes, with a range of from 17 to 229 minutes.[105] This is very different from the usual times of several minutes commonly reported in adults. The reasons for this increased time are several, including the common preference for the groin as a site of entry in small children, with the more difficult twisting pathway required of a catheter from this entry site to traverse the cardiac chambers, compared to the route from the jugular vessels. Number 5 French catheters are commonly used in children due to their small size, instead of 7 French catheters. The smaller diameter multilumen catheter tends to be stiffer than its larger counterpart, making the catheterization process more difficult in the child. The child's vessels are usually small and often difficult to cannulate when compared to the large femoral or jugular veins in the adult. Finally, the cardiac output of a small child in absolute terms is much less than that of an adult. Thus, less blood flow is available as a motive force to carry the balloon and catheter through the heart on its journey into the pulmonary circuit. Because of the increased time required to place a pulmonary artery catheter in the child, there is a direct risk to the child during the procedure because the physicians and nurses become so involved with the technical aspects of placing the catheter and achieving procedural success that they tend to ignore the child under the surgical drapes. This tends to place the child at risk during the period of placement for unrecognized hemodynamic or respiratory compromise. To minimize the likelihood of this occurring, it is our practice to require two teams of nurses and physicians at the bedside during pulmonary artery catheterizations. One team attends to the technical procedure of catheter placement and verification, while the other team is solely responsible for monitoring the patient and maintaining hemodynamic and respiratory stability.

The catheter balloon is made of latex rubber. It has a limited effective lifetime within the bloodstream. Raphaely found that the average effective lifetime of the balloon was only 44 hours.[104,105] The distribution of balloon integrity is shown in Fig. 3.5. Note that some balloons ruptured on the first day, actually within several hours of placement, while others survived up to 120 hours of use. Another problem discovered by Raphaely was that even when a catheter of appropriate diameter

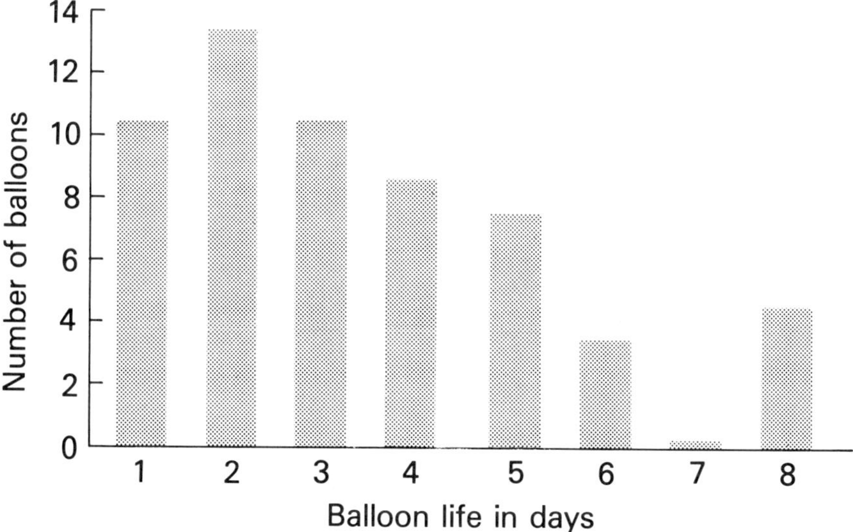

Fig. 3.5. Pulmonary artery catheter balloon life in a series of children reported by Raphaely.[105] Note that while some balloons lasted as long as 8 days, many lasted only 1 day, and in some cases, only hours.

was used according to the age of the patient, 28 percent of the catheters placed via the groin resulted in location of the proximal CVP port below the diaphragm, outside of the thoracic cavity. Thus, the CVP port was not useful for measurement of right sided filling pressure. Special catheters can be obtained for any age group with the CVP port placed at any desired location (for an additional reasonable charge). The recommendations for catheter size and CVP port location from Raphaely's study are shown in Table 3.1.

Once the catheters are placed, the pressure must be measured. Water manometers are simple, reliable, inexpensive, and require no special set up or skill to use. They deliver estimates of mean pressure only. Transducer-amplifier combinations allow the user to display the pressure waveform for diagnostic purposes and also provide a continuous digital or analog display of the measured pressure. Systolic and diastolic pressures may be displayed along with mean pressure in the case of pulmonary artery catheters. For these reasons, the routine when using pulmonary artery catheters has become continuous display of the pressure waveform and processed pressures.

Table 3.1. Recommendations for Catheter Size and CVP Port Placement using Femoral Insertion Site

Age	Size and CVP Location
Newborn–3 years	5 French, 10 cm
3–8 years	5 French, 15 cm
8–14 years	7 French, 20 cm
>14 years	7 French, 30 cm

Cardiac Output/Cardiac Index

The cardiac output (CO) is the amount of blood pumped to the peripheral tissues per unit time, usually given in units of liters/minute. There are several technologies available for the measurement of cardiac output.[103] It is often normalized to body weight or body surface area and is represented as cardiac index (CI), which is simply the cardiac output divided by body surface area, CI = CO/BSA in units of liters/minute/meter^2 (L/min/m^2). Use of the normalized cardiac index allows the evaluation of cardiac performance without regard to body size, since the normal range for cardiac index is the same in all age groups and patient sizes. The usual resting value for CI is between 3.5 and 4.5 L/min/m^2. Shock, or low flow state, is usually considered to exist when the cardiac index falls below 2.2 L/min/m^2.

Fick principle technique

Most cardiac output measurement techniques are modifications of the Fick principle, which essentially states that in conditions of steady state, the quantity of a substance entering a structure minus the quantity of the substance leaving a structure is equal to the quantity of the substance either consumed or produced within that structure, depending on whether the resultant difference is positive or negative in value. If the substance is metabolically inert, and is neither consumed or produced, then the quantity of substance entering a structure over time is equal to the quantity leaving the structure.

The classic method of estimating cardiac output, and still the standard against which new methods are tested, is the Fick method involving total body oxygen consumption ($\dot{V}O_2$), and the oxygen contents of arterial (C_aO_2) and mixed venous ($C_{\bar{v}}O_2$) blood. The relationship between the three values is:

$$\text{in} - \text{out} = \text{consumed}$$

$$CO \times C_aO_2 - CO \times C_{\bar{v}}O_2 = \dot{V}O_2$$

Solving for CO, one gets:

$$CO = \dot{V}O_2/(C_aO_2 - C_{\bar{v}}O_2)$$

or

$$CO = \dot{V}O_2/(a\text{-}\bar{v})DO_2$$

To use the Fick technique, one measures the total body oxygen consumption ($\dot{V}O_2$), and the oxygen contents of arterial and mixed venous blood. The problem with this technique is that the measurement of the total body oxygen consumption is a very difficult measurement to make accurately. One needs to collect exhaled gas from the child without contamination or loss, and to compare the oxygen content of exhaled gas with that of the inhaled gas. Accurate measures of inhaled and exhaled minute volume are also required, since inhaled and exhaled gas volumes are not usually identical due to nonequal production of carbon dioxide and consumption of oxygen. The typical difference in oxygen concentrations between inspired and exhaled gas in patients requiring supplemental oxygen for respiratory failure may be only 1 to 3 percent. Unfortunately, this is the limit of accuracy that can be provided by most clinically available oxygen analyzers. Thus, the crucial measurement of oxygen concentration difference is destroyed by the lack of adequate precision in that measurement.

A second major problem with the Fick method is that it requires access to the central circulation for mixed venous blood oxygen content measurement. If estimates are made of mixed venous oxygen content, then the value of the resulting estimate is no better than guessing the value of the cardiac output itself. Even when mixed venous blood is actually sampled, the presence of small inaccuracies in the primary measurements may render the resulting calculated cardiac output unreliable. As an example, consider the following situation. If the total body oxygen consumption could be measured and were found to be 300 ml/min, and the arterial oxygen content were 15 vol%, with a mixed venous oxygen content of 10 vol%, then the resulting calculated cardiac output would be 6 L/min. If, however, one considers usual measurement errors in the measurement of oxygen content the following might occur: assume that the accuracy of the oxygen content measurement were 5 percent overall, not an unreasonable error in clinical lab measurements. Then, in a worst case scenario, the reported arterial oxygen content might be 15.25 vol% and the mixed venous oxygen content might be 10.5 vol%. Using the original total body oxygen consumption figure of 300 ml/min, the calculated cardiac output using the new reported figures, each subject to a 5 percent error, is now 8 L/min. The cumulative effect of two independent measures of oxygen content, of 5 percent each, is to create a 60 percent error in the final calculation. The reason for this is that the arterial and mixed venous oxygen contents are subtracted from each other, and are generally close in value to each other prior to subtraction. Small primary errors under such conditions give rise to large secondary errors. It can be shown that if the errors in O_2 content are 10 percent, then the worst case error is 100 percent in the final calculation. In general terms, experience with the Fick technique of cardiac output measurement typically results in a precision of about 20 percent.[139]

Indicator dilution method

The next method introduced to estimate cardiac output was the indicator dilution method, which depends on the Stewart-Hamilton equation,[56,58] itself a modification of the classic Fick principle. In this technique, the indicator is an inert substance which is not metabolized on its first pass through the venous circulation. The indicator is injected as a bolus in the central circulation, usually through a centrally placed intrathoracic catheter. The indicator travels to the heart, where it mixes with the venous return to the heart. It continues mixing as it travels through the right atrium, right ventricle, the lungs, and the left atrium and ventricle. Immediately after the injection, the concentration of indicator is sampled from a peripheral location. The resultant concentration versus time curve of the indicator is shown in Figure 3.6. Usually, the concentration of indicator is measured and recorded by a microcomputer that facilitates calculation of the time averaged concentration and final computation of the cardiac output. Note that there is a lag time between dye injection and its appearance at the peripheral artery. This is the time required to traverse the central circulation.

In this method, it is dilution of the indicator by venous return that is being measured, not cardiac output. If there are no shunts between the left and right

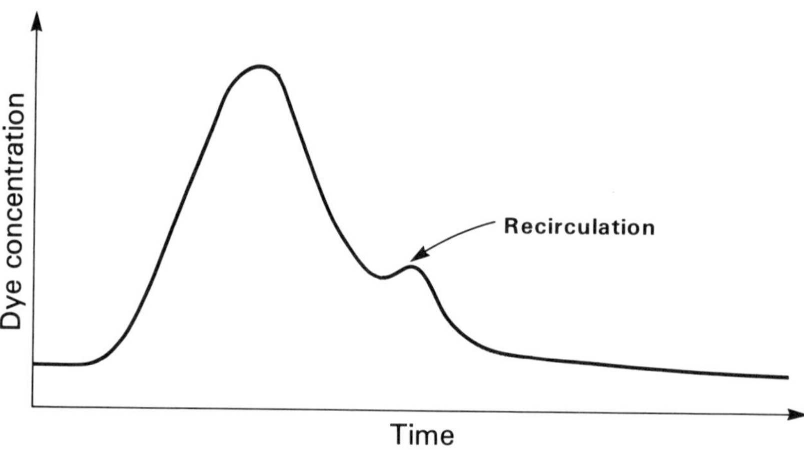

Fig. 3.6. A typical dye dilution cardiac output curve. Important features include: a stable baseline, a brisk and smooth upstroke suggesting bolus injection of dye into the central circulation, an exponential downstroke necessary for most computers to analyze the data, and a recirculation hump on the downstroke as dye returns to the central circulation for a second pass.

side of the heart, there will be no difference, in the steady state, between venous return and cardiac output. If there were, the heart would either empty or explode, and it does neither. If, on the other hand, there are intracardiac or extracardiac shunts between the left and right sides of the heart, the assumption that venous return equals cardiac output no longer applies, and the indicator dilution method is invalid.

The two major methods of the indicator dilution method are those using indocyanine green dye or thermal energy for the indicator.

Indocyanine green dye In the traditional green dye dilution method, the green dye is injected as a bolus in the central circulation.[36,79] Arterial blood is then withdrawn at a distal location into an optical cuvette where the concentration of dye in the arterial blood over time is measured. The system requires access to arterial blood and the withdrawal of approximately 15 to 25 ml of blood from the patient. The blood may be reinfused if the tubing, connections, and cuvette are sterile, but the logistics of keeping sterile cuvettes and the potential breakdown in asepsis make reinfusion uncommon. Thus, the method is limited to infrequent measurements and use in children large enough to tolerate a loss of 15 to 20 ml of blood. The optical measuring system needs to be calibrated each time with a sample of the patient's blood, adding greatly to the inconvenience of use. Since indocyanine green dye does recirculate, it will reappear in the central circulation after one passage through the body. This manifests in a "recirculation hump" on the downstroke of the time versus concentration curve measured in the arterial blood. The microcomputer must account for the recirculation in its calculations. Examination of the curve will often demonstrate a technical problem with injection or analysis that invalidates the data. Several examples of curves are shown in Figure 3.7 with accompanying legends describing the underlying events.

Thermodilution technique An alternative to the indocyanine green dye technique is the thermodilution technique.[24,29,50,84,85] This system takes advantage of the

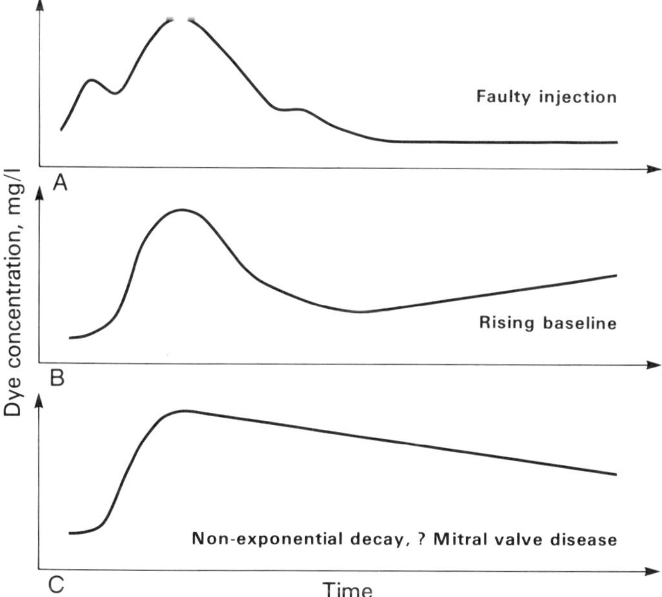

Fig. 3.7. Examples of dye dilution curves showing (A) a faulty injection technique, (B) a rising baseline due to photodetector drift, and (C) a poor downstroke suggesting sluggish circulation, perhaps mitral disease. With curves such as these, the measurement of cardiac output is unreliable.

fact that negative thermal energy (cold) can be injected in the form of cold water into the central circulation and that venous return (hence, cardiac output by inference) may be estimated by examining the dilution of cold water with warm blood.

Temperature is measured with a rapidly responding thermistor on a pulmonary artery catheter in the main or branch pulmonary artery. Knowing the specific heat of the injected water, the temperature of the injectate, the blood temperature of the patient prior to injection, and the rates of heat transfer along the catheter and between blood and injectate, a modified Stewart-Hamilton equation is used to calculate the cardiac output. Cold water, in volumes of 3 to 10 ml at a temperature of 0 to 22°C, can be injected into the central circulation and venous return estimated from analysis of the temperature vs. time curve in the pulmonary artery. Since the thermal transfer is complete in one pass through the lungs, there is no recirculation and no accumulation of indicator with which to contend. Thus, the measurement may be repeated at frequent intervals, and is, in fact, often done in duplicate or triplicate to improve precision. In addition, no withdrawal of blood is necessary to accomplish the measurement, and no calibration is required.

Disadvantages of the thermodilution technique include the necessity of having a pulmonary artery catheter with a thermistor, and the fact that the estimate of venous return is averaged over a small number of heartbeats and is thus quite dependent on the timing of injection with respect to respiratory cycle. To reduce the impact of this latter problem, most investigators now recommend that the injection be performed in the same phase of the respiratory cycle each time that it is done, and most recommend that injection should occur with the end of passive exhalation, prior to mechanical inflation.[67,131]

Oxygen Assessment

Historically, the major emphasis in terms of oxygen assessment in clinical situations was placed on arterial oxygen content and saturation rather than on oxygen gas tension. Virtually all of classic physiology was based on measurements of oxygen content and saturation. The routine measurement of oxygen tension awaited the introduction in the 1950s of the polarographic Clark electrode and its miniaturized versions. The rationale for saturation as a primary oxygen monitoring variable rather than oxygen tension lies in the relationship between the content and oxygen saturation on the one hand, and the content and gas tension on the other. The relationship between content, saturation, hemoglobin concentration, and oxygen tension is expressed as follows[91]:

$$CaO_2 = 1.39 \times Hgb \times O_2Sat + 0.0031 \times PaO_2$$

This relationship is depicted graphically in Figure 3.8, which demonstrates the intimate agreement between O_2Sat and oxygen content compared with the non-linear relationship between the P_aO_2 and the content.

Oxygen saturation may be measured invasively in a continuous fashion with fiberoptic devices implanted in catheter material placed in the vascular space.[41,86] Such fiberoptic systems are available on umbilical artery catheters for use in newborns and on multilumen pulmonary artery catheters of 5 and 7 French for use in the pediatric and adult population. The devices are stable, and allow many hours and even days of continuous and reliable oxygen saturation measurements until the catheters become coated with fibrin depositions which interfere with their ability to accurately track O_2Sat.

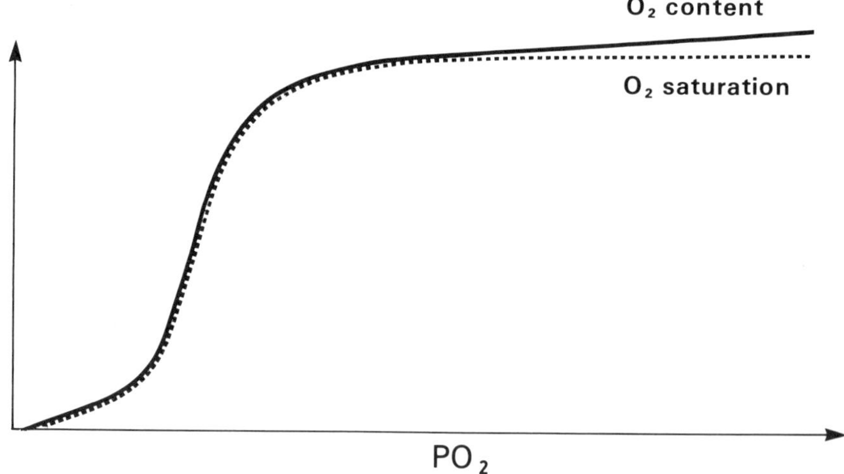

Fig. 3.8. Relationship between O_2 saturation, O_2 content, and arterial oxygen tension. Note the close relationship between saturation and content, and the nonlinear relationship between tension and content. The divergence of the content and saturation after the blood is fully saturated is due to small amounts of dissolved oxygen.

Once the microminiature Clark electrode was introduced in the 1950s, the measurement of oxygen tension in the blood became practical. The technology for arterial P_aO_2 monitoring is available in two major forms for children and newborns, intermittent sampling from percutaneous sticks or indwelling catheters, and continuous indwelling catheters with microminiaturized Clark electrodes that are inserted directly into the blood stream.[97,107]

Intermittent sampling suffers from the problem common to most noncontinuous monitoring techniques, that is, one is never certain that the event for which one is searching occurs at precisely the time of sampling. Continuous invasive monitoring of P_aO_2 is far from perfected however. Like its counterpart, O_2Sat monitoring, the indwelling Clark electrode suffers from limitation of size and duration of use due to fibrin deposition on the polarographic membrane used to cover the electrode. Fluorescent methods depending on chemical reactions of dyes placed on indwelling catheters sensitive to changes in P_aO_2 are now being developed, and we may see these applied in clinical situations in the near future.

Because the arterial oxygen content is fairly constant in conditions of typical gas exchange, the major reflection of alterations in tissue oxygen extraction is the mixed venous oxygen saturation (O_2Sat) and tension ($P_{\bar{v}}O_2$).[69,121] If the oxygen delivery is compromised to the periphery, the tissues will increase their extraction of oxygen to compensate.[20] The venous oxygen content will fall, resulting in a mixed venous O_2Sat of less than 70 vol%, corresponding to a mixed venous PO_2 of approximately 40 mmHg. Thus, in an indirect manner, the venous O_2Sat and $P_{\bar{v}}O_2$ are both useful indicators of the adequacy of peripheral oxygen delivery. The relationship between cardiac output (CO), oxygen utilization and the cross body difference for oxygen content $(a\text{-}\bar{v})DO_2$ is:

$$\dot{V}O_2 = (a\text{-}\bar{v})DO_2 \times CO$$

Rearranging the equation provides the following relationship:

$$(a\text{-}\bar{v})DO_2 = \dot{V}O_2/CO$$

Thus, the $(a\text{-}\bar{v})DO_2$ represents the ratio between demand ($\dot{V}O_2$) and supply which is dominated by CO if we assume that pulmonary gas exchange is adequate and that the arterial blood is nearly fully saturated. A larger than normal value for $(a\text{-}\bar{v})DO_2$ implies a demand in excess of supply, either because the demand is high, or the supply is low. Such may occur during profound hyperthermia, or more commonly during conditions in which cardiac reserves are inadequate to meet even normal demands of the body at rest or mild exercise in cases of cardiomyopathy, trauma, etc. Low $(a\text{-}\bar{v})DO_2$ and concomitant high mixed venous O_2Sat and P_vO_2 may occur whenever the supply is in excess of demand, such as in (1) systemic poisoning with cyanide intoxication, (2) early septic shock with interference of peripheral oxygen utilization, (3) death of peripheral tissues with continued perfusion, and (4) the presence of excessive exogenous catecholamines with cardiac output in excess of peripheral tissue demand.

The methods available for invasive monitoring of venous oxygen saturation and/ or mixed venous oxygen tension are fiberoptic catheters and microminiaturized Clark electrodes fitted to special balloon tipped pulmonary artery catheters for flotation into the main or branch pulmonary artery. No continuous noninvasive means are yet available for this purpose.

Tissue pH Monitoring

In the same sense that mixed venous oxygen content or $P_{\bar{v}}O_2$ monitoring provides an assessment of the *adequacy* of the supply and demand relationship rather than the absolute cardiac output, the monitoring of tissue pH also provides insight into the adequacy of supply vs. demand.[31,114] If sufficient substrate is delivered to the tissue, then the tissue pH will be normal. If the substrate delivery to the tissue is not adequate, either because of inadequate substrate concentration or because the cardiac output itself is low, then the tissues will shift into anaerobic metabolism with the local production of excess acid and hydrogen ion H^+, and there will be a drop in local tissue pH. If the flow to the tissue is low, then the excess production of H^+ will not be swept away by nutritive flow, and the H^+ will accumulate. Tissue pH will drop still further.

Thus, on theoretical grounds, an excellent indicator of the adequacy of local nutritive flow would be the local tissue pH. In fact, such a relationship does exist, at least in the animal model. Sagy demonstrated a close relationship between local tissue pH and total cardiac output in dogs given sublethal doses of endotoxin to induce a syndrome of endotoxin induced shock.[118] He found that the agreement between tissue pH and cardiac output was better than those between cardiac output and arterial or venous pH, heart rate, mean arterial blood pressure, or urine output. Figure 3.9 demonstrates a fairly typical relationship in one animal between the local tissue pH and the cardiac output determined by classic thermodilution technique. Other investigators have used this technique in neonates and children and

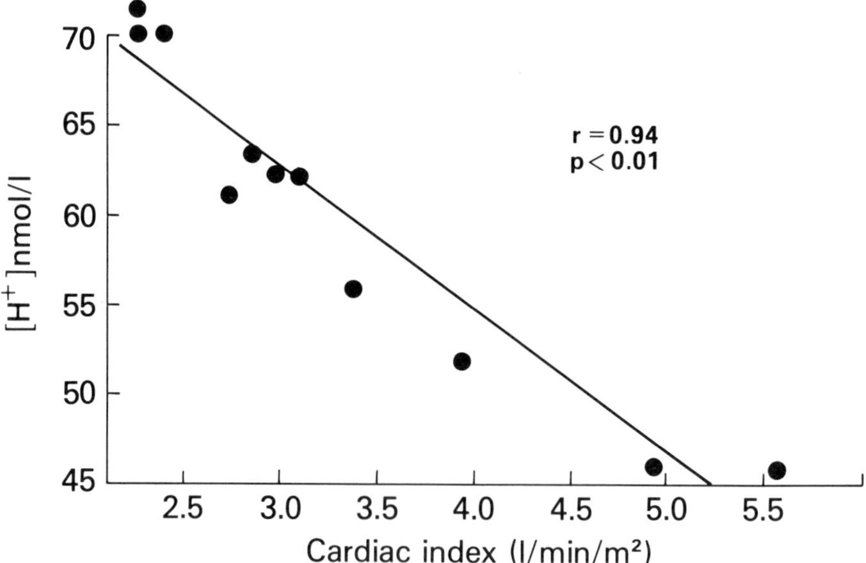

Fig. 3.9. Relationship between cardiac index and tissue hydrogen ion concentration $[H^+]$ in a dog given a sublethal dose of endotoxin.

have found it to be a useful monitor for assessing the adequacy of local perfusion.[17,46,47] One would naturally expect that this variable would be a sensitive indicator of nutritive perfusion in the compromised child, since the skin will be one of the first organs to have its perfusion sacrificed during periods of low flow state as the body tries to defend perfusion to vital organs such as the heart and brain.

CALCULATED HEMODYNAMIC PERFORMANCE VARIABLES

Systemic Vascular Resistance

Invasive monitoring provides the clinician with the primary variables necessary to understand and manipulate the failing circulation in the critically ill child. Several additional variables can be calculated or derived from the primary variables that may give additional insight into the pathophysiologic process and allow the clinician to "fine tune" the circulation.

A major determinant of left ventricular afterload is the impedance to ejection of blood from the left ventricle into the aorta. Contributing to the impedance to ejection is the total peripheral vascular resistance of the body. In simple terms, if the body is tightly vasoconstricted, presenting a high resistance circuit to the cardiac pump, then the myocardium will have to work harder to pump blood through the high resistance circuit. The systemic vascular resistance (SVR) is altered by endogenous and exogenous catecholamines, the renin-angiotensin system, and vasodilators.

Measuring the peripheral resistance allows one to adjust catecholamines and vasodilators to optimize the ventricular afterload by reducing the peripheral resistance. The physiology and pharmacology of afterload reduction is covered elsewhere in this volume. The technology of the measurement is quite simple. One measures the mean arterial pressure (MAP), the central venous pressure (CVP), and the cardiac output (CO), usually with a thermodilution cardiac output pulmonary artery catheter, and calculates the SVR according to the relationship:

$$\text{SVR} = \frac{\text{MAP} - \text{CVP}}{\text{CO}} \times 79.92 \text{ dyne·sec·cm}^{-5}$$

In order to normalize the specific values from a particular child so that comparisons to normal may be made, the raw number calculated as above is usually divided by the estimated body surface area (BSA) to yield the systemic vascular resistance *index* (SVRI):

$$\text{SVRI} = \frac{\text{SVR}}{\text{BSA}} \text{ dyne·sec·cm}^{-5}/\text{meter}^2$$

The normal values usually quoted[124] for SVRI are 1760 to 2600. SVRI values in excess of 3000 usually signify excessive vasoconstriction.

Pulmonary Vascular Resistance

The SVR is a useful measurement of the degree of peripheral vasoconstriction that the pumping of the left ventricle must overcome to eject blood, and hence, a prime determinant of left ventricular afterload. In the same sense, the pulmonary vascular resistance (PVR) is a measure of the pulmonary vascular state of health and a major determinant of right ventricular afterload. In severe pulmonary parenchymal disease, however, such as in sepsis or ARDS, the pulmonary microvasculature becomes obstructed to a greater or lesser degree by agglutination of white cells, platelets, and thrombin deposition.[62,140,145] The microthrombi eventually occupy a sizeable fraction of the available pulmonary vascular bed. The result is an elevation in PVR and afterload to right ventricular ejection. The PVR is defined in a parallel fashion to the SVR according to the formula:

$$\text{PVR} = \frac{\text{Mean PAP} - \text{Left atrial pressure}}{\text{CO}} \times 79.92 \text{ dyne}\cdot\text{sec}\cdot\text{cm}^{-5}$$

In order to compare patients of all different sizes, the raw PVR is usually normalized to body surface area:

$$\text{PVRI} = \text{PVR/BSA dyne}\cdot\text{sec}\cdot\text{cm}^{-5}/\text{meter}^2$$

The normal PVRI (pulmonary vascular resistance index) is usually taken as 45 to 225.[124] Shoemaker and Zapol demonstrated that in ARDS, the PVRI follows the clinical severity of the illness and is often a good predictor of outcome.[124,145] When PVRI remains low or only slightly elevated, the prognosis for pulmonary recovery is usually good, whereas, in situations in which the PVRI rises to very high numbers, there is so much microthrombotic occlusion of the small vessels in the lung that recovery is less likely. One problem with the interpretation of PVRI as a measure of pulmonary vascular damage occurs when positive end-expiratory pressure (PEEP) is being used to support diminished lung volumes in these patients with very sick lungs. Initially, the high PVR associated with collapse of lung parenchyma and air-containing lung volume results in hypoxia. As PEEP is applied, the airways are pulled open by recruitment of collapsed airways, oxygen exchange improves, and the PVR falls. As PEEP is elevated above some "optimal" value, however, the effective PVR may actually rise if the elevated airway pressure is transmitted to the perivascular space to the extent that the pulmonary vessel caliber is compromised by the elevated airway pressure. In this condition, a type of starling resistor phenomenon occurs in which the PVRI will rise as additional airway pressure compromises vessel patency.[7,23,81,90,101,142] Figure 3.10 demonstrates this phenomenon.

It is obvious that the measurement of PVRI requires a pulmonary artery catheter and estimation of mean left atrial pressure, along with an estimate of cardiac output, to perform the calculation. While separate PA and LA catheters are sometimes available in the postoperative cardiothoracic surgical patient, the medical or general surgical patient usually will require a thermodilution Swan-Ganz pulmonary artery catheter in place to make the above measurement. The mean left atrial pressure is usually estimated by the pulmonary artery occluded pressure (PAOP) and the formula becomes:

$$\text{PVR} = \frac{\text{PAPmean} - \text{PAOP}}{\text{CO}} \times 79.92 \text{ dyne}\cdot\text{sec}\cdot\text{cm}^{-5}$$

The value is again normalized to the PVRI by dividing the raw value by the body surface area.

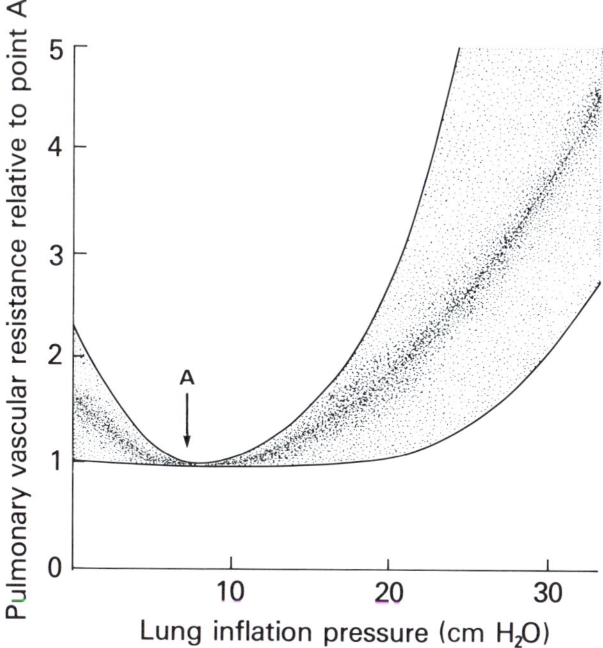

Fig. 3.10. Relationship between pulmonary vascular resistance (PVR) and lung inflation pressure. Note that PVR first falls as positive end expiratory pressure (PEEP) is increased and then begins to rise as pulmonary vessels are constricted by the rising inflating pressure. (Redrawn by permission of the publisher from Nunn JF, Applied Respiratory Physiology, 2nd edn. London: Butterworths (Publishers) Ltd. 1977.)

Pulmonary Venous Admixture

The pulmonary venous admixture, often called the intrapulmonary shunt, and denoted by the symbol $\dot{Q}s/\dot{Q}t$, is a hypothetical quantity calculated from oxygen contents of the pulmonary and systemic arterial blood and pulmonary end-capillary blood. The $\dot{Q}s/\dot{Q}t$ estimates the fraction of the total cardiac output $\dot{Q}t$ that would have to flow through a nongas-exchanging intrapulmonary shunt $\dot{Q}s$ to account for the observed desaturation found in arterial blood. When considering the intrapulmonary venous admixture, the user should realize that the quantity of shunt blood calculated is not really a well defined localized anatomic shunt, but rather a mathematical representation of the total amount of nonexchanging or suboptimally exchanging blood flow. The actual physiology accounting for the hypoxemia is usually a result of maldistributed ventilation and perfusion throughout the diseased lung, along with any true anatomic shunts that may exist. The $\dot{Q}s/\dot{Q}t$ is calculated by the relationship:

$$\dot{Q}s/\dot{Q}t = \frac{C_{c'}O_2 - C_aO_2}{C_{c'}O_2 - C_{\bar{v}}O_2}$$

where $C_c'O_2$ is the oxygen content of pulmonary end-capillary blood and C_aO_2 and $C_{\bar{v}}O_2$ are the arterial and mixed venous oxygen contents, respectively. Arterial and mixed venous O_2 contents are easily sampled and measured using arterial and pulmonary artery blood. However, the pulmonary end-capillary blood is impossible to sample under any condition. The only option is to estimate the end-capillary blood oxygen content by using various forms of the alveolar gas equation to estimate the alveolar PO_2 (P_AO_2), assume total O_2Hgb saturation if the P_AO_2 is high enough, and calculate the end-capillary blood oxygen content from the formula for estimating oxygen content:

$$C_{c'}O_2 = Hgb \times 1.39 \times O_2Sat + 0.0031 \times P_AO_2$$

The normal value of $\dot{Q}s/\dot{Q}t$ is approximately 0.08, and is accounted for by some true anatomic shunt, and some $\dot{V}/\dot{Q}$ maldistribution that occurs even in the normal lung.[124] As gas exchange worsens, the calculated $\dot{Q}s/\dot{Q}t$ rises until at about a $\dot{Q}s/\dot{Q}t$ value of 0.15, respiratory failure usually is considered to exist.[51,52] In severe ARDS, the calculated $\dot{Q}s/\dot{Q}t$ may approach or even exceed 0.50 in value. One scheme for managing PEEP in cases of severe ARDS is to manipulate the PEEP and measure the $\dot{Q}s/\dot{Q}t$ after each change in PEEP. The goal of such therapy is to minimize the $\dot{Q}s/\dot{Q}t$, usually to a value below 0.15.

Critics of $\dot{Q}s/\dot{Q}t$ calculations point to the fact that the value of $\dot{Q}s/\dot{Q}t$ actually gives no additional information to the clinician than knowledge of the P_aO_2 and the simultaneous F_IO_2 required to achieve it. However, the $\dot{Q}s/\dot{Q}t$ calculation does provide a convenient shorthand notation that implies a physiologic process rather than just describing severe hypoxemia on high supplemental oxygen. The user should not become overly enamored of the technology, however, for it is fraught with several technical problems interfering with its accuracy and hence, the certainty that it seems to confer on the system of measurement. For example, in the formula above for the calculations of $\dot{Q}s/\dot{Q}t$, the user can see that the numerator of the equation is the difference between the O_2 content of end-capillary blood and arterial blood. In the usual situation, these two numbers may be very close to each other, and hence, the difference is a very small number. If one accepts the fact that all measurements are prone to error, one sees that the error applied to each of the primary data elements may distribute in such a manner that the difference is affected greatly. For example, let us assume that the F_IO_2 is such that the end capillary blood is fully saturated and that the hemoglobin concentration and P_aO_2 are such that the *true* arterial O_2 content is 12 vol% and the calculated end-capillary O_2 content is 12.2 vol%. In this situation, if the end-capillary to mixed venous O_2 content difference is the normal value of 5 vol%, then the calculated $\dot{Q}s/\dot{Q}t$ is 0.2/5.0 = 0.04, a normal value. If, on the other hand, the errors in O_2 content measurement and the calculation of end-capillary measurements were only 5 percent, *and the errors were in opposite directions*, then the following might occur. The arterial O_2 content might be *measured* at 12.6 vol%, and the end-capillary blood O_2 content might be calculated at 11.59. The $\dot{Q}s/\dot{Q}t$ now calculates to:

$$\dot{Q}s/\dot{Q}t = \frac{12.6 - 11.59}{5.0}$$

or 20.2%, a calculated answer *5 times* greater than truth! If the errors in measurement and calculation were of equal magnitude but merely in the opposite direction than the above example, then the calculated $\dot{Q}s/\dot{Q}t$ might be:

$$\dot{Q}s/\dot{Q}t = \frac{11.59 - 12.6}{5.0}$$

or $\dot{Q}s/\dot{Q}t = -20.2\%$, a *negative* shunt. We have just created a calculation that tells us that the lung *creates oxygen*! Thus, the value of the $\dot{Q}s/\dot{Q}t$ calculation is dominated by the accuracy of the primary measurements. The user should take care not to read too much into the calculated values.

SUMMARY

We have explored the technology of measurement and several primary and secondary variables that may be of interest when confronted with the child with a failing circulation. Some of the variables lend themselves to noninvasive measurement or assessment, whereas others can only be approached by invasive means. When considering any variable and its measurement by invasive means, the clinician must finally address the same question: "Do I need this data enough to justify the increased risk and cost that I and the child must pay to acquire it?" When the answer to the question is "yes," then the invasive means should be employed. When the answer is "no," it should not. Of course, it is the different way people view the need and the cost that makes the clinical practice of critical care medicine so interesting.

One additional principle is worth remembering when considering invasive monitoring. *Children are entitled to the same quality of care as adults.* Technology now exists that provides the means to extend the same level of monitoring and physiologic intervention for children as has existed for many years in the adult population. Physicians caring for children should apply the same basic principles of good care and patient consideration as they would employ for their adult patients. Children need be therapeutic orphans no more.

REFERENCES

1. Agostini E 1972 Mechanics of the pleural space. Physiological Reviews 52: 57
2. Alderman EL, Glantz SA 1976 Acute hemodynamic interventions shift the diastolic pressure-volume curve in man. Circulation 54: 662
3. Allen EV 1929 Thromboangiitis obliterans: methods of diagnosis of chronic occlusive arterial lesions distal to the wrist with illustrative cases. American Journal of Medical Sciences 178: 237
4. Asler DC, Bryan-Brown CW 1973 Use of the axillary artery for intravascular monitoring. Critical Care Medicine 1: 148
5. Aziz EM, Robertson AF 1973 Paraplegia: a complication of umbilical artery catheterization. Journal of Pediatrics 82: 1051
6. Band JD, Maki D 1979 Infections caused by arterial catheters used in hemodynamic monitoring. American Journal of Medicine 67: 735
7. Banister J, Torrance RW 1960 The effects of the tracheal pressure upon flow:pressure relations in the vascular bed of isolated lungs. Quarterly Journal of Experimental Physiology 45: 352
8. Bar-Joseph G, Galvis AG 1983 Perforation of the heart by central venous catheters in infants: guidelines to diagnosis and management. Journal of Pediatric Surgery 18: 284
9. Barnes RW, Peterson JL, Krugmire RB, Strandness DE 1974 Complications of percutaneous femoral arterial catheterization: prospective evaluation with the Doppler ultrasonic velocity detector. American Journal of Cardiology 33: 259
10. Bauer SB, Feldman SM, Gellis SS, Retik AB 1975 Neonatal hypertension a complication of umbilical-artery catheterization. New England Journal of Medicine 293: 1032
11. Beardsmore CS, Helms P, Stocks J, Hatch DJ, Silverman M 1980 Improved esophageal balloon technique for use in infants. Journal of Applied Physiology: Respiratory, Environmental and Exercise Physiology 49: 735
12. Bedford RF 1975 Percutaneous radial-artery cannulation-increased safety using teflon catheters. Anesthesiology 42: 219

13. Bedford RF 1978 Long-term radial artery cannulation: effects on subsequent vessel function. Critical Care Medicine 6: 64
14. Bedford RF 1978 Wrist circumference predicts the risk of radial-arterial occlusion after cannulation. Anesthesiology 48: 377
15. Bedford RF, Wollman H 1973 Complications of percutaneous radial artery cannulation: an objective prospective study in man. Anesthesiology 38: 228
16. Belani KG, Buckley JJ, Gordon JR, Castanada W 1980 Percutaneous cervical central venous line placement: a comparison of the internal and external jugular vein routes. Anesthesia and Analgesia 59: 40
17. Bhat R, Vidyasagar D, Asonye UO, Papazafiratou C 1980 Continuous tissue pH monitoring in critically ill neonates. Journal of Pediatrics 97: 445
18. Bloom JD, Mozersky DJ, Buckley CJ, Hagood CO 1974 Defective limb growth as a complication of catheterization of the femoral artery. Surgery, Gynecology, and Obstetrics 138: 524
19. Brodsky JB 1973 A simple method to determine patency of the ulnar artery prior to radial-artery cannulation. Anesthesiology 42: 626
20. Bryan-Brown CW 1975 Tissue blood flow and oxygen transport in critically ill patients. Critical Care Medicine 3: 104
21. Bryan-Brown CW 1977 Wrecking the machinery? Critical Care Medicine 5: 163
22. Buda AJ, Pinsky MR, Ingels NB, Daughters GT, Stinson EB, Alderman EL 1979 Effect of intrathoracic pressures. New England Journal of Medicine 301: 453
23. Burton AC, Patel DJ 1958 Effects on pulmonary vascular resistance of inflation of the rabbit lungs. Journal of Applied Physiology 12: 239
24. Callaghan ML, Weintraub WH, Coran AG 1976 Assessment of thermodilution cardiac output in small subjects. Journal of Pediatric Surgery 11: 629
25. Calvin JE, Driedger AA, Sibbald WJ 1981 Does the pulmonary capillary wedge pressure predict left ventricular preload in critically ill patients? Critical Care Medicine 9: 437
26. Cassidy SS, Eschenbacher WL, Robertson CH, Nixon JV, Blomqvist G, Johnson RL 1979 Cardiovascular effects of positive-pressure ventilation in normal subjects. Journal of Applied Physiology: Respiratory, Environmental and Exercise Physiology 47: 453
27. Cliffe P 1982 Transducers for the measurement of pressure. In: Scurr C and Feldman S (ed) Scientific Foundations of Anaesthesia. Year Book, Chicago
28. Coleman SS, Anson BJ 1961 Arterial patterns in the hand based upon a study of 650 specimens. Surgery, Gynecology, and Obstetrics 113: 409
29. Colgan FJ, Stewart S 1977 An assessment of cardiac output by thermodilution in infants and children following cardiac surgery. Critical Care Medicine 5: 220
30. Cote CJ, Jobes DR, Schwartz AJ, Ellison N 1979 Two approaches to cannulation of a child's internal jugular vein. Anesthesiology 50: 371
31. Cough NP, Dmochowski JR, van de Water JM, Harken DW, Moore FD 1971 Muscle surface pH as an index of peripheral perfusion in man. Annals of Surgery 173: 173
32. Cullen DJ 1977 Results and costs of intensive care. Anesthesiology 47: 203
33. Davis FM, Stewart JM 1980 Radial artery cannulation: a prospective study in patient undergoing cardiothoracic surgery. British Journal of Anesthesia 52: 41
34. Davis RF 1985 Clinical comparison of automated auscultatory and oscillometruc and catheter-transducer measurements of arterial pressure. Journal of Clinical Monitoring 1: 114
35. DeAngelis J 1976 Axillary artery monitoring. Critical Care Medicine 4: 205
36. Dow P 1956 Estimations of cardiac output and central blood volume by dye dilution. Physiological Reviews 36: 77
37. Downs JB 1976 A technique for direct measurement of intrapleural pressure. Critical Care Medicine 4: 207
38. Downs JB, Rackstein AD, Klein EF, Hawkins IF 1973 Hazards of radial-artery catherization. Anesthesiology 38: 283
39. Downs JB, Douglas ME 1980 Assessment of cardiac filling pressure during continuous positive-pressure ventilation. Critical Care Medicine 8: 285
40. Enge I, Flatmark A 1973 Percutaneous removal of intravascular foreign bodies by the snare technique. Acta Radiologica Diagnostica 14: 747
41. Enson Y, Briscoe WA, Polanyi ML, Cournand A 1962 In vivo studies with an intravascular and intracardiac reflection oximeter. Journal of Applied Physiology 17: 552
42. Ersoz CJ, Hedden M, Lain L 1979 Prolonged femoral arterial catheterization for intensive care. Anesthesia and Analgesia 49: 160
43. Essop AR, Frolich J, Moosa MR, Miller M, Ming RC 1984 Risk factors related to bacterial contamination of indwelling vascular catheters in non-infected hosts. Intensive Care Medicine 10: 193

44. Feeley TW 1977 Re-establishment of radial-artery patency for arterial monitoring. Anesthesiology 46: 73
45. Fibuch EE, Tuohy GF 1980 Intracardiac knotting of a flow-directed balloon-tipped catheter. Anesthesia and Analgesia 59: 217
46. Filler RM, Das JB 1971 Muscle surface pH: a new parameter in the monitoring of the critically ill child. Pediatrics 47: 880
47. Filler RM, Das JB, Espinosa HM 1972 Clinical experience with continuous muscle pH monitoring as an index of tissue perfusion and oxygenation and acid-base status. Surgery 72: 23
48. Finnie KJC, Watts DG, Armstrong PW 1984 Biases in the measurement of arterial pressure. Critical Care Medicine 12: 965
49. Forrester JS, Diamond G, McHugh TJ, Swan HJC 1971 Filling pressures in the right and left sides of the heart in acute myocardial infarction a reappraisal of central-venous pressure monitoring. New England Journal of Medicine 285: 190
50. Freed MD, Keane JF 1978 Cardiac output measured by thermodilution in infants and children. Journal of Pediatrics 92: 39
51. Gallagher TJ, Civetta JM, Kirby RR 1978 Terminology update: optimal PEEP. Critical Care Medicine 6: 323
52. Gallagher TJ 1982 Acute respiratory failure: rationale of therapy. Respiratory Care 27: 1527
53. Groff DB, Ahmed N 1974 Subclavian vein catherization in the infant. Journal of Pediatric Surgery 9: 171
54. Gaash 1976 Left ventricular compliance: mechanics and clinical implications. American Journal of Cardiology 38: 645
55. Grace MP Greebaum DM 1982 Cardiac performance in response to PEEP in patients with cardiac dysfunction. Critical Care Medicine 10: 358
56. Hamilton WF, Moore JW, Kinsman JM, Spurling RG 1928 Simultaneous determination of the pulmonary and systemic circulation times in man and of a figure related to the cardiac output. American Journal of Physiology 84: 338
57. Hamilton WF, Dow P 1939 An experimental study of the standing waves in the pulse propagated through the aorta. American Journal of Physiology 125: 48
58. Hamilton WF, Riley RL, Attyah AM, Cournand A, Fowell DM, Himmelstein A, Noble RP, Remington JW, Richards DW, Wheeler NC, Witham AC 1948 Comparison of the Fick and dye injection methods of measuring the cardiac output in man. American Journal of Physiology 153: 309
59. Hewlett-Packard 1977 Guide to Physiological Pressure Monitoring. Application note AN739 Hewlett-Packard Company, Waltham, Massachusetts, p 57
60. Hewlett-Packard 1977 Guide to Physiological Pressure Monitoring. Application note AN739 Hewlett-Packard Company, Waltham, Massachusetts, p 33
61. Higgs BD, Behrakis PK, Bevan DR, Milic-Emili J 1983 Measurement of pleural pressure with esophageal balloon in anesthetized humans. Anesthesiology 59: 340
62. Hinson JM, Hutchison AA, Ogletree ML, Brigham KL, Snapper JR 1983 Effect of granulocyte depletion on altered lung mechanics after endotoxemia in sheep. Journal of Applied Physiology: Respiratory, Environmental, Exercise Physiology 55: 92
63. Hoar PF, Stone JG, Wicks AE, Edie RN, Scholes JV 1978 Thrombogenesis associated with Swan-Ganz catheters. Anesthesiology 48: 445
64. Hoar PF, Wilson RM, Mangano DT, Avery GJ, Szarnicki RJ, Hill JD 1981 Heparin bonding reduces thrombogenicity of pulmonary-artery catheters. New England Journal of Medicine 305: 993
65. Hoyt AB 1985 A surgeon's view: the subclavian vein. Journal of Clinical Monitoring 1: 61
66. Husum B, Palm T 1978 Arterial dominance in the hand. British Journal of Anaesthesia 50: 913
67. Jansen JRC, Schreuder JJ, Boggaard JM, van Rooyen W, Versprille A 1981 Thermodilution technique for measurement of cardiac output during artificial ventilation. Journal of Applied Physiology: Respiratory, Environmental, Exercise Physiology 50: 584
68. Johnstone RE, Greenhow DE 1973 Catherization of the dorsalis pedis artery. Anesthesiology 39: 654
69. Kandel G, Aberman A 1983 Mixed venous oxygen saturation: its role in the assessment of the critically ill patient. Archives of Internal Medicine 143: 1400
70. Katz AM, Birnbaum M, Moylan J, Pellet J 1974 Gangrene of the hand and forearm: a complication of radial artery cannulation. Critical Care Medicine 2: 270
71. Kitterman JA, Phibbs RH, Tooley WH 1970 Catherization of umbilical vessels in newborn infants. Pediatric Clinics of North America 17: 895
72. Kroeker EJ, Wood EH Comparison of simultaneously recorded central and peripheral arterial pressure pulses during rest, exercise and tilted position in man. Circulation Research 3: 623

73. Lappas D, Lell WA, Gabel JC, Civetta J, Lowenstein E 1973 Indirect measurement of left-atrial pressure in surgical patients—pulmonary-wedge and pulmonary-artery diastolic pressures compared with left-atrial pressure. Anesthesiology 38: 394
74. Linos DA, Mucha P, van Heerden JA 1980 Subclavian vein: a golden route. Mayo Clinic Proceeding 55: 315
75. Lipp H, O'Donoghue K, Resnekov L 1971 Intracardiac knotting of a flow-directed balloon catheter. New England Journal of Medicine 284: 220
76. Lowenstein E, Little JW, Har Lo H 1971 Prevention of cerebral embolization from flushing radial-artery cannulas. New England Journal of Medicine 285: 1414
77. Marshall AG, Erwin DC, Wyse RKH, Hatch DJ 1984 Percutaneous arterial cannulation in children: concurrent and subsequent adequacy of blood flow at the wrist. Anaesthesia 39: 27
78. Michenfelder JD, Martin JT, Altenburg BM, Rehder K 1969 Air embolism during neurosurgery: 229 evaluation of right-atrial catheters for diagnosis and treatment. Journal of the American Medical Association 208: 1353
79. Miller DE, Gleason WL, McIntosh HD 1962 A comparison of the cardiac output determination by direct Fisk method and the dye-dilution method using indocyanine green and a cuvette densitometer. Journal of Laboratory and Clinical Medicine 59: 345
80. Miller MJ 1982 Tissue oxygenation in clinical medicine: an historical view. Anesthesia and Analgesia 61: 527
81. Mitzner W 1983 Resistance of the pulmonary circulation. Clinics in Chest Medicine 4: 127
82. Miyasaka K, Edmonds JF, Conn AW 1976 Complications of radial artery lines in the paediatric patient. Canadian Anaesthetists Society Journal 23: 914
83. Mokrohisky ST, Levine RL, Blumhagen JD, Wesenberg RL, Simmons MA 1978 Low positioning of umbilical-artery catheters increases associated complications in newborn infants. New England Journal of Medicine 299: 561
84. Moodie DS 1980 Measurement of cardiac output by thermodilution in pediatric patients. Pediatric Clinics of North America 27: 513
85. Moodie DS, Feldt RH, Kaye MP, Strelow DA, van der Hagen LJ 1978 Measurement of cardiac output by thermodilution: development of accurate measurements at flows applicable to the pediatric patient. Journal of Surgical Research 25: 305
86. Mook GA, Osypka P, Strum RE, Wood EH 1968 Fibre optic reflection photometry on blood. Cardiovascular Research 2: 199
87. Morgan C, Downs JB, Weled BJ 1980 Accurate measurement of intrapleural pressure. Anesthesiology 53: S187
88. Mortensson W, 1980 Effects of percutaneous femoral artery catheterization on leg growth in infants and children. Acta Radiologica Diagnosis 21: 297
89. Nicolson SC, Sweeney MF, Moore RA, Jobes DJ 1985 Comparison of internal and external jugular cannulation of the central circulation in the pediatric patient. Critical Care Medicine, 13: 747
90. Nunn JF 1977 Applied Respiratory Physiology, 2nd edn. Butterworths, London, p 259
91. Nunn JF 1977 Applied Respiratory Physiology, 2nd edn. Butterworths, London, p 390
92. Package insert R10/80, Nosogastric tube with esophogeal balloon. National Catheter Company, Argyle, New York
93. Pape KE, Armstrong DL, Fitzhardinge PM 1978 Peripheral median nerve damage secondary to brachial arterial blood gas sampling. Journal of Pediatrics 93: 852
94. Pape LA, Haffajee MB, Markis JE, Ockene IS, Paraskos JA, Dalen JE, Alpert JS 1979 Fatal pulmonary hemorrhage after use of the flow-directed balloon-tipped catheter. Annals of Internal Medicine 90: 344
95. Park MK, Robotham JL, German VF 1983 Systolic pressure amplification in pedal arteries in children. Critical Care Medicine 11: 286
96. Pokora TJ, Boros SJ, Brennom WS, Huseby TL, Galliani CA 1981 Fatal neonatal thrombosis associated with a pulmonary arterial catheter. Critical Care Medicine 9: 618
97. Pollitzer MJ, Soutter LP, Reynolds EOR, Whitehead MD 1980 Continuous monitoring of arterial oxygen tension in infants: four years of experience with an intravascular oxygen electrode. Pediatrics 66: 31
98. Poole JL 1980 Subclavian vein catheterization for cardiac surgery in children. Anaesthesia and Intensive Care 8: 81
99. Pottecher T, Forrler M, Picardat P, Krause D, Bellocq JP, Otteni JO 1984 Thrombogenicity of central venous catheters: prospective study of polyethylene, silicone and polyurethane catheters with phlebography or post-mortem examination. European Journal of Anaesthesiology 1: 361
100. Powers SR, Mannal R, Neclerio M, English M, Marr C, Leather R, Ueda H, Williams G, Custead W, Dutton R 1973 Physiologic consequences of positive end-expiratory pressure (PEEP) ventilation. Annals of Surgery 178: 265

101. Powers SR, Dutton R 1975 Correlation of positive end-expiratory pressure with cardiovascular peformance. Critical Care Medicine 3: 64
102. Prian GW, Wright GB, Rumack CM, O'Meara OP 1978 Apparent cerebral embolization after temporal artery catheterization. Journal of Pediatrics 93: 1115
103. Prys-Roberts C 1969 The measurement of cardiac output. British Journal of Anaesthesia 41: 751
104. Raphaely R 1983 Shock. In: Fleisher GR and Ludwig S (ed) Textbook of Pediatric Emergency Medicine. Williams & Wilkins, Baltimore
105. Raphaely R, Swedlow D, Kettrick R, Godinez R, Heiser M 1980 Experience with pulmonary artery catheterizations in critically ill children. Critical Care Medicine 8: 265
106. Richman KA, Kim YL, Marshall BE 1979 Thrombocytopenia induced by Swan-Ganz catheters. Anesthesiology 51: S161
107. Rithalia SVS, Bennett PJ, Tinker J 1981 The performance characteristics of an intra-arterial oxygen electrode. Intensive Care Medicine 7: 305
108. Robertson JT, Schick RW, Morgan F, Matson DD Accurate placement of ventriculo-atrial shunt for hydrocephalus under electrocardiographic control. Journal of Neurosurgery 18: 255
109. Rosen M, Latto IP, Shang W 1981 The internal jugular vein. In: Handbook of Percutaneous Vein Catherizations, WB Saunders, London, p. 76
110. Rosen M, Latto IP, Shang W 1981 The arm veins. In: Handbook of Percutaneous Vein Catherizations. WB Saunders, London, p. 35
111. Rosen M, Latto IP, Shang W 1981 The subclavian vein. In: Handbook of Percutaneous Vein Catherizations. WB Saunders, London, p. 51
112. Rosen M, Latto IP, Shang W 1981 The femoral vein. In: Handbook of Percutaneous Vein Catherizations. WB Saunders, London, p. 121
113. Rothe CF, Kim KC 1980 Measuring systolic arterial blood pressure: Possible errors from extension tubes or disposable transducer domes. Critical Care Medicine 8: 683
114. Rozkovec A, Rithalia SVS 1984 Clinical applications of continuous pH monitoring. Intensive Care Medicine 10: 3
115. Rull JR, Aguirre JL, de la Puerta E, Millan EM, Maldonado LP, Clausell CP 1984 Thrombocytopenia induced by pulmonary artery flotation catheters: a prospective study. Intensive Care Medicine 10: 29
116. Runciman WB, Rutten AJ, Isley AH 1981 An evaluation of blood pressure measurement. Anaesthesia and Intensive Care 9: 314
117. Ryan JF, Raines J, Dalton BC, Mathieu A 1973 Arterial dynamics of radial artery cannulation. Anesthesia and Analgesia 52: 1017
118. Sagy M, Swedlow DB, Schaible D, Fleischer G 1984 Tissue pH reliably follows cardiac index during endotoxemia. Anesthesiology 61: A165
119. Sanford TJ 1985 An anesthesiologist's view: the right internal jugular vein. Journal of Clinical Monitoring 1: 58
120. Sarnoff SJ 1955 Myocardial contractility as described by ventricular functional curves: observations on Starling's law of the heart. Physiological Reviews 35: 107
121. Schmidt CR, Frank LP, Forsythe SB, Estafanous FG 1984 Continuous SvO_2 measurement and oxygen transport patterns in cardiac surgery patients. Critical Care Medicine 12: 523
122. Seldinger SI 1952 Catheter replacement of the needle in percutaneous arteriography: a new technique. Acta Radiologica 39: 368
123. Shinozaki T, Deane RS, Mazuzan JE 1980 The dynamic responses of liquid-filled catheter systems for direct measurements of blood pressure. Anesthesiology 53: 498
124. Shoemaker WC 1980 Pathophysiology, monitoring and therapy of shock syndromes. In: Shoemaker WC, Thompson WL (eds) Critical Care: State of the Art. Society of Critical Care Medicine, Fullerton, CA
125. Siegel JH, Greenspan M, Del Guercio LRM 1967 Abnormal vascular tone, defective oxygen transport and myocardial failure in human septic shock. Annals of Surgery 165: 504
126. Simmons MA, Levine RL, Lubchenco LO, Guggenheim MA 1978 Warning: serious sequelae of temporal artery catheterization. Journal of Pediatrics 922: 284
127. Sise MJ, Hollingsworth P, Brimm JE, Peters RM, Virgilio RW, Shackford SR 1981 Complications of flow-directed pulmonary-artery catheter: a prospective analysis in 219 patients. Critical Care Medicine 9: 315
128. Spahr RC, MacDonald HM, Holzman IR 1979 Catherization of the posterior tibial artery in the neonate. American Journal of Diseases of Children 133: 945
129. Smith-Wright DL, Green TP, Lock JE, Egar MI, Furhman BP 1984 Complications of vascular catherization in critically ill children. Crit Care Med 12: 1015
130. Starling EH 1918 The Linacre lecture on the law of the heart. Longmans, Green and Company, London

131. Stevens JH, Raffin TA, Mihm FG, Rosenthal MH, Stetz CW 1985 Thermodilution cardiac output measurement effects of the respiratory cycle on its reproducibility. Journal of the American Medical Association 253: 2240
132. Swedlow D, Kim Y, Richman K, Marshall B 1980 Thrombocytopenia associated with prolonged pulmonary artery catheterization in children. Critical Care Medicine 8: 273
133. Todres ID, Rogers MC, Shannon DC, Moylan FMB, Ryan JF 1975 Percutaneous catheterization of the radial artery in the critically ill neonate. Journal of Pediatrics 87: 273
134. Tooley WH, Myerberg DZ 1978 Should we put catheters in the umbilical artery? Pediatrics 62: 853
135. Warwick R, Williams PL (ed) 1973 Gray's Anatomy, 35th ed. WB Saunders, Philadelphia, p 653
136. Warwick R, Williams PL (ed) 1973 Gray's Anatomy, 35th ed. WB Saunders, Philadelphia, p 647
137. Webre DR, Arens JF 1973 Use of cephalic and basilic veins for introduction of central venous catheters. Anesthesiology 38: 389
138. Weil MH 1978 Principles of fluid challenge for routine treatment of shock. In: Weil MH and Daluz PL (ed) Critical Care Medicine Manual. Springer-Verlag, New York
139. Wesseling KH 1976 The pulse contour cardiac output computer probably as accurate as clinical Fick or indicator dilution methods. Progress Report of Institute Medicine and Physics, Utrecht, Netherlands 5: 63
140. Wilson JW 1975 Some effects of shock on the lung's cellular components. The Proceedings of a Symposium on Recent Research Developments and Current Clinical Practice in Shock. Upjohn
141. Wilson JA 1976 Infection control in intravenous therapy. Heart and Lung 5: 430
142. Whittenberger JL, McGregor M, Berglund E, Borst HG 1960 Influence of state of inflation of the lung on pulmonary vascular resistance. Journal of Appplied Physiology 15: 878
143. Wyatt R, Glaves I 1974 Proximal skin necrosis after radial-artery cannulation. Lancet 1: 1135
144. Youngberg JA, Miller ED 1976 Evaluation of percutaneous cannulations of the dorsalis pedis artery. Anesthesiology 44: 80
145. Zapol WM, Snider MT 1977 Pulmonary hypertension in severe acute respiratory failure. New England Journal of Medicine 296: 476

4

Anesthesia Considerations for Patients Undergoing Palliative or Reparative Operations for Congenital Heart Disease

Roger A. Moore

INCIDENCE OF CONGENITAL HEART DISEASE

The reported incidence of congenital heart disease varies depending on the age of the children studied, the geographical location of the patient population, and many other factors. The New England Regional Infant Cardiac Program report indicated that only 0.24 percent of live births resulted in children diagnosed as having congenital heart disease in the first year of life,[51] while others have found an incidence closer to 0.8 percent.[40,113] A study by the National Center of Health Statistics[138] revealed that as many as 2 percent of children had congenital heart disease and 4 percent of adolescents had some form of heart disease. No matter what the actual incidence, the child born with congenital heart disease is at risk. Without effective therapeutic intervention as many as 50 percent of these children will die within the first year of life,[51,112] and one third of these deaths can be expected within the first month.[109,112] These dramatic statistics underline the driving force that has led to the major advances in pediatric cardiovascular surgery and pediatric cardiovascular anesthesia over the past few decades. Surgery and anesthesia have been closely linked, with innovations in one field initiating and complementing advances in the other. There is no better illustration of this than the incidents surrounding the first cardiac surgical procedure. In 1937 Graybiel successfully ligated a patent ductus arteriosus only to have the patient die from aspiration of gastric contents.[65] The use of endotracheal tubes and muscle relaxants provided better control of the airway and ventilation for patients requiring thoracotomy.[52,169]

Gibbon's development of the heart-lung machine and its first successful use for an 18-year-old girl undergoing closure of an atrial septal defect at the Thomas Jefferson Medical College in Philadelphia[56] paved the way for the present development of cardiothoracic surgery and anesthesia. Complete cardiac repairs for congenital heart defects are being performed at earlier and earlier ages without the use of intervening palliative procedures.[21,27,58,78,103,158] Though technical difficulties are certainly greater with smaller children, the benefits of early complete correction, including the elimination of the psychological and physical stresses that a second operation later in life produces, outweigh the technical difficulties. However, continual reassessment of the mortality associated with complete repair at an early age compared to the morbidity and mortality of combining an early palliative operation with a later complete corrective procedure must be made.[27,103] In addition, children with early, complete repairs must be followed closely to determine if revisions or enlargements of the initial operation are necessary, possibly defeating the purpose of the early, complete repair.

PREOPERATIVE EVALUATION

Anatomic, physiologic and pharmacokinetic features of infants and children require special management techniques when providing anesthesia for these patients. The pediatric patient with congenital heart disease has additional requirements caused by the cardiac lesion and the severity of cardiac decompensation. The patient's management will be largely directed by the findings during the preoperative evaluation. The primary goals of this evaluation are to (1) gain a detailed understanding of the patient's general physical condition, (2) develop a special understanding of a child's cardiac lesions, (3) prepare the child and family psychologically for the operative procedure, and (4) determine an anesthetic plan appropriate for that patient's specific needs.

Medical History

The history-taking portion of the preoperative visit is used to gather pertinent medical information needed to prepare an anesthetic plan and to reduce the anxiety of the child and the family.[41,79] The anesthesiologist's primary role is to provide comfort and safety to the child during the operative procedure, thereby making him the child's protector and friend. The often unstated fear children have prior to surgery is that they will be awake during the operation, and the anesthesiologist needs to firmly address this issue with each child. The other major fear that some children have prior to cardiac surgery is that of dying.[11] These children need confident reassurance so they can approach the surgical procedure with a positive outlook. Some evidence suggests that severe anxiety and feelings of doom may increase the risk of a morbid result.[86,87] Persistence of the child's feeling of impending death may be an indication for delaying surgery until appropriate psychological support can be obtained. A simple nonthreatening explanation of what will occur in the operating room will dispel most of the fear generated from facing the unknown. Allowing the child to take a familiar toy or security object to the operating room also serves as added reassurance.

The medical history should include routine questions concerning allergies, medications, past medical history, and previous anesthetic experiences. Questions should be asked about the child's activity level to get some indication of the patient's cardiac reserve. An increase in the number or duration of cyanotic episodes, increasing fatigability and shortness of breath, or increasing feeding difficulties, especially in the infant, all point to a deteriorating cardiorespiratory state.

Medications

The pediatric cardiac patient may be taking a variety of drugs preoperatively. Diuretics may be given to the patient with congestive heart failure while digitalis is used for both congestive heart failure and arrhythmia control. Patients with idiopathic hypertrophic subaortic stenosis or infundibular pulmonic stenosis may be taking beta-blockers such as propranolol. In general, if the patient requires medication for prevention of cardiac decompensation preoperatively, the drug should be continued up to the time of surgery. The major exception to this rule is digitalis, which should be discontinued at least 24 hours prior to an operation requiring cardiopulmonary bypass. Studies of serial serum digitalis levels following bypass indicate an unexplained increase in the serum digitalis level.[26,31,119] This elevation, in conjunction with the fall in serum potassium that occurs frequently following bypass, can lead to potentially fatal ventricular and supraventricular arrhythmias.[26,119] Patients who have undergone recent digitalization may be at even greater risk for arrhythmias.[91]

Prophylactic antibiotics are also frequently given to the congenital heart patient in the preoperative period for subacute bacterial endocarditis prophylaxis and as a means to decrease postoperative wound infection.[48,123] The American Heart Association recommends subacute bacterial endocarditis prophylaxis for any patient undergoing cardiac surgery, and specific recommendations are indicated in Table 4.1.[83] In addition, any child who has a cardiac lesion or who has had either palliative or reparative cardiac surgery should receive subacute bacterial endocarditis prophylaxis for the remainder of his life for any surgery or manipulation performed on his oral cavity, upper airway, gastrointestinal tract, genital urinary tract, or infected sites.[83] The only exceptions to this rule are those patients who have undergone an uncomplicated secundum atrial septal defect closure or patent ductus arteriosus ligation. For these patients, subacute bacterial endocarditis prophylaxis need be provided for only the 6 month period following the cardiac operation.[80,84,120]

Physical Examination

A good indication of how the child is physically withstanding his cardiac disease is the location on the growth grids of his height, weight, and head circumference. Since 8.5 percent of children with symptomatic congenital heart disease fall into a specific syndrome category,[67] an attempt should be made to identify what, if any, syndrome each child may have. It is important to make this identification to anticipate associated anesthetic problems which may affect the patient's anesthetic management. An example of this is the increased anticholinergic sensitivity that may occur with Down's syndrome patients[71] or the airway management problems that children with Treacher Collins or Pierre Robin syndromes can present. The child's heart rate and blood pressure should be noted and considered in relation to his age (Figs. 4.1 and 4.2). Since infants depend on increases in heart rate rather than stroke volume to increase cardiac output, the presence of bradycardia usually indicates a critically ill child that needs immediate attention. Bradycardia, with its attendant low output, can rapidly lead to hypoxemia, acidosis, and cardiac arrest.

Particular attention should be placed on the child's upper airway. Teeth first begin to erupt between 7 and 9 months of age, and the child begins losing primary teeth between 6 and 8 years of age. A large tongue, narrow palate, and mandibular hypoplasia are all conditions that can lead to difficulty in airway management. The higher metabolic requirements of children, in conjunction with their relatively small functional residual lung capacity,[121] put them at risk for the development

Table 4.1. Subacute Bacterial Endocarditis Prophylaxis for Children

I. Dental procedures and instrumentation or surgery of the upper respiratory tract
  A. For most congenital and rheumatic cardiac defects
    1. *Parenteral-oral combination*
       Aqueous crystalline penicillin G (30,000 U/kg IM) mixed with procaine penicillin G (600,000 U IM) given 30 minutes to 1 hour prior to procedure and penicillin V 250 mg (for children less than 60 lbs.) or 500 mg (for children over 60 lbs.) orally every 6 hours for 8 doses.
    2. *Oral only*
       Penicillin V 2 g orally 30 minutes to 1 hour prior to procedure and then 500 mg orally every 6 hours for 8 doses for children over 60 lbs. If less than 60 lbs. use initial dose of 1 g with 250 mg maintenance doses.
    3. *Allergy to penicillin*
       Vancomycin 20 mg/kg IV over 30 minutes to 1 hour prior to procedure (maximum dose of 44 mg/kg/24 hours) followed by erythromycin 10 mg/kg orally every 6 hours for 8 doses, *OR* 20 mg/kg erythromycin orally 90 minutes to 2 hours prior to procedure and then 10 mg/kg every 6 hours for 8 doses.
  B. For children with prosthetic valves or on long-term oral penicillin therapy
    1. Aqueous crystalline penicillin G (30,000 U/kg IM) mixed with procaine penicillin G (600,000 U IM) plus streptomycin (20 mg/kg IM given 30 minutes to 1 hour prior to the procedure) then penicillin V 500 mg (for children over 60 lbs.) or 250 mg (for children less than 60 lbs.) orally every 6 hours for 8 doses.
    2. *Allergy to penicillin*
       Combination of intravenous vancomycin and oral erythromycin as indicated above.

II. Genitourinary tract and gastrointestinal tract instrumentation or surgery
    1. Aqueous crystalline penicillin G (30,000 U/kg IM or IV) or ampicillin (50 mg/kg IM or IV) plus gentamycin (2.0 mg/kg IM or IV not to exceed 80 mg) or streptomycin (20 mg/kg IM). Initial doses should be given 30 minutes to 1 hour prior to procedure. If gentamycin is used, then give a similar dose of gentamycin and penicillin (or ampicillin) every 8 hours for two additional doses. If streptomycin is used, then give a similar dose of streptomycin and penicillin (or ampicillin) every 12 hours for two additional doses.
    2. *Allergy to penicillin*
       Vancomycin (20 mg/kg IV over 30 minutes to 1 hour) plus streptomycin (20 mg/kg IM). A single dose of these antibiotics begun 30 minutes to 1 hour prior to the procedure is probably sufficient but the same dose may be repeated in 12 hours.

III. Cardiac Surgery
    1. A penicillinase resistant penicillin or cephalosporin antibiotic started shortly before the operative procedure and continued for no more than 3–5 days postoperatively.

(Adapted from Kaplan E, Anthony B, Bisno A, Durack D, House H, Millard H, Sanford J, Shulman S, Stillerman M, Taranta A, Wenger N 1977. Prevention of bacterial endocarditis. Circulation 56: 139A–143A, by permission of the American Heart Association, Inc.)

of hypoxemia during airway obstruction. This is particularly true for those children with cyanotic congenital heart disease and hyperactive pulmonary vasculature. The child's airway normally differs from the adult's in a number of important ways.[39,106] The epiglottis is more elongated, and the larynx is located higher in the neck (C3 to C4 compared to C7 in the adult). The cricoid ring limits the diameter of the child's airway, and an endotracheal tube, which passes through the vocal cords, may not pass into the trachea. The relatively small length of the trachea in the infant can lead to displacement of the endotracheal tube, either into a mainstem bronchus or out of the trachea, with movement of the child's head.[164]

Pulses should be checked in all extremities. Patients who have undergone Blalock-Taussig operations will be missing the arm pulses on the shunted side. The remainder of the examination should be directed toward assessing the severity

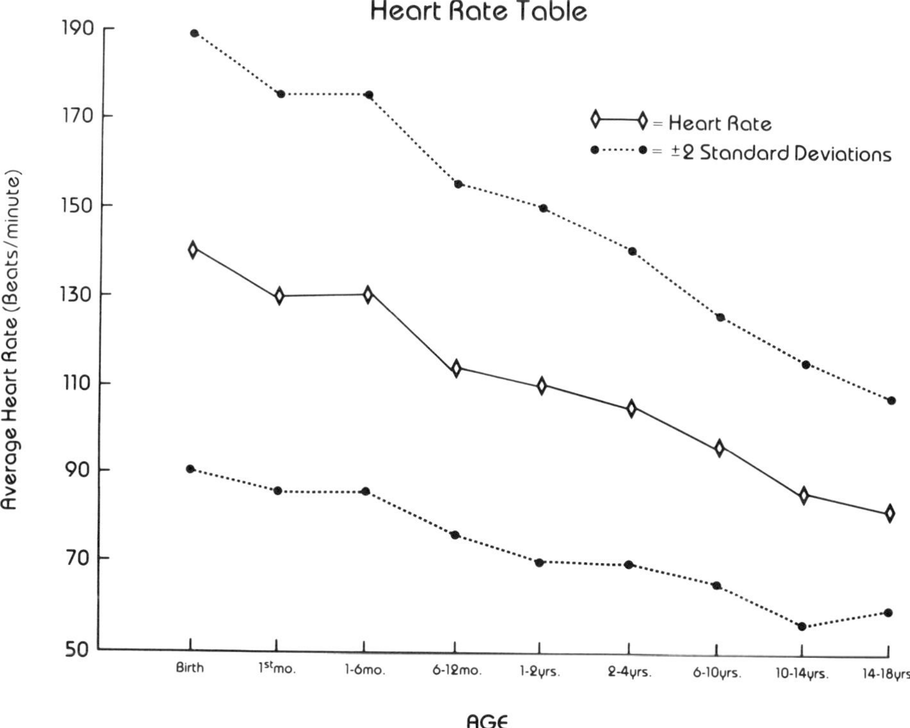

Fig. 4.1. Changes in resting heart rate with age in normal children. (Data from Lowrey GH 1986 Growth and Development of Children, 8th edn., Year Book Medical Publishers, Inc., Chicago.)

of congestive heart failure. When heart failure occurs in a child, it is usually biventricular, and nonspecific signs such as anorexia, irritability, and excessive perspiration may be the predominant findings. Hepatomegaly, jugular venous distension, tachypnea and rales are commonly found.[124]

Laboratory Studies

Review of the chest roentgenogram, electrocardiogram, and blood analysis should be undertaken to discover any major deviations from normal. Particular attention should be placed on the complete blood count. The hypoxic stimulation in cyanotic heart disease leads to an increase in erythropoesis. The physiologic effect of this for the child is not only a marked increase in hematocrit—occasionally to values over 70 percent—but also expansion of the patient's blood volume.[112] Significant hypervolemia may result from the increased red cell volume. As the red cell mass increases, the blood viscosity also increases, producing sheering forces great enough to impede peripheral tissue perfusion.[89] This state exists when a hematocrit is over 70 percent and may lead to a progressive metabolic acidosis. Transient periods of dehydration, normally tolerated by a child with a lower hematocrit, can lead to end organ thrombosis and infarction. Infarctions are particularly common in the pulmonary[46] and cerebral[132] vascular beds. Polycythemia is also associated with

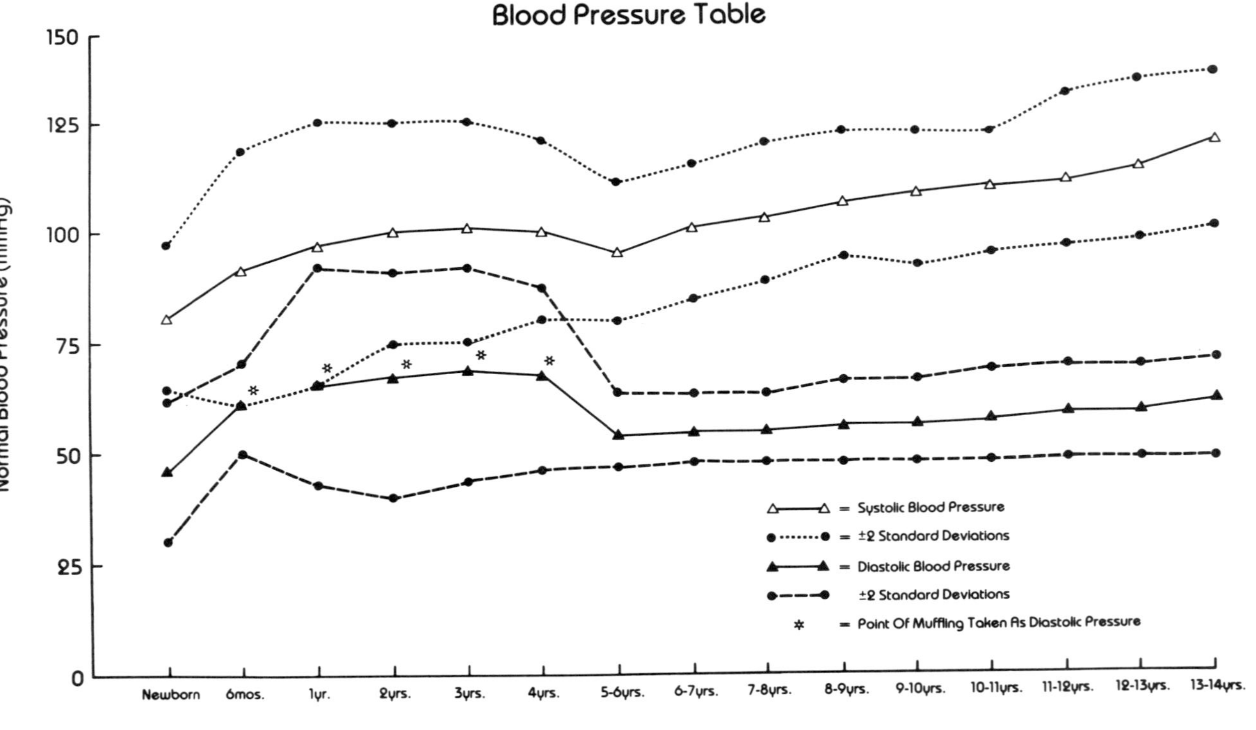

Fig. 4.2. Change in resting systolic and diastolic blood pressures with age in normal children. (Data from Nadas AS, Fyler DC 1972 Pediatric Cardiology, 3rd edn., WB Saunders, Philadelphia.)

an altered state of coagulation. Decreased clotting factors, increased fibrinolysis, and both quantitative and qualitative platelet dysfunction may occur in the congenital cardiac patient.[44,59,88,90] Prolongation of the prothrombin time and partial thromboplastin time may be seen as part of the coagulation profile.

Children with significant polycythemia who are scheduled for cardiac surgery may benefit from a preoperative red blood cell pheresis. For children having cardiac lesions with pulmonary blood flow independent of the systemic circuit, a reduction in blood viscosity will produce an increase in both total and effective pulmonary blood flow.[98,143] However, when the pulmonary blood flow is primarily derived from the systemic circuit, a drop in hematocrit may actually lead to a fall in pulmonary blood flow and a further reduction in systemic oxygenation.[143] Red blood cell pheresis is of benefit in correcting the abnormal coagulopathies of pediatric cardiac patients. Immediately following a blood volume exchange of 20 ml/kg with fresh-frozen plasma, platelet abnormalities improve; and normal platelet function returns within 3 days.[108] If red blood cell pheresis is not performed, consideration must be given to preoperative intravenous hydration during the period when oral fluids are withheld. Newborns may have bleeding problems on the basis of reduced liver-dependent coagulation factors. These children may benefit from an intramuscular or intravenous dose of vitamin K.

The absolute platelet count should be noted. Although the increased intravascular volume in children who are severely polycythemic[142] and the decreased volume in children on diuretic therapy for congestive heart failure can affect the absolute platelet count, the count is still of use in indicating the general quantity of platelets available. For patients undergoing cardiopulmonary bypass, platelets should be readily available for transfusion if (1) the platelet count is less than 120,000 platelets/mm^3, (2) the child has a cyanotic congenital heart defect, (3) the thoracic cavity is being entered for a second time, or (4) the child has been taking an aspirin-containing medication within the week prior to the operation.

Children with congestive heart failure, particularly infants, are prone to the development of hypoglycemia[17,170] and hypocalcemia.[21] These children will occasionally show signs of jitteriness, tachypnea, and tachycardia, but most have no pathognomonic signs. Therefore, these laboratory values need to be noted preoperatively for the child at risk, and continually assessed throughout the intraoperative and postoperative periods.

Serum electrolytes should be checked with particular attention to a low serum potassium in the digitalized patient. Finally, an arterial blood gas analysis in cyanotic children can be helpful in determining the amount of oxygen reserve. An oxygen saturation less than 75 percent indicates that the child has little reserve and that meticulous airway management will be necessary during induction.

Valuable data are derived from the cardiac catheterization. The written report may provide information helpful in planning the anesthetic, but does not substitute for a direct evaluation of the angiogram to obtain a better understanding of the contractile state of the heart, the various chamber sizes, and the severity of outlet obstruction. This evaluation is best performed in the presence of both the cardiologist and surgeon, thereby providing an opportunity for interdisciplinary exchange of ideas for the optimal management of the patient.

Table 4.2. Various Factors Affecting the Hemodynamic State

Preload:	
Increase:	Intravascular volume expansion
	Capacitance vessel constriction—phenylephrine
Decrease:	Intravascular volume depletion—third space losses, bleeding
	Capacitance vessel dilation—nitroglycerin, trimethaphan, nitroprusside
Pulmonary vascular resistance:	
Increase:	↑ PCO_2, ↓ PO_2, acidosis
	Arteriolar constrictors—ketamine
Decrease:	↓ PCO_2, ↑ PO_2, alkalosis
	Arteriolar dilators—tolazoline, nitroprusside
Systemic vascular resistance:	
Increase:	Arteriolar constrictors—phenylephrine
	Anesthetics—ketamine, nitrous oxide
Decrease:	Arteriolar dilators—nitroprusside, isoproterenol
	Anesthetics—droperidol, isoflurane
	Relaxants—curare
	Calcium channel blockers
Heart rate:	
Increase:	Anticholinergics—atropine, scopolamine, glycopyrrolate
	Relaxants—pancuronium, gallamine
Decrease:	Digoxin, propranolol, verapamil
Contractility:	
Increase:	Inotropes—epinephrine, dopamine, dolbutamine, isoproterenol
	Calcium
Decrease:	β blockers and calcium channel blockers
	All inhalational anesthetics

CARDIAC GRID

Following the preoperative visit, a safe plan for managing the child's intraoperative course should be formulated. Deciding how to best manage a critically ill patient may be extremely confusing. The stability of the child's cardiovascular state may be altered by a wide spectrum of pharmacologic and physiologic manipulations. (Table 4.2) The goal of a safe and stable operative course can be unintentionally thwarted by inducing an undesired change in the patient's hemodynamic status that is contradictory to his cardiovascular needs. This may lead to cardiovascular decompensation ending in death. Because of this, a hemodynamic profile or a cardiac grid should be made for each patient before formulation of an anesthetic plan.[116] The cardiac grid should take into consideration a number of factors, including the patient's age, cardiac lesion, and associated medical problems. The purpose of the cardiac grid is to show how the five hemodynamic factors—preload, systemic vascular resistance, pulmonary vascular resistance, heart rate, and contractility—can best be manipulated to optimize intraoperative hemodynamic stability. A number of commonly encountered congenital defects are listed in Table 4.3 with suggestions on how each of the hemodynamic factors can be changed to optimize cardiovascular stability. From such a grid, one can begin to predict which pharmacologic and physiologic manipulations might help a given patient. For example, a child with tetralogy of Fallot has a cardiac lesion made up of four com-

Table 4.3. Cardiac Grid for Common Congenital Heart Diseases (Desired Hemodynamic Changes)

	Preload	Pulmonary Vascular Resistance	Systolic Vascular Resistance	HR	Contractility
ASD (L → R)	↑	↑	↓	N	N
VSD (R → L)	N	↓	↑	N	N
VSD (L → R)	↑	↑	↓	N	N
IHSS	↑	N	N – ↑	*↓	*↓
PDA	↑	↑	↓	N	N
Coarct.	↑	N	↓	N	N
Valvular PS	↑	↓	N	↓	↑
Infundibular PS	↑	↓	N	↓	*↓
AS	↑	N	*↑	*↓	N – ↑
MS	↑	N – ↓	N	*↓	N – ↑
AR	↑	N	↓	N – ↑	N – ↑
MR	↑	N – ↓	↓	N – ↑	N – ↑

* An overriding consideration.

Key: ASD = atrial septal defect; VSD = ventricular septal defect; IHSS = idiopathic hypertrophic subaortic stenosis; PDA = patent ductus arteriosus; PS = pulmonary stenosis; AS = aortic stenosis; AR = aortic regurgitation; MR = mitral regurgitation; MS = mitral stenosis; N = normal. (Adapted from Moore R 1981 Anesthesia for the pediatric congenital heart patient for noncardiac surgery. Anesthesiology Review 8: 23.)

ponents—overriding aorta, right ventricular hypertrophy, ventricular septal defect with right-to-left shunting, and pulmonic stenosis (usually infundibular). The effect of the overriding aorta on the child's total hemodynamic state is insignificant until the heart has been repaired, at which time there may be a component of left ventricular outflow tract obstruction. As for right ventricular hypertrophy, a higher preload may be necessary in order for the ventricle to function on an optimal portion of the Starling curve. To reduce the arterial desaturation resulting from right-to-left shunting across the ventricular septal defect, hemodynamic manipulation should include a reduction in pulmonary vascular resistance and augmentation of the systemic vascular resistance. Finally, the presence of infundibular pulmonic stenosis requires the control of heart rate and contractility. Increases in either of these hemodynamic parameters can cause a dramatic fall in pulmonary blood flow. Therefore, this patient should be managed intraoperatively with the preload augmented with fluid, use of pharmacologic agents which increase peripheral vascular resistance, and avoidance of positive chronotropes and inotropes, until the pulmonary outflow obstruction is surgically relieved.

Obviously, modifications of this hemodynamic matrix will be necessary when the changing intraoperative state of the patient introduces new variables. Once the child's palliative, closed heart, or complete cardiac repair is performed, the anesthetist is dealing with a new hemodynamic state. Therefore, a new cardiac grid must be considered. The reasoning necessary to produce each cardiac grid creates a more comprehensive approach to the intraoperative management.

PREMEDICATION

The child's anesthetic begins with the preoperative visit where the development of trust and reassurance can pave the way for a quiet and cooperative child arriving in the operating room.[79] Not only will induction of anesthesia be aided by this psychological preparation, but the patient's postoperative course may also be smoother.[41]

The pharmacologic beginning of the anesthetic is premedication. Numerous agents have been used as premedicants, but they all fall into three basic categories: (1) anticholinergics, (2) sedative-hypnotics, and (3) analgesics.

The purpose of the anticholinergic is to provide a dry airway, thereby reducing secretions that can lead to aspiration or laryngeal spasm. Another purpose is to prevent vagally induced bradycardia during laryngoscopy and intubation. This feature is particularly important for the infant who depends on his heart rate for maintenance of cardiac output. The most widely used anticholinergic is atropine (0.02 mg/kg with a minimum dose of 0.15 mg and a maximum dose of 0.4 mg IM). Within 15 minutes of an intramuscular dose of atropine the antisialagogic effects are evident. The vagolytic cardiac effects may need supplementation at the time of intubation. Scopolamine is also frequently used (0.01 mg/kg, maximum dose 0.4 mg IM). Its major advantages over atropine are a more intensive antisialagogic effect and a greater sedation, reversible with physostigmine. Scopolamine, however, does not block vagally induced bradycardia as well as atropine.[49] Glycopyrrolate (0.01 mg/kg IM) is a quaternary ammonium anticholinergic which does not cross the blood-brain barrier. It has an intense antisialagogic action of longer duration than either atropine or scopolamine, while the vagolytic effects are less intense, as indicated by less tachycardia with intravenous injection.[35] Paradoxically, glycopyrrolate may be more protective than atropine against bradyarrhythmias when given in combination with an anticholinesterase, such as neostigmine for reversal of muscle relaxants.[173] It also provides a greater reduction in gastric volume and acidity[148] than other anticholinergics.

A wide range of sedative hypnotic drugs have been used and are still being developed as premedicants. The large variety indicates that no particular agent is optimal. The more commonly used drugs include secobarbitol (4 mg/kg, maximum 100 mg IM), pentobarbitol (4 mg/kg, maximum 100 mg IM), hydroxyzine (2 mg/kg IM or PO, maximum 50 mg),[141] promethazine (1 mg/kg IM, maximum 25 mg),[149] and diazepam (0.6 mg/kg PO, maximum 10 mg).[141] In addition, rectal administration of a short-acting barbiturate such as methohexital (20 mg/kg) has been advocated for premedication of pediatric cardiac patients.[102] If barbiturates are used as premedicants, half the calculated dose is frequently used in unstable patients because of their potential for myocardial depression.

Agents used for analgesia include the narcotics morphine (0.1 to 0.2 mg/kg IM, maximum 10 mg)[137] and meperidine (1 mg/kg IM, maximum 100 mg) and the combination of 75 μg/kg droperidol and 1.5 μg/kg fentanyl (Innovar). All narcotics produce a dose-related respiratory depression so they should be used carefully in children with signs of respiratory insufficiency or the potential for airway obstruction. Inadvertant intravenous administration can lead to severe tachycardia with meperidine or hypotension in the case of morphine or a fentanyl-droperidol combination.

The choice of premedicant will be based in part on the child's disease and in part on the anesthesiologist's preference. One view is that premedicants should be as light as possible to prevent adverse physiologic effects during a time when the child is not under the anesthesiologist's direct supervision. For cardiac surgery, a

Table 4.4. Recommendation for Premedication*

0–6 months	Atropine, 0.02 mg/kg (min. 0.15 mg)
6–12 months	Atropine, 0.02 mg/kg Pentobarbitol, 2 mg/kg
Over 12 months	Scopolamine, 0.01 mg/kg (max. 0.4 mg) or atropine, 0.02 mg/kg (max. 0.4 mg) Pentobarbitol, 2 mg/kg (max. 100 mg) Morphine, 0.2 mg/kg (max. 10 mg)

* The premedicant should be given intramuscularly 1 hour prior to the time the child is expected to arrive in the operating room. Modification of the morphine dose downward is advised for children with preexisting airway problems.

more widely held view is that a potent premedicant should be given to lessen stress in the preinduction period that may lead to cardiovascular deterioration.[69] A proven premedication to produce a quiet, often sleeping child is indicated in Table 4.4.

PREOPERATIVE PREPARATION AND MONITORING

Prior to the arrival of the child, the operating room must be prepared. Appropriate for any operative procedure is the checking of the suction apparatus, anesthesia circuit, and anesthesia machine, as well as the selection of airway and endotracheal intubation equipment. For a pediatric cardiac operation, a selection of drugs must be prepared in advance, in concentrations appropriate for the child's weight. A list of drugs and dosages that should be available for a child undergoing heart surgery is shown in Table 4.5. Only one inotropic infusion need be prepared ahead of time (usually dopamine or isoproterenol). A simple, easy, and fast method of preparing an infusion of dopamine or dobutamine is to place the number of milligrams of drugs equal to the child's weight in kilograms into 100 ml of 5 percent dextrose. The resulting concentration will provide 5 μg/kg/min of the drug when run at a rate of 0.5 ml/min. In children under 10 kg of body weight this concentration will give too large a fluid load, so the concentration can be increased by a factor of 10 with a corresponding decrease in infusion rate.

Precautions must be taken to prevent introduction of air when giving any intravenous injection to a child with an intracardiac shunt. The same warning applies for the insertion of intravascular cannulae. The reason for this precaution is that air may cross the intracardiac shunt into the systemic circulation and produce brain, kidney, or other organ infarction. Even children with predominantly left-to-right shunts are at risk for systemic embolization since a shunt is rarely entirely unidirectional throughout the cardiac cycle. Some precautions to minimize the chance of air bubble embolization are listed in Table 4.6.

Decisions concerning the type, extent, and location of monitoring for the operation should be made prior to the child's arrival to the operating room. All children should have minimum monitoring including an electrocardiogram, blood pressure cuff, rectal thermistor, and esophageal or precordial stethoscope. Children undergoing palliative or closed cardiac procedures should usually have an arterial cannula placed as well. The location of the arterial cannula is determined by the

Table 4.5. Nonanesthetic Drugs Used Frequently During Pediatric Open Heart Surgery

Agent	Initial Intravenous Dose
Drugs to be prepared for each case	
Atropine sulfate	0.02 mg/kg
Calcium chloride or	10 mg/kg
calcium gluconate	30 mg/kg
Lidocaine	1 mg/kg
Sodium bicarbonate (mEq)	$\frac{0.3 \times \text{body weight (kg)} \times \text{base deficit}}{2}$
Phenylephrine	1 μg/kg (double subsequent doses to effect)
Trimethaphan	10 μg/kg (double subsequent doses to effect)
Epinephrine	1.0–10 μg/kg (use higher dose for cardiac arrest)
Heparin	0.5–1 mg/kg for partial heparinization, 4 mg/kg for full heparinization
Protamine Sulfate	1 mg/100 U active heparin
One inotropic infusion	
Epinephrine	0.1 μg/kg/min (increase to effect)
Dopamine	5 μg/kg/min (increase to effect)
Isoproterenol	0.05 μg/kg/min (increase to effect)
Dolbutamine	5 μg/kg/min (increase to effect)
Drugs to have available but not prepared	
Glycopyrrolate	0.01 mg/kg
Scopolamine	0.01 mg/kg
Edrophonium	0.01 mg/kg
Neostigmine	0.07 mg/kg
Nitroglycerin	0.5 μg/kg/min (increase to effect)
Sodium nitroprusside	0.1 μg/kg/min (increase to effect but do not exceed 10 μg/kg/min)
Chloropromazine	0.1 mg/kg slowly
Propranolol	10 μg/kg slowly
Procainamide	2 mg/kg slowly
Bretylium	5 mg/kg slowly
Diphenylhydantoin	4 mg/kg slowly
Verapamil	0.05 mg/kg slowly (max. 2.5 mg, repeated to effect)
Glucogon	0.05 mg/kg
Glucose (50%)	250 mg/kg
Hydrocortisone	20 mg/kg
Theophylline	4 mg/kg slowly
Naloxone	0.01 mg/kg
Potassium chloride (mEq)	$\frac{0.3 \times \text{body weight (kg)} \times [\text{desired } K^+ \text{ (mEq)} - \text{serum } K^+ \text{ (mEq)}]}{2}$
Diphenhydramine	0.3 mg/kg
Mannitol	0.5 gm/kg
Furosemide	0.05 mg/kg (double subsequent doses to effect)
Ethacrynic	0.5 mg/kg
ε-Amino caproic acid	70 mg/kg

procedure. If a shunt using the right subclavian artery is to be performed, the right radial artery should not be the site used for arterial cannula insertion. For patent ductus arteriosus ligations or repair of aortic coarctation, the right radial is preferred over the left due to potential dampening of the trace during periods of compression or partial cross-clamping of the left subclavian. Two intravenous cannulae are suggested for palliative and closed heart procedures, should rapid volume replacement be required.

For open heart procedures, further monitoring should include additional tem-

Table 4.6. Precautions for the Prevention of Intravascular Air Bubbles

1. Clear all air bubbles from intravenous tubing (especially at injection ports) prior to use.
2. Insure a free flow of blood and intravenous fluid from intravascular cannula and intravenous tubing during connection.
3. Inject small amount of solution from syringe before giving intravenous injection in order to clear air from needle and syringe hub.
4. Avoid injecting last milliliter from syringe due to air bubbles on plunger.
5. Use air bubble detectors and air traps on intravenous tubing whenever possible.
6. Never leave central venous pressure cannula open to air when patient can develop a negative intrathoracic pressure.

perature probes (nasopharyngeal and toe), urinary catheter, and central venous pressure catheter. After discussion with the surgeons, transducers should also be prepared for use when intraoperative left atrial, right atrial or pulmonary artery catheters are to be inserted. A discussion of these monitoring devices for the purpose of making therapeutic decisions can be found in other chapters. Finally, a defibrillator with paddles appropriate to the age and size of the child should be available and ready for use.

Anesthetic Systems

The routine circle system, which recirculates gases and eliminates carbon dioxide, is adequate for children over 15 kg.[147] This system has a number of disadvantages for the smaller child, including increased air-flow resistance due to valves, increased dead space predisposing the patient to carbon dioxide retention, and bulkiness, especially at the endotracheal tube connection. Numerous alternative systems have been devised based on modifications of the Ayers T-piece. One particularly useful system is the Mapleson D circuit.[104]

The Mapleson D system provides direct fresh gas inflow at the point of connection to the endotracheal tube, thereby decreasing dead space (Fig. 4.3A). The expiratory limb of this system extends from the endotracheal connector, allowing one to modify the amount of rebreathing and therefore the amount of carbon dioxide retention by adjusting fresh gas flow. An expiratory gas valve and gas reservoir are placed at the end of the expiratory limb. The Bain modification of the Mapleson D system redirects the fresh gas flow through a small tube situated inside the expiratory limb (Fig. 4.3B).[6] This serves to decrease the bulkiness of the system and decreases the chance of intraoperative extubation. Adjustment of the fresh gas inflow during controlled ventilation without adjustment of minute ventilation can produce marked changes in carbon dioxide elimination. Too low a flow can lead to excessive rebreathing and accumulation of carbon dioxide. Suggested fresh gas flows for children less than 10 kg is at least 2 L/min while children over 10 kg should have 3.5 L/min or more total gas flow.[7,8,68]

Fresh gas is constantly presented to the patient when using the Mapleson D circuit. Gases supplied from a central system are not humidified and can produce tracheal hyperemia, thickening of bronchial secretions, and ineffectual cilliary action.[133] For this reason, humidification of inspired gases is suggested; a number of reliable methods are available.[45]

A.

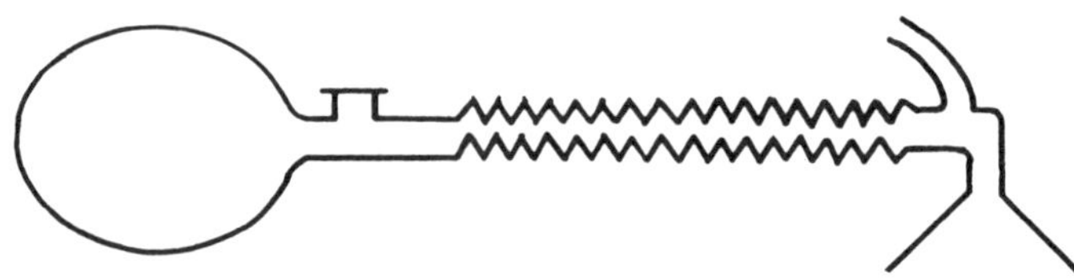

B.

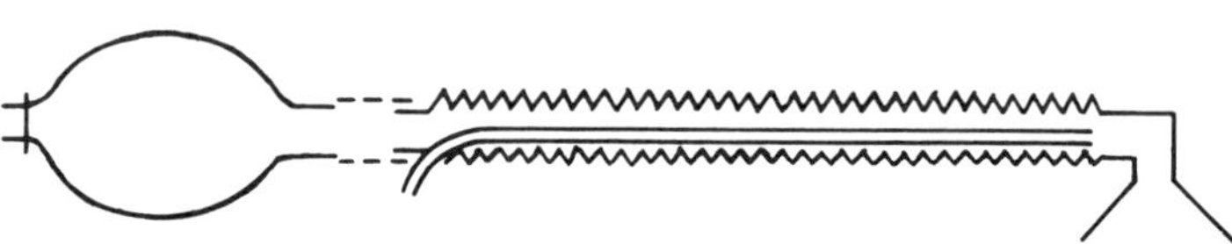

Fig. 4.3. Anesthetic breathing systems: (A) Mapleson-D anesthetic breathing system. Note gas supply enters system near endotracheal tube connector. (Mapleson WW 1954 The elimination of rebreathing in various semi-closed anaesthetic systems. British Journal of Anaesthesia 26: 323.) (B) Modified Mapleson-D (Bain). Note gas supply enters system near reservoir bag, travels through expiratory tubing, and releases the gas at endotracheal tube connector. (Bain JA, Spoerel W 1972 A streamlined anaesthetic system. Canadian Anaesthetists' Society Journal 19: 426.)

ANESTHETIC INDUCTION

The choice of anesthetic for induction will be based on a number of factors, including the hemodynamic requirements indicated by the cardiac grid, the child's level of awareness and anxiety on arrival in the operating room, the severity of the child's illness, associated medical problems, and the presence or absence of an intravenous cannula. The primary goal is to induce anesthesia with the least possible cardiovascular and psychological stress.

Anesthetic induction agents fall into two major classifications: parenteral and inhalational. Of the parenteral group the most commonly used drugs are thiopental, ketamine, morphine, and fentanyl. Although thiopental (4 mg/kg) is one of the drugs most frequently used for anesthesia induction during general surgical procedures, its use in cardiac surgery is limited. Direct cardiac depression as well as a decrease in systemic vascular resistance may produce a fall in blood pressure. A child with a right-to-left shunt may develop increased shunting and increased hypoxemia. In addition, the preinduction placement of an intravenous cannulae is required, which in the pediatric group can be a stressful experience for both patient and anesthesiologist. At present, thiopental's use in pediatric cardiac anesthesia is limited to the older and more stable child.[149]

Ketamine (1 to 4 mg/kg IV, or 4 to 10 mg/kg IM) is a "dissociative" agent which may provide excellent cardiovascular support in the critically ill patient.[47] The direct myocardial depressive effects are offset by central sympathetic stimulation, which can produce significant increases in heart rate, cardiac work, and systemic vascular resistance.[38,47] Because of these properties, some have found ketamine especially advantageous for use in cyanotic patients for both induction[134] and maintenance.[72] Increases in pulmonary vascular resistance, however, can also occur secondary to an increase in the cardiac output.[54,166] Induction with ketamine may be faster in patients with right-to-left shunting if the pulmonary circuit is partially bypassed. Other advantages include the ability to use higher inspired oxygen concentrations, antiarrhythmogenic actions,[38] and antibronchospastic properties in asthmatics.[5] Disadvantages include the need to give the drug parenterally, and the occurrence of respiratory depression,[177] as well as the potential for extensor spasm[135] and postoperative hallucinations.

Morphine sulfate (1 to 2 mg/kg IV) became popular in pediatric cardiac anesthesia after Lowenstein et al introduced high dose morphine as a sole anesthetic agent in adult cardiac patients.[100] Morphine has minimal cardiac depressant activity and it is not arrhythmogenic. It provides continued postoperative analgesia and allows the use of a high oxygen technique. Its primary disadvantage is the rapid drop in systemic vascular resistance mediated through direct arteriolar dilitation and histamine release. This could lead to sudden deterioration in a child with cyanotic heart disease. Also, bronchoconstriction due to histamine release,[5] prolonged postoperative respiratory depression,[72] and the need for an intravenous cannula prior to induction, all have limited its present use for pediatric cardiac anesthesia. Narcotics with fewer hemodynamic side effects have largely replaced morphine as a cardiac anesthetic.

Fentanyl (50 to 100 μg/kg IV) is a synthetic narcotic which has rapidly gained acceptance for cardiac anesthesia in adults due to its limited effects on the circulation.[153] It still has some of the disadvantages of all narcotics, such as prolonged respiratory depression and the need for preinduction placement of an intravenous cannulae. The cardiovascular stability maintained by the drug in the critically ill child, however, outweighs these disadvantages.[139] Rapid infusion of the drug can lead to chest wall spasm and bradycardia unless a vagolytic muscle relaxant such as pancuronium bromide is given early in the induction.

Inhalational anesthetics used frequently in cardiovascular surgery include nitrous oxide, halothane, and isoflurane. Nitrous oxide (minimum alveolar concentration—amount of anesthetic to prevent movement to stimuli—105 percent) was one of the earliest anesthetics used in pediatric cardiac surgery in combination with another inhalational agent.[70] As indicated by the minimum alveolar concentration (MAC), nitrous oxide alone is insufficient as a sole anesthetic in spite of the frequent use of a nitrous-oxide relaxant technique in neonatal surgery.[128,139] In neonates, its advantages are relative preservation of myocardial function and the ability to regulate inspired oxygen to prevent retrolental fibroplasia. Nitrous oxide is not innocuous however, expecially when used in combination with other agents. With morphine, nitrous oxide causes an increase in systemic vascular resistance, pulmonary vascular resistance, central venous pressure, and peak inspiratory pressure. It causes a decrease in heart rate, stroke volume, and blood pressure.[9,94,171] These effects are in part due to its inhibition of sympathetic tone.[163] Therefore, a patient with right heart failure might undergo further decompensation with nitrous oxide alone.[94] Other disadvantages include the inability to provide a high oxygen concentration, the enlargement of any embolized intravascular air bubbles, and the need for associated agents in order to provide adequate anesthesia. Because of these disadvantages, nitrous oxide is rarely used except to smooth the initial portion of an induction.

Halothane (MAC 0.8 percent) is a halogenated hydrocarbon which has been one of the most frequently used induction agents for pediatric cardiac anesthesia. It has a relatively pleasant odor and therefore is well tolerated by children during induction. The major disadvantage of halothane is its direct dose-related myocardial depressant effect.[9,110] In young children where MAC requirements approach the toxic dose of the drug, halothane can produce significant myocardial depression.[34,66,126] The heart is also sensitized to catecholamine-induced arrhythmias.[81] Systemic and pulmonary vascular resistances are maintained at fairly stable levels with the drug, however.[110,43] In spite of its disadvantages, halothane continues to be frequently used.[50,97] Its advantages include an atraumatic induction without the need for an intravenous cannula, ability to use a high oxygen technique, easy regulation of anesthetic dose, beta-blockade for patients with infundibular valvular stenosis, and the potential for early extubation. In patients who are critically ill or very young, halothane must be used with great care.[50]

Isoflurane (MAC 1.2 percent) is one of the newest widely used inhalational agents. Isoflurane causes less myocardial depression than halothane,[157] though at high concentrations cardiovascular collapse can occur.[155] Decreases in stroke volume due to cardiac depression are compensated for by an increase in heart rate leading to a stable cardiac output.[157] A reduction in systemic vascular resistance by the agent can lead to a fall in blood pressure.[77,155] Though the heart is sensitized to catecholamine-induced arrhythmias with isoflurane, this effect is less severe than seen with halothane.[81] A disadvantage of the drug is its noxious odor, which complicates its use in children. The increased heart rate and decreased peripheral vascular resistance can be undesirable hemodynamic changes for patients with some congenital heart defects.

One factor that determines which induction agent is best suited for a specific child is the child's level of consciousness upon arrival in the operating room. If the child arrives in the operating room sleeping peacefully, unless he is severely compromised hemodynamically, a "steal" technique can be used. Prior to moving the patient from the stretcher to the operating room table, an inhalational induction is performed without awakening the child. As soon as consciousness is lost, the child is moved to the operating room table and full monitoring is established. Obviously, the experience of the anesthesiologist is important in determining the depth of anesthesia in these cases. On the other hand, if the child enters the operating room awake and combative, either intramuscular ketamine or thiopental through a 25 gauge intravenous cannula will facilitate a relatively smooth induction. In both situations, once a good intravenous catheter has been inserted and the child is stable, a decision based on the patient's cardiovascular state can be made concerning the anesthetic agent to be used for maintenance.

Orotracheal intubation, rather than nasotracheal, is performed on most patients scheduled for open heart surgery. Trauma produced during a nasal intubation can lead to severe epistaxis following heparinization. If prolonged intubation is anticipated, the orotracheal tube can be exchanged for a nasotracheal tube at the conclusion of the operation.

Significance of Hemodynamic Factors During Induction

The rate of induction for an inhalational anesthetic can be affected by numerous factors, including minute ventilation, cardiac output, cerebral blood flow, and anesthetic solubility. With all children, and in particular the group with critical

Table 4.7. Blood/Gas Solubilities of a Number of Anesthetics

Nitrogen	0.01	Lowest Solubility
Cyclopropane	0.42	↓
Nitrous oxide	0.47	
Isoflurane	1.41	
Enflurane	1.78	
Halothane	2.36	
Ether (Diethyl)	12.1	Highest Solubility

cardiac defects, lessening the stress and length of induction can benefit the child's total intraoperative course. In order to have a rapid, smooth induction of anesthesia, an understanding of the principles of anesthesia uptake are necessary.

Ventilation

As blood flows through the pulmonary capillaries, inhalational anesthetics are taken up causing their alveolar concentration to fall. The more rapid the alveolar ventilation, the faster the replacement of the anesthetic in the alveoli, resulting in a relatively higher alveolar concentration. Therefore, a higher blood concentration can be achieved earlier leading to a faster induction. The solubility of the anesthetic agent also effects the speed of induction for patients with increased minute ventilation. The more soluble the anesthetic, the greater the effect ventilatory changes have on induction.[42] Table 4.7 lists the common anesthetic agents in order of their solubilities. An increase in minute ventilation has minimal effect on induction speed for an insoluble gas such as nitrous oxide but can be very important for a soluble agent such as ether. Another factor to be considered is the effect of hyperventilation on cerebral blood flow. Normally, a fall in carbon dioxide due to hyperventilation will lead to cerebral vascular constriction and a decrease in cerebral blood flow, thus decreasing the amount of anesthetic getting to the brain. In the case of poorly soluble agents, this effect on the cerebral blood vessels may even slow the onset of anesthesia. For more highly soluble agents, however, the effect of hyperventilation in providing increased alveolar concentrations predominates and induction speed is increased.[42,122] Another factor is that anesthetic agents themselves may directly effect the vasoactivity of the cerebral vasculature. The same factors are pertinent if hypoventilation occurs during induction. With soluble anesthetic agents, the induction time would be significantly slowed while little effect would be observed when insoluble anesthetics were used.

Cardiac output

The small child is directly dependent on heart rate for maintenance of cardiac output. During induction, estimation of changes in the child's cardiac output can be based upon changes in heart rate—particularly if bradycardia occurs. Increases in cardiac output produce increases in pulmonary blood flow (in the absence of major intracardiac shunts) which in turn lead to a more rapid uptake of anesthetic gases and a fall in alveolar anesthetic concentration. In spite of quantitatively more anesthetic being taken up, the concentration of the agent reaching the brain is lower. Therefore, increases in cardiac output tend to slow induction. Again, the solubility of the gas plays a major role; the more soluble agents are more greatly affected by changes in cardiac output than the insoluble agents.[42,122] In regard to intravenous induction agents, the higher the cardiac output is, the faster the delivery of the anesthetic agent will be to the brain. Thus, increasing cardiac output with intravenous inductions has a tendency to increase the induction speed.

Intracardiac shunts

Children with major congenital cardiac defects frequently have cardiac shunts which can influence induction time. Children with cyanotic lesions normally have right-to-left shunting of blood that bypasses the lungs leading to hypoperfusion of the pulmonary circuit. Acyanotic cardiac lesions with the existence of intracardiac shunts usually have a left-to-right flow of blood in which oxygenated blood is recirculated through the lungs, leading to an increased total pulmonary blood flow. Rarely does a child have a pure right-to-left or left-to-right shunt, however, since changing pressure relationships during the cardiac cycle produce bidirectional flow. Overall, however, the shunt usually is predominantly in one direction or the other. A change in the hemodynamic state of the child can lead to a change in this balance of shunting. A sudden drop in the systemic vascular resistance in a child with a balanced shunt could rapidly lead to a right-to-left shunt and cause a sudden drop in systemic oxygenation.

Right-to-left shunts Theoretically, with right-to-left shunting of blood in the heart, the blood which has traveled through the lungs and picked up anesthetic is diluted with blood which has bypassed the lungs and is relatively anesthetic-free. The blood leaving the heart would have a relatively lower anesthetic concentration, which would increase the induction time for an inhalational anesthetic.[42] This has been partially substantiated in a dog model where right-to-left shunting was produced by clamping the left mainstem bronchus.[160] Increases in arterial concentrations of insoluble anesthetics was delayed, though no change was seen for soluble agents. Clinical correlation was also obtained by showing a slower rate of rise of arteriolar halothane concentrations in patients with tetralogy of Fallot.[160] For intravenous induction agents, the speed of induction is slightly increased due to the time saved in bypassing the pulmonary circuit.

Left-to-right shunts Children with left-to-right shunts have blood which has already picked up inhaled anesthetic undergoing recirculation through the lungs. The recirculated blood picks up an even higher blood level of anesthetic,[42] causing a higher anesthetic concentration to exist in the blood leaving the heart. Theoretically, the speed of induction would be increased.[114] However, a computer model of left-to-right shunting indicates that this increased rate of induction would be clinically insignificant unless there was a coexistent, large right-to-left shunt.[161] In this situation, the induction speed for insoluble anesthetic agents would be significantly increased. Induction with an intravenous agent for a patient with a left-to-right shunt would be slowed since there would be a delay in the agent reaching the brain due to pulmonary recirculation.

Another factor which affects the amount of left-to-right shunting is the hematocrit. An increase in hematocrit without change in blood volume leads to a significant increase in pulmonary and systemic vascular resistances as well as a decrease in left-to-right shunting.[98] Higher hematocrits in critically ill patients with left-to-right intracardiac shunts may decrease the shunt and the degree of congestive heart failure.

Muscle Relaxants

Muscle relaxation is an integral part of pediatric cardiovascular anesthesia. Whether a depolarizing agent such as succinylcholine or a nondepolarizing agent such as d-tubocurarine, pancuronium, metocurine, or gallamine is used, the child's response to the drug differs from that of an adult. There is a continued maturation of the myoneural junction after birth.[61] Newborns seem to have less neuromuscular reserve to tetanic stimulation,[28] which would seem to predispose the child to increased susceptibility to muscle relaxants. However, evidence seems to point toward an increased requirement for both depolarizing and nondepolarizing muscle relaxants in the newborn and young child.[28,34,62,64,162] The relatively increased extracellular fluid space of the infant may explain the apparent resistance to muscle relaxants. This may also explain the wide variability of responses observed in different infants with the same drug dose.[25,127,145] One important observation is that depression of the respiratory muscles of infants seems to occur in parallel with peripheral muscle depression.[29] Therefore, in a child (as opposed to an adult) sparing of the respiratory muscles does not occur, predisposing the child to early respiratory depression.

The choice of muscle relaxant for the child with a cardiac lesion will depend in part on the child's hemodynamic needs, as indicated by the cardiac grid. One possible choice is succinylcholine (1 to 2 mg/kg IV, 4 mg/kg IM), which is a rapidly acting depolarizing muscle relaxant with a short duration of action. Due to the rapid metabolism by serum pseudocholinesterase, succinylcholine's duration of action is only 5 to 10 minutes. In older children, succinylcholine can produce intense muscle fasiculations. Fasiculations are not usually observed in children less than 8 years old. In addition, serum potassium is routinely increased 0.5 mEq/L after succinylcholine, and this may be an important consideration for the child who is already hyperkalemic.[168] Finally, following repeated doses of succinylcholine, a profound and sustained bradycardia can occur in infants and young children.[36,96] This may progress to cardiac arrest, especially when repeated doses of succinylcholine are given. This relaxant is at present rarely used for the pediatric cardiac patient.

D-turbocurarine (0.5 mg/kg) is a nondepolarizing muscle relaxant which can cause hypotension through ganglionic blockade and histamine release. A 26 percent fall in arterial blood pressure has been observed in infants following a 0.6 mg/kg dose.[34] Because of this potential for hypotension, d-turbocurarine is infrequently used in pediatric cardiac anesthesia. Metocurine (0.4 mg/kg) is a pharmacologic relative of d-turbocurarine with less histamine releasing properties. At therapeutic doses, a fall in blood pressure can be observed, however. Metocurine is used for pediatric cardiac patients when afterload reduction is desired or not contraindicated.

The most popular muscle relaxant for pediatric cardiac surgery is pancuronium bromide (0.1 mg/kg). This is a long acting nondepolarizing agent with relatively little effect on the cardiovascular system in children.[30,107] An increase in heart rate occurs either through vagolytic effects or increases in the speed of atrioventricular conduction.[14,55,159] The increased heart rate is accompanied by a stable stroke volume and increased cardiac output.[159]

When tachycardia and hypotension are both undesired clinical hemodynamic actions—limiting the usefulness of either pancuronium or metocurine alone—an effective alternative is the combined use of low doses of both drugs[95] (pancuronium 0.025 mg/kg, metocurine 0.1 mg/kg). This provides a solid neuromuscular block while avoiding adverse hemodynamic effects.

SPECIAL INTRAOPERATIVE CONSIDERATIONS

Infants

On a miligram/kilogram basis, neonates require larger amounts of a drug than older children to produce the same therapeutic result. This seems true whether the drug is a depolarizing or nondepolarizing muscle relaxant[28,33,62,64,162] or an intravenous anesthetic agent like ketamine.[99] They also require a higher concentration of inhalational anesthetic agent such as halothane.[66,126] With increasing age, the concentration of an inhalational anesthetic needed to produce anesthesia decreases. The reduction in requirements occurs most rapidly in the first 6 months of life (Fig. 4.4).[66] A number of explanations for this observation have been proposed. Neonates have a proportionally larger amount of total body water (approximately 80 percent of body weight) and extracellular water (approximately 45 percent of body weight). Any drug that is water soluble would be distributed through a larger amount of fluid and thus diluted in concentration. Another explanation is that younger children have a proportionally greater cerebral blood flow, cerebral metabolism, and cerebral neuronal density. This may increase the

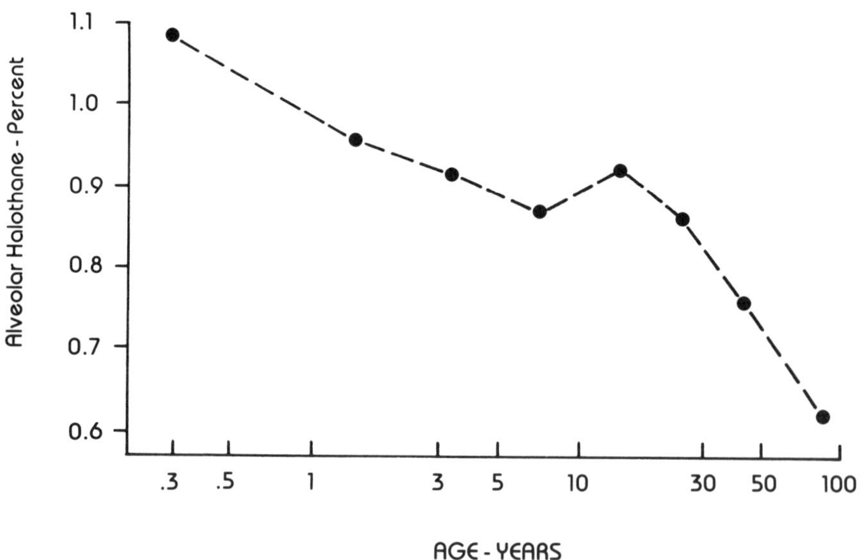

Fig. 4.4. Change with age in the minimum alveolar concentration of halothane required to induce anesthesia. (Gregory GA, Eger E II, Munson E 1969 The relationship between age and halothane requirement in man. Anesthesiology 30: 488.)

dosage of an anesthestic needed to obtain an effective result.[66,126] No matter what the reason, the effective MAC of halothane is 30 to 50 percent higher in neonates than adults.[33]

In addition, the neonate's alveolar concentration of an inhaled anesthetic reaches a steady state more rapidly than that of older children.[146] This is most likely due to the neonate's higher cardiac output, greater alveolar ventilation, and proportionally larger amount of vessel-rich tissue.[146] The increased anesthetic requirement and more rapid rise in alveolar concentration would not be of major clinical significance if the toxic dose of the agent was very high. Unfortunately, the cardiovascular tolerance to halothane falls with decreasing age.[34] This observation is substantiated clinically by the relatively rapid onset of significant hypotension in neonates when therapeutic anesthetic levels are provided.[50,126] Therefore, in spite of the neonate's increased requirement for anesthetic concentrations, they cannot tolerate the high concentration as well as older children. This is of particular importance for the neonate whose cardiovascular system is already compromised by a congenital heart defect. Therefore, potent inhalational agents must be used with caution in neonates with cardiac disease. If an intravenous agent is chosen, drug requirements may need to be increased up to four times the adult dose in milligrams per kilogram.[99]

Prior to induction of anesthesia in neonates, awake intubation is usually performed. The reason for this is to secure the airway while the child is still able to breathe spontaneously. An anesthetized neonate's airway can be difficult to manage without an endotracheal tube. The child's small functional residual capacity and increased metabolic requirements make it imperative that adequate ventilation be maintained. Recently, some authors have suggested that particularly vigorous neonates should be anesthetized prior to intubation.[73,154] Obviously, if this method is used, meticulous care must be taken to insure adequacy of the airway.

Thermal Homeostasis

Prevention of hypothermia

If therapeutic hypothermia is not being used in conjunction with cardiopulmonary bypass, a major concern when working with small children is maintenance of body temperature. This is especially important in the operating room setting where environmental temperatures are low, the child may be naked, and the anesthetic has reduced the child's ability to generate heat by shivering or to conserve heat by vasoconstriction. Though hypothermia may have beneficial effects in specific circumstances (i.e., cardiopulmonary bypass) the usual consequences of hypothermia are progressive metabolic acidosis,[53] increased oxygen consumption,[75] and cardiorespiratory depression.[18]

The small child is especially at risk for the development of hypothermia. The child's larger surface area to body weight ratio and greater body curvature leads to greater heat loss by the four mechanisms of heat exchange—convection, conduction, evaporation, and radiation.[2] The infant who is cooled will increase heat production by increasing his metabolic rate in an attempt to warm himself. However, this increased metabolic requirement creates a stress on a child who may already be critically ill. The increase in stress is directly proportional to the temperature gradient occurring between the child's body surface and the environment.[1]

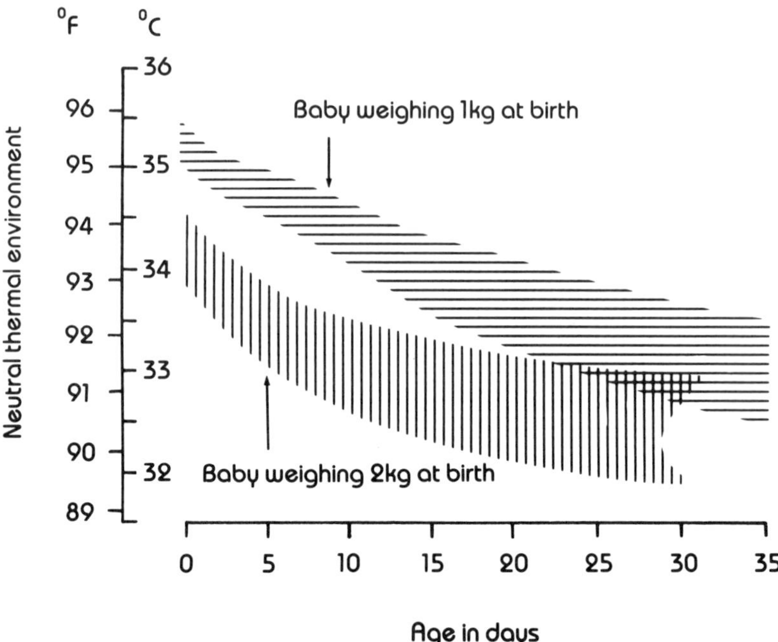

Fig. 4.5. The environmental temperature ranges in which the least metabolic stress is placed on the infant (neutral thermal environment). (Hey EN, Katz G 1970 The optimum thermal environment for naked babies. Archives of Diseases in Childhood. 45: 328. Reproduced by permission of the Authors and Editors of the Archives of Diseases in Childhood.)

The term "neutral thermal environment" has been used to describe the environmental temperature range over which the infant has the least thermal stress. Within this temperature range, the child has minimal metabolic demands placed upon him for temperature regulation (Fig. 4.5) at both reduced and elevated temperatures.[1,75]

Thermal stress in the operating room can come from many sources.

Evaporation In the normal infant, evaporative heat loss accounts for only 10 percent of total metabolic heat production; this figure is even less in the older child. A number of factors increase the importance of evaporative heat loss in the operating room, however. Use of volatile antiseptic solutions has been directly related to significant intraoperative heat loss in children.[140] Following the surgical procedure, these thermally stressed children reveal a prolonged increase in oxygen requirement. Because of this, use of less volatile antiseptic solutions (i.e., betadine rather than alcohol), which are prewarmed and wiped off following application, is recommended. In addition, blood and fluid seepage from the wound onto the child may contribute to evaporative losses and can be easily prevented by using plastic or nonabsorbant drapes. Increasing environmental humidification from 25 to 75 percent saturation can reduce heat loss from skin and respiratory tract evaporation by 50 percent.[75] Heating of humidified inspired gases can further reduce the caloric heat loss.[18]

Conduction Loss of heat due to direct contact with surrounding solid objects normally accounts for only a small proportion of the total thermal requirement.

In the operating room this can become more important, especially for infants with relatively thin skin and less fatty insulation.[2] The heating blanket is an effective means of maintaining intraoperative body temperature, especially for children who weigh less than 10 kg.[63] Prewarming of infused solutions is also very important. One hundred milliliters of fluid at 5°C infused into a 3 kg infant can reduce the child's temperature by 1°C.[140]

Convection Heat loss by convection occurs when the surrounding air currents take away the surface body heat. This is determined by air movement and air temperature. Convection is the primary source of heat loss in children over 2 years old and accounts for approximately 30 percent of heat loss in infants. The operating room environment, which has been traditionally cold and drafty, is conducive to major convective heat losses. The use of plastic drapes during the operation and blankets in the preoperative and postoperative periods can reduce this loss.[63] Increasing the ambient room temperature appropriate for the child's age and weight will also reduce convective heat loss (Fig. 4.5).[1,75]

Radiation The primary source of heat loss in infants and a major source of heat loss in older children is radiation to surrounding cooler objects. Adequate increases in ambient temperature will reduce this loss.[15] In addition, wrapping portions of the body not involved in the operation, particularly the head, in reflective material such as aluminum foil will decrease radiant heat loss. Overhead radiant warmers and infrared lamps also will aid in maintaining an adequate body temperature.[152]

Induction of hypothermia for cardiopulmonary bypass

Following Bigelow's initial evaluation of the beneficial effects of deep hypothermia and circulatory arrest for cardiac surgery in dogs,[20] anesthesiologists began applying the techniques of surface cooling to humans. With the advent of the heart-lung machine[50] came the ability to maintain circulation and the ability to rapidly cool or warm the patient. Because of this, the use of surface cooling was nearly abandoned. In spite of the improved techniques of extracorporeal circulation, mortality from open heart surgery performed on neonates, especially for complex intracardiac lesions, continued to be high. Surgery was technically difficult during routine cardiopulmonary bypass since the heart did not remain completely quiet and blood continued to flood the operative field.[12] This led to a return to profound hypothermic techniques using combined surface and bypass cooling followed by cardiac arrest during the reparative portion of the operation. This technique decreased operative morbidity and mortality.[12,118,158] The degree of hypothermia achieved was directly related to the length of time circulatory arrest could be continued without adverse end-organ sequelae.[20]

The technique of combined surface cooling and hypothermic cardiopulmonary bypass has been described by many groups, with slight modifications.[12,27,78,118,158,172] Basically, the technique entails packing the child in ice after induction of anesthesia and the establishment of monitoring. Ice is not placed over the heart due to the increased risk of cardiac depression and arrhythmias. The hands, feet, and ears are not covered to avoid thermal injury and necrosis. Hypothermic skin injuries are prevented by periodically changing the location of the ice packs over the body and by wrapping the ice packs in damp towels. When a rectal temperature of 32°C is reached, the surgical procedure is begun. By the time cannulation has been accomplished, the rectal temperature has normally drifted to 30°C. Particular attention should be paid to the potassium and pH values during the prebypass period since spontaneous ventricular fibrillation can occur.[58] Following cannulation, hypothermic cardiopulmonary bypass is initiated and the child's core temperature is reduced to 20° to 22°C. At this point cardiopulmonary bypass is discontinued, and the intracardiac repair is performed. Following the repair, cardiopulmonary bypass is resumed and the child rewarmed to a rectal temperature of at least 35°C.

The advantages of surface cooling in combination with hypothermic cardiopulmonary bypass include a more uniform decrease in temperature throughout the body, a decrease in total metabolic requirements prior to the decrease in cardiac output with manipulation of the heart during cannulation, and a reduction in the time required on cardiopulmonary bypass.[158] Numerous studies have been undertaken to assess impairment of neurologic and intellectual function following periods of hypothermic arrest. An inherent problem in the design of these studies is the lack of an accurate and reproducible method of quantitating intellectual function in the neonate. Another approach has been to measure the children's intelligence many years after the hypothermic arrest, comparing their levels with those of a control nonarrest group. Unfortunately, in these studies separation of intellectual impairment due to hypothermic arrest as opposed to multiple other causes is impossible. At present, evidence seems to point to a lack of intellectual impairment with up to 60 minutes of arrest during profound hypothermia.[12,37]

Retrolental Fibroplasia

The retinal vessels of the fetus reach maturity between 36 and 42 weeks of gestation. Until then, the child remains at risk for developing retrolental fibroplasia (RLF) during exposure to elevated oxygen concentrations. Periods of hyperoxia lead to constriction of the immature peripheral retinal vessels, which become obliterated, leading to formation of fibrotic membranes. Unfortunately, the critical arterial partial pressure of oxygen (P_aO_2) and duration of exposure required to produce RLF in susceptible infants is unknown.[150] In fact, RLF has been reported in an infant with cyanotic congenital heart disease, the least likely candidate to acquire RLF if blood oxygen tension was the only determining factor.[82] At present a P_aO_2 below 70 mmHg is considered safe.[32]

Infants are being brought to the operating room at increasingly early gestational ages for both palliative and total corrective cardiac surgery.[12,172] A report exists of an infant developing RLF after exposure to an elevated P_aO_2 only during surgery.[19] It is recommended that all potentially susceptible children have an ophthalmologic examination before surgery. The examination should be repeated after surgery and at weekly intervals until the child is gestationally older than 44 weeks or no longer exposed to increased inspired oxygen concentrations. If the child is not cyanotic, an oxygen-air or oxygen–nitrous oxide mixture can be provided to achieve an appropriate level of arterial oxygenation during surgery and transport to and from the operating room. Blood samples for gas analysis should be drawn from a right radial or right temporal artery. This will prevent the sample from being contaminated with blood shunted from a patent ductus arteriosus. Since many intraoperative events can change the P_aO_2, a transcutaneous oxygen monitor can be very valuable in helping prevent accidental hypoxemia.[131]

Oxyhemoglobin Dissociation Curve

Visual assessment and quantitation of cyanosis in children with congenital heart defects is extremely difficult. In order for central cyanosis to be observed, 5 g/dl of arterial hemoglobin needs to be desaturated.[13] A child with a serum hemoglobin of 10 g/dl would require half his hemoglobin to be desaturated before cyanosis became evident while a child with a hemoglobin of 20 g/dl would require only 25 percent desaturation. Children with high hemoglobins are therefore more likely to show cyanosis. The point where one half of the hemoglobin is desaturated (the P_{50}) occurs at an oxygen tension of 27.5 mmHg for patients with hemoglobin A (adult hemoglobin). Infants with hemoglobin F (fetal hemoglobin) have an even lower P_{50} (16.8 mmHg) due to an increased affinity of this hemoglobin for oxygen. This leads to a leftward shift of the oxyhemoglobin dissociation curve (Fig. 4.6). Therefore, infants require an even greater reduction in arterial oxygen tension than adults before central cyanosis becomes evident.

In addition to different hemoglobins, the oxyhemoglobin dissociation curve is

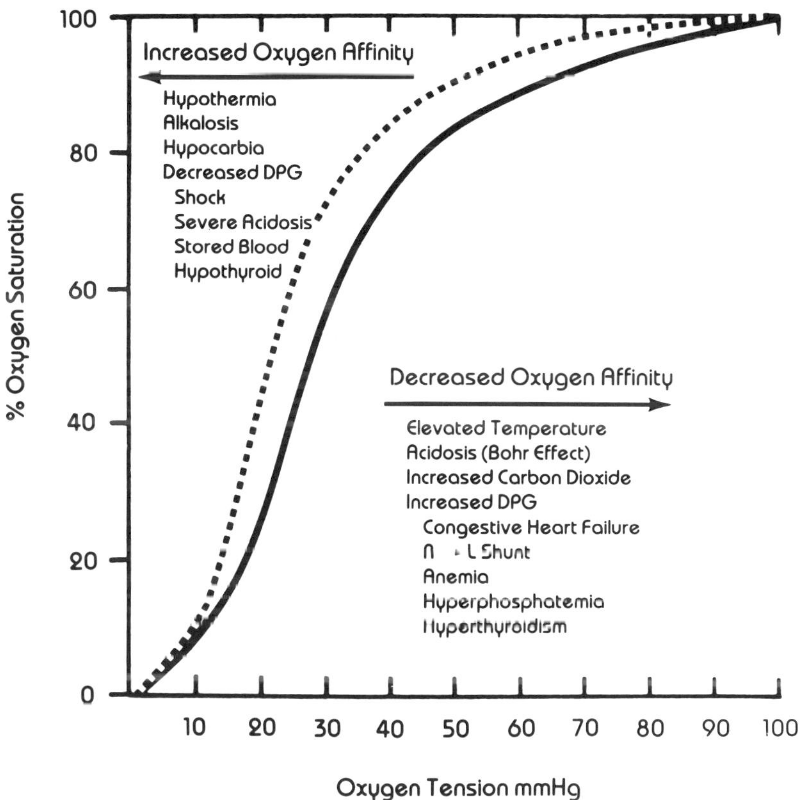

Fig. 4.6. Hemoglobin dissociation curve for both adult hemoglobin (————) and fetal hemoglobin (■■■■■). Factors effecting hemoglobin's affinity for oxygen are listed.

influenced by a number of other factors (Fig. 4.6).[151] These factors are interdependent and a change in one leads to variations in the others. The oxyhemoglobin dissociation curve is influenced the most by the Bohr effect. An increase in hydrogen ions causes an immediate decrease in the hemoglobin's affinity for oxygen, leading to a rightward shift of the curve. Increases in carbon dioxide also lead to a rightward shift, which is independent of any pH change. This is accomplished through binding of the carbon dioxide molecule to the N terminal amino acid on the deoxyhemoglobin molecule—the carbamino effect.[85] A rightward shift can also be induced with hyperthermia, and the physiologic effect is that oxygen becomes more available to the tissues during periods of temperature elevation (i.e., exercise and fever).[151] Finally, serum organic phosphates also play a major role, especially 2,3 diphosphoglycerate (DPG). An elevation of this compound induces an immediate rightward shift of the oxyhemoglobin dissociation curve. This may be significant for children with cyanotic heart disease since the hypoxemic state induces an elevation in serum DPG levels, thereby allowing easier oxygen availability.[136,144,174] Following corrective cardiac surgery, the DPG levels in these children return toward normal. DPG levels progressively fall in stored bank blood. A cyanotic child requiring a massive transfusion with stored blood may only be receiving partial benefit for peripheral tissue oxygenation since his oxyhemoglobin dissociation curve would be undergoing a major leftward swing.[151]

Fluid Requirements

Fluid management begins during the preoperative evaluation. Obviously, a hypervolemic child in congestive heart failure responds to anesthetic induction much differently than a child in congestive heart failure who is hypovolemic due to intensive diuretic therapy. The duration of time the child will tolerate the withholding of fluids prior to surgery needs to be assessed for each patient. Normally, a child less than 6 months of age can have clear fluids 4 hours prior to surgery. This period is extended to 6 hours for children between 6 and 12 months of age. For children over 12 months of age, 8 hours of withholding fluids is usually well-tolerated. Modifications of these suggestions are occasionally necessary, especially for severely polycythemic infants who may require an intravenous infusion preoperatively to achieve adequate hydration.

For children undergoing open heart surgery, it is more difficult to predict the type and amount of fluids that will be necessary than for children undergoing palliative or closed heart procedures. Congenital cardiac lesions, with their attendant differing hemodynamic requirements, dictate that a fluid management plan be developed for each patient.[116] The goal of fluid management is to produce adequate urine output (1 ml/kg/hour is satisfactory) without fluid overload. An adequate hematocrit should also be maintained (greater than 40 percent in newborns, and greater than 30 percent in older children). During the relatively stable prebypass period, infusions of 10 percent dextrose and 0.225 percent saline for the newborn or 5 percent dextrose and 0.225 percent saline for the older child are usually provided at maintenance levels through a peripheral intravenous catheter. Additional fluids in the form of Ringer's lactate can be used for preload augmentation, replacement of third space losses (up to 4 ml/kg/hour for intrathoracic procedures) and blood loss. While on bypass, major shifts in fluids occur and hemodilution from pump prime may decrease the hematocrit to the 20 to 25 percent range. This lowered hematocrit helps to compensate for the increased blood viscosity associated with hypothermia.[60]

At termination of bypass, the hematocrit should be returned toward normal. Fresh-frozen plasma and platelets may be necessary for hemostasis. In the postbypass period, it is impossible to predict fluid requirements. Patients who have undergone right atrial to pulmonary artery anastomosis or who have had a right ventriculotomy may have two or three times normal postbypass fluid requirements. In addition, use of inotropic agents and afterload reducers will affect the amount of fluids required by a particular patient. Because of this, decisions concerning fluid management are often based on invasive monitoring. Changes in central venous pressure, particularly after a fluid challenge, can be very helpful. A good indicator of relative hypovolemia is the amount of respiratory variation seen on the arterial pressure trace (Fig. 4.7).

The fluid management for palliative and closed cardiac surgical procedures is much more predictable. One should be prepared, however, for rapid volume replacement in the event of hemorrhage.

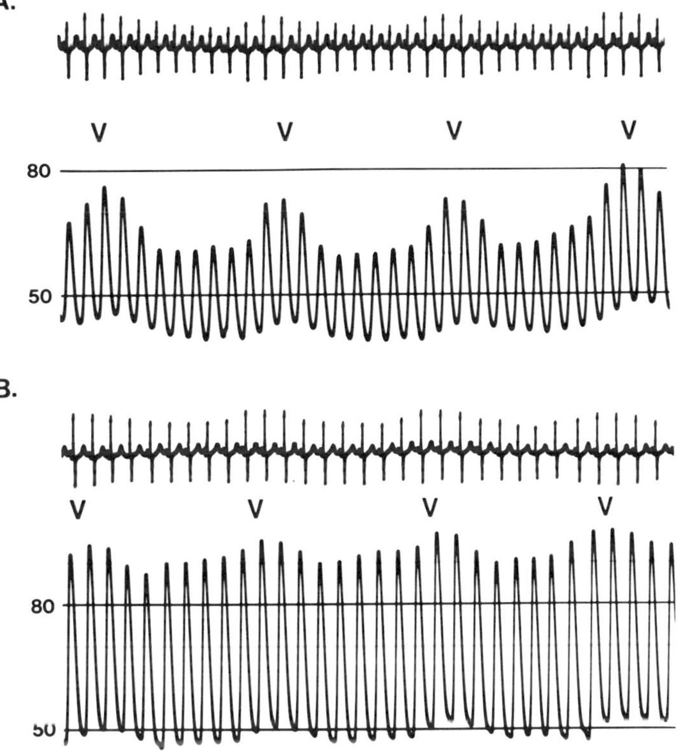

Fig. 4.7. The electrocardiogram, arterial blood pressure trace, and timing of positive pressure ventilations (V) are shown for a 7-year-old male undergoing repair of partial anomalous pulmonary venous return. (A) Obtained when the child was hypovolemic (central venous pressure of 2). Note marked variations in blood pressure with ventilation. (B) Obtained 10 minutes later after a rapid fluid infusion of 20 ml/kg (central venous pressure of 12). Note the wider pulse pressure and smaller variations in arterial blood pressure with ventilation.

Coagulation

A major concern of the cardiac anesthesiologist is adequate anticoagulation before insertion of the extracorporeal cannulae. Without anticoagulants, the oxygenator will clot and the patient will die. With inadequate anticoagulation, ongoing consumption of clotting factors and platelets predisposes the patient to bleeding problems after bypass. Many methods have been developed for monitoring intraoperative anticoagulation but the activated clotting time (ACT) continues to be the simplest and most widely used method.[74] The ACT is the time a sample of blood takes to clot when activated by celite. A baseline ACT is normally in the range of 110 to 130 seconds.

Bull et al[23,24] described a linear relationship between the ACT and the unit/kg dose of heparin. Individual patients may have a wide variation in response to heparin, but the response is linear. From a plot made of the preheparin ACT and post 200 units/kg heparin ACT, an accurate prediction of the heparin dosage needed for adequate anticoagulation can be made. Since fibrin monomer production is found with ACTs less than 400 seconds,[176] the level of adequate heparinization has been arbitrarily placed at 480 seconds to provide some reserve. A basic principle in all open heart surgery is that it is always better to overanticoagulate than underanticoagulate.

After termination of cardiopulmonary bypass, an ACT is drawn. Based on its location on the Bull curve, the amount of active heparin remaining and thus the amount of protamine necessary for heparin reversal can be determined. The protamine should be given slowly through a peripheral intravenous, since histamine may be released during its passage through the lungs, producing a fall in systemic vascular resistance. In addition, calcium chelation by protamine can decrease the inotropic state of the heart. The result of both the cardiac depression and peripheral dilatation can be profound hypotension.[117,129,167] There may be less of a hypotensive response to protamine if it is infused through the left atrium or aorta.[4]

Hemostasis in the postbypass period is essential, especially for children with cyanotic heart disease. Right sided filling pressures are commonly elevated following repair in these children, and adequate coagulation is necessary for venous hemostasis. Children with congenital heart disease frequently have quantitative and qualitative platelet abnormalities, decreased clotting factors, and increased fibrinolysis.[44,59,88,90] During bypass, dilution of the clotting factors by pump prime, destruction of platelets by the perfusion apparatus, splenic sequestration of platelets due to hypothermia, and augmented fibrinolysis from tissue damage all predispose the patient to bleeding. If bleeding persists after reversal of the heparin, laboratory evaluation of coagulation should be done to suggest replacement of coagulation factors. This may include the use of fresh-frozen plasma, cryoprecipitate, and platelets. If the fibrin split products are less than 40 μg/ml, epsilon aminocaproic acid is given to reverse any fibrinolysis that may be ongoing.[22,92,101,111,156] This drug can be particularly helpful for the child with cyanotic congenital heart disease. If a fibrin split product level is greater than 40 μg/ml, disseminated intravascular coagulation is suspected and epsilon aminocaprioc acid is contraindicated.[125] Usual indicators of disseminated intravascular coagulation are not very useful in the postbypass period, due to the major derangement of all clotting factors that can occur. Following chest closure, positive end expiratory pressure may be helpful in decreasing mediastinal bleeding.[76]

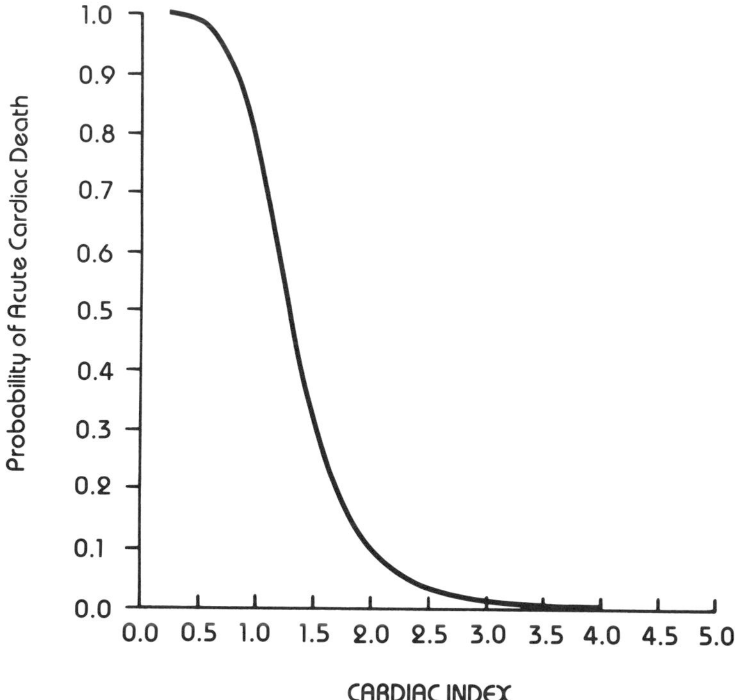

Fig. 4.8. The relationship between the cardiac index in children following open heart surgery and the probability of acute cardiac death. Note the marked increase in mortality with cardiac indexes less than 2 L/m^2. (Parr G, Blackstone E, Kirklin J 1975 Cardiac performance and mortality early after intracardiac surgery in infants and young children. Circulation 51: 867, by permission of the American Heart Association, Inc.)

Cardiac Output

Measurement of cardiac output is helpful in patient management following cardiopulmonary bypass. Though Swan-Ganz catheters are rarely placed in children, a 2 or 3 French thermistor catheter has been developed which can be placed in the pulmonary artery during surgery.[115,175] A right atrial catheter is used for injection of cold saline to determine cardiac output. These cardiac output values correlate well with outputs obtained through dye dilution techniques.[115,175] The amount of injectate is adjusted to the age of the child. With smaller injectate volumes, however, errors in cardiac output of 25 percent can occur if the dead space of the catheter is not taken into consideration.[105] A small amount of injectate should first be flushed through the catheter to clear it prior to injection of the measured amount of injectate.

The value of cardiac output measurement was shown by Parr et al.[130] A significant increase in mortality occurred in their study for those children with cardiac indexes less than 2 L/m^2 in the 72 hour period following cardiac surgery (Fig. 4.8). A mixed venous oxygen partial pressure less than 30 mmHg was another ominous indicator. Others confirmed this finding and indicated that children less than 2 years old were particularly prone to the development of a low cardiac output syndrome.[165]

When treating a child in a low cardiac output state, initial efforts to improve forward flow should be directed at augmentation of preload. Following open heart surgery, particularly when a right ventriculotomy has been done, children require increased preload, even to the point of elevations in right atrial pressure higher than those of left atrial pressure. Bradycardia should be treated either pharmacologically or with a pacemaker. Acidosis from poor tissue perfusion should be corrected since this can further impair myocardial function and decrease the effectiveness of inotropic support. If all of these measures fail to increase the child's cardiac index, a trial of afterload reduction with agents such as nitroprusside may help if systemic vascular resistance is elevated.[3] Nitroprusside, however, may cause a further decrease in cardiac output, in which case an inotrope can be added.[16] The inotrope should increase systemic blood pressure and cardiac index without changing right atrial pressure, left atrial pressure, pulmonary vascular resistance, or systemic vascular resistance. Dopamine has these properties[93] while providing increased renal blood flow by stimulation of renal vascular dopaminergic receptors.

Extubation

The time of tracheal extubation is critical. The child's age, condition, and the type of surgical procedure performed will be major determining factors. After a closed cardiac or palliative procedure, most children can be extubated following reversal of the anesthetic and muscle relaxant. The decision for the child who has undergone an open heart procedure is more difficult, however, Some view the extension of intubation by even a few hours as potentially detrimental.[10] However, others have found the rate of reintubation and morbidity associated with early extubation of open heart pediatric patients to be significant.[57] Since bleeding is common in the first few hours following open heart surgery in children, a child extubated prematurely would have to undergo the stress of another induction period and reintubation. In addition, during the first few hours following open heart surgical procedures rapid changes in the patient's hemodynamic state can occur, which can be further confused by a changing respiratory state. For these reasons, electing to delay extubation at least 2 hours following an open heart procedure would seem to be the safest approach.

CONCLUSION

The anesthetic management of the pediatric cardiac patient requires a fine integration of technical skill, specialized knowledge, and extreme vigilance. A firm foundation in the sciences of pediatric physiology and pharmacology are necessary before the comprehensive care of these children should be undertaken. There is little reserve for error in the care of these children since relatively small manipulations of the cardiovascular, respiratory, or fluid managements can lead to rapid clinical deterioration. On the other hand, few areas of anesthesia provide both the challenge and fulfillment found with the pediatric cardiovascular patient.

ACKNOWLEDGMENTS

I would like to acknowledge the assistance of Donald Clark, M.D. for his critical review of this chapter as well as Mary Pintye and Deanna Kerns for all their help.

REFERENCES

1. Adamson K, Gandy G, James L 1965 Influence of thermal factors upon oxygen consumption of the newborn human infant. Journal of Pediatrics 66: 495
2. Adamson K, Towell M 1965 Thermal homeostasis in the fetus and newborn. Anesthesiology 26: 531
3. Appelbaum A, Blackstone E, Kouchoukos N, Kuklin J 1977 Afterload reduction and cardiac output in infants early after intracardiac surgery. American Journal of Cardiology 39: 445
4. Aris A, Solanes H, Bonnin J, Garin R, Caralps J 1981 Intraaortic administration of protamine: method for heparin neutralization after cardiopulmonary bypass. Cardiovascular Diseases, Bulletin of the Texas Heart Institute 8: 23
5. Aviado D 1975 Regulation of bronchomotor tone during anesthesia. Anesthesiology 42: 68
6. Bain J, Spoerel W 1972 A streamlined anaesthetic system. Canadian Anaesthetists' Society Journal 19: 426
7. Bain J, Spoerel W 1973 Flow requirements for a modified Mapleson D system during controlled ventilation. Canadian Anaesthetists' Society Journal 20: 629
8. Bain J, Spoerel W 1977 Carbon dioxide output and elimination in children under anaesthesia. Canadian Anaesthetists' Society Journal 24: 533
9. Barash P, Glanz S, Katz J, Taunt K, Talner N 1978 Ventricular function in children during halothane anesthesia. Anesthesiology 49: 79
10. Barash P, Lescovich F, Katz J, Talner N, Stansel H 1980 Early extubation following pediatric cardiothoracic operation: a viable alternative. Annals of Thoracic Surgery 29: 228
11. Barnes C, Kenny F, Call T, Reinhart J 1972 Measurement in management of anxiety in children for open heart surgery. Pediatrics 49: 250
12. Barratt-Boyes B, Simpson M, Neutze J 1971 Intracardiac surgery in neonates and infants using deep hypothermia with surface cooling and limited cardiopulmonary bypass. Circulation 43–44(Supplement I): I25
13. Behrman R 1983 The Respiratory System. In: Fanaroff A, Martin R (eds) Neonatal-Perinatal Medicine, 3rd edn. C.V. Mosby Company, St. Louis
14. Bennett E, Bowyer D, Giesecke A, Stephen C 1973 Pancuronium bromide: a double blind study in children. Anesthesia and Analgesia 52: 12
15. Bennett E, Patel K, Grundy E 1977 Neonatal temperature and surgery. Anesthesiology 46: 303
16. Benzing G III, Helmsworth J, Schreiber J, Kaplan S 1979 Nitroprusside and epinephrine for treatment of low output in children after open heart surgery. Annals of Thoracic Surgery 27: 523
17. Benzing G III, Schubert W, Hug G, Kaplan S 1969 Simultaneous hypoglycemia and acute congestive heart failure. Circulation 40: 209
18. Berry F, Hughes-Davies D, DiFazio C 1973 A system for minimizing respiratory heat loss in infants during operation. Anesthesia and Analgesia 52: 170
19. Betts E, Downes J, Schaffer D, Johns R 1977 Retrolental fibroplasia and oxygen administration during general anesthesia. Anesthesiology 47: 518
20. Bigelow W, Lindsay W, Greenwood W 1950 Hypothermia. Annals of Surgery 132: 849
21. Bove E, Behrendt D 1980 Open heart surgery in the first week of life. Annals of Thoracic Surgery 29: 130
22. Brodsky I, Gill D, Lusch C 1967 Fibrinolysis in congenital heart disease. Preoperative treatment with ϵ-aminocaproic acid. American Journal of Clinical Pathology 51: 51
23. Bull B, Huse W, Brauer F, Korpman R 1975 Heparin therapy during extracorporeal circulation, Part II. Journal of Thoracic and Cardiovascular Surgery 69: 685
24. Bull B, Korpman R, Huse W, Biggs B 1975 Heparin therapy during extracorporeal circulation, Part I. Journal of Thoracic and Cardiovascular Surgery 69: 674
25. Bush G, Stead A 1962 Use of D-tubocurarine in neonatal anaesthesia. British Journal of Anaesthesia 34: 721
26. Carruthers S, Cleland T, Kelly T, Lyons S, McDevitt D 1975 Plasma and tissue digoxin concentrations in patients undergoing cardiopulmonary bypass. British Heart Journal 37: 313
27. Castaneda A, Lamberti J, Sade R, Williams R, Nadas A 1974 Open heart surgery during the first three months of life. Journal of Thoracic and Cardiovascular Surgery 68: 719
28. Churchill-Davidson H, Wise R 1963 Neuromuscular transmission in the newborn infant. Anesthesiology 24: 271
29. Churchill-Davidson H, Wise R 1964 Response of the newborn infant to muscle relaxants. Canadian Anaesthetists' Society Journal 11: 1
30. Cohen N 1980 Hemodynamic effects of pancuronium in critically ill children. Anesthesiology 53: S159

31. Coltart D, Chamberlain D, Howard M, Kettlewell M, Mercer J, Smith T 1971 Effect of cardiopulmonary bypass on plasma digoxin concentration. British Heart Journal 33: 334
32. Committee on Retrolental Fibroplasia 1976 Retrolental fibroplasia. Pediatrics (supplement) 57: 591
33. Cook D 1981 Muscles relaxants in infants and children. Anesthesia and Analgesia 60: 335
34. Cook D, Brandom B, Shiu G, Wolfson B 1981 The inspired median effective dose, brain concentration at anesthesia, and cardiovascular index for halothane in young rats. Anesthesia and Analgesia 60: 182
35. Cozanitis D, Dundee J, Khan M 1980 Operative study of atropine and glycopyrrolate on suxamethonium induced changes in cardiac rate and rhythm. British Journal of Anaesthesia 52: 291
36. Craythorne N, Tundorf H, Dripps R 1960 Changes in pulse rate and rhythm associated with the use of succinylcholine in anesthetized children. Anesthesiology 21: 465
37. Dickinson D, Sambrooks J 1979 Intellectual performance in children after circulatory arrest with profound hypothermia in infancy. Archives of Disease in Childhood 54: 1
38. Dowdy E, Kaya K 1968 Studies of the mechanism of cardiovascular responses to CI-581. Anesthesiology 29: 931
39. Eckenhoff J 1951 Some anatomic considerations of the infant larynx influencing endotracheal anesthesia. Anesthesiology 12: 401
40. Editor 1975 Congenital heart-disease: incidence and aetiology. Lancet 2: 692
41. Egbert L, Battit G, Turndorf H, Beecher H 1963 Value of the preoperative visit by an anesthetist. Journal of the American Medical Association 185: 553
42. Eger E II 1974 Circulation and uptake and effect of ventilation/perfusion abnormalities. In: Anesthetic Uptake and Action, Williams & Wilkins, Baltimore
43. Eger E II, Smith N, Stoelting R, Cullen D, Kadis L, Whitcher C 1970 Cardiovascular effects of halothane in man. Anesthesiology 32: 396
44. Ekert H, Sheers M 1974 Preoperative and postoperative platelet function in cyanotic congenital heart disease. Journal of Thoracic and Cardiovascular Surgery 67: 184
45. Epstein R 1971 Humidification during positive pressure ventilation of infants. Anesthesiology 35: 532
46. Ferencz C 1960 The pulmonary vascular bed in Tetralogy of Fallot. I. Changes associated with pulmonic stenosis. Bulletin of Johns Hopkins Hospital 106: 81
47. Folts J, Afonso S, Rowe G 1975 Systemic and coronary haemodynamic effects of ketamine in intact anaesthetized and unanaesthetized dogs. British Journal of Anaesthesia 47: 686
48. Fong I, Baker C, McKee D 1979 The value of prophylactic antibiotics in aorta-coronary bypass operations. Journal of Thoracic and Cardiovascular Surgery 78: 908
49. Freeman A, Bachman L 1959 Pediatric anesthesia: an evaluation of preoperative medication. Anesthesia and Analgesia 38: 429
50. Friesen R, Lichtor J 1982 Cardiovascular depression during halothane anesthesia in infants: a study of three induction techniques. Anesthesia and Analgesia 61: 42
51. Fyler D 1980 Report on the New England regional infant cardiac program. Pediatrics (supplement) 65: 376
52. Gale J, Waters R 1931 Closed endobronchial anesthesia in thoracic surgery. Journal of Thoracic Surgery 1: 432
53. Gandy G, Adamson K, Cunningham N, Silverman W, James L 1964 Thermal eenvironment and acid-base homeostasis in human infants during the first few hours of life. Journal of Clinical Investigation 43: 751
54. Gassner S, Cohen M, Aygen M, Levy E, Ventura E, Shashdi J 1974 Effect of ketamine on pulmonary artery pressure. Anaesthesia 29: 141
55. Geha D, Rozelle B, Raessler K, Groves B, Wightman M, Blitt C 1977 Pancuronium bromide enhances atrioventricular conduction in halothane-anesthetized dogs. Anesthesiology 46: 342
56. Gibbon J 1954 Application of a mechanical heart and lung apparatus to cardiac surgery. Minnesota Medicine 37: 171
57. Glenn J, Don H, Ebert P, Cohen N, Matthay M 1980 Tracheal extubation after cardiac surgery in children. Anesthesiology 53: S158
58. Glover W 1977 Management of cardiac surgery in the neonate. British Journal of Anaesthesia 49: 59
59. Goldschmidt B 1969 Fibrinolysis in children with congenital heart-disease (letter). Lancet 1: 677
60. Gordon R, Ravin M, Daicoff G, Rawitscher R 1975 Effects of hemodilution on hypotension during cardiopulmonary bypass. Anesthesia and Analgesia 54: 482
61. Goudsouzian N 1980 Maturation of neuromuscular transmission in the infant. British Journal of Anaesthesia 52: 205

62. Goudsouzian N, Donlon J, Savarese J, Ryan J 1975 Re-evaluation of dosage and duration of action of d tubocurarine in the pediatric age group. Anesthesiology 43: 416
63. Goudsouzian N, Morris R, Ryan J 1973 The effects of a warming blanket on the maintenance of body temperatures in anesthetized infants and children. Anesthesiology 39: 351
64. Goudsouzian N, Ryan J, Savarese J 1974 Neuromuscular effects of pancuronium in infants and children. Anesthesiology 41: 95
65. Graybiel A, Strieder J, Boyer N 1938 An attempt to obliterate the patent ductus arteriosus in a patient with subacute bacterial endarteritis. American Heart Journal 15: 621
66. Gregory GA, Eger E II, Munson E 1969 The relationship between age and halothane requirement in man. Anesthesiology 30: 488
67. Greenwood R, Rosenthal A, Parisi L, Fyler D, Nadas A 1975 Extracardiac abnormalities in infants with congenital heart disease. Pediatrics 55: 485
68. Gwilt D, Goat V, Maynard P 1978 The Bain system: gas flows in small subjects. British Journal of Anaesthesia 50: 127
69. Harmel M, Lamont A 1946 Anesthesia in the surgical treatment of congenital pulmonic stenosis. Anesthesiology 7: 477
70. Harris A 1950 The management of anesthesia for congenital heart operations in children. Anesthesiology 11: 328
71. Harris W, Goodman R 1968 Hyper reactivity to atropine in Down's syndrome. New England Journal of Medicine 279: 407
72. Hatano S, Keane D, Boggs R, El-Naggar M, Sadove M 1976 Diazepam-ketamine anaesthesia for open heart surgery a "micro-mini" drip administration technique. Canadian Anaesthetists' Society Journal 23: 648
73. Hatch D, Gumner E 1981 Neonatal anaeesthesia. In: Feldman S, Scurr C (eds) Current Topics in Anaesthesia. Year Book Medical Publishers, Chicago
74. Hattersley P 1966 Activated coagulation time of whole blood. Journal of the American Medical Association 196: 150
75. Hey EN, Katz G 1970 The optimum thermal environment for naked babies. Archives of Diseases in Childhood 45: 328
76. Hoffman W, Tomasello D, MacVaugh H 1982 Control of postcardiotomy bleeding with PEEP. Annals of Thoracic Surgery 34: 71
77. Homi J, Konchigeri H, Eckenhoff J, Linde H 1972 A new anesthetic agent—Forane: preliminary observation in man. Anesthesia and Analgesia 51: 439
78. Ingersoll I, Lell W, Allarde R, Corssen G 1975 The role of profound hypothermia in infants undergoing surgical correction of complicated heart defects. Anesthesia and Analgesia 54: 660
79. Jackson K 1951 Psychologic preparation as a method of reducing the emotional trauma of anesthesia in children. Anesthesiology 12: 293
80. Johnson D, Rosenthal A, Nadas A 1975 A forty-year review of bacterial endocarditis in infancy and childhood. Circulation 51: 581
81. Johnston R, Eger E II, Wilson C 1976 Comparative interaction of epinephrine with enflurane, isoflurane, and halothane in man. Anesthesia and Analgesia 55: 709
82. Kalina R, Hodson W, Morgan B 1972 Retrolental fibroplasia in a cyanotic infant. Pediatrics 50: 765
83. Kaplan E, Anthony B, Bisno A, Durack D, House H, Millard H, Sanford J, Shulman S, Stillerman M, Taranta A, Wenger N 1977 Prevention of bacterial endocarditis. Circulation 56: 139A
84. Kaplan E, Rich H, Gersony W, Manning J 1979 A collaborative study of infective endocarditis in the 1970's. Circulation 59: 327
85. Kilmartin JV, Rossi-Bernardi L 1969 Inhibition of CO_2 combination and reduction of the Bohr effect in haemoglobin chemically modified at its α-amino groups. Nature 222: 1243
86. Kilpatrick D, Miller W, Allain A, Huggins M, Lee W 1975 The use of psychological test data to predict open-heart surgery outcome: a prospective study. Psychosomatic Medicine 37: 62
87. Kimball CP 1969 Predictive study of adjustment to cardiac surgery. Journal of Thoracic and Cardiovascular Surgery 58: 891
88. Komp D, Sparrow A 1970 Polycythemia in cyanotic heart disease—a study of altered coagulation. Journal of Pediatrics 76: 231
89. Kontras S, Bodenbender J, Craenen J, Hosier D 1970 Hyperviscosity in congenital heart disease. Journal of Pediatrics 76: 214
90. Kontras S, Sirak H, Newton W 1966 Hematologic abnormalities in children with congenital heart disease. Journal of the American Medical Association 195: 611
91. Krasula R, Hastreiter A, Levitsky S, Yanagi R, Soyka L 1974 Serum, atrial, and urinary digoxin levels during cardiopulmonary bypass in children. Circulation 49: 1047
92. Lambert C, Marengo-Rowe A, Leveson J, Green R, Thiele JP, Geisler G, Adam M, Mitchel B

1979 Treatment of postperfusion bleeding using ε-aminocaproic acid, cryoprecipitate, fresh frozen plasma, and protamine sulfate. Annals of Thoracic Surgery 28: 440
93. Lang P, Williams R, Norwood W, Castaneda A 1980 Hemodynamic effects of dopamine in infants after corrective cardiac surgery. Journal of Pediatrics 96: 630
94. Lappas D, Buckley M, Laver M, Daggett W, Lowenstein E 1975 Left ventricular performance and pulmonary circulation following addition of nitrous oxide to morphine during coronary-artery surgery. Anesthesiology 43: 61
95. Lebowitz P, Ramsey F, Savarese J, Ali H, deBros F 1981 Combination of pancuronium and metocurine: neuromuscular and hemodynamic advantages over pancuronium alone. Anesthesia and Analgesia 60: 12
96. Leigh M, McCoy D, Belton M, Lewis G 1957 Bradycardia following intravenous administration of succinylcholine chloride to infants and children. Anesthesiology 18: 698
97. Levin R, Seleny F, Streczyn M 1975 Ketamine-pancuronium narcotic technic for cardiovascular surgery in infants—a comparative study. Anesthesia and Analgesia 54: 800
98. Lister G, Hellenbrand W, Kleinman C, Talner N 1982 Physiologic effects of increasing hemoglobin concentration in left-to-right shunting in infants with ventricular septal defects. New England Journal of Medicine 306: 502
99. Lockhart C, Nelson W 1974 The relationship of ketamine requirement to age in pediatric patients. Anesthesiology 40(5): 507
100. Lowenstein E, Hallowell P, Levine F, Daggett W, Austen G, Laver M 1966 Cardiovascular response to large doses of intravenous morphine in man. New England Journal of Medicine 281: 1389
101. McClure P, Izsak J 1974 Use of epsilon-aminocaproic acid to reduce bleeding during cardiac bypass in children with congenital heart disease. Anesthesiology 40: 604
102. Maguire H, Webb G, Rees A, Gattinella J 1979 Noninvasive evaluation of cardiovascular effects of preoperative sedation in children. Canadian Anaesthetists' Society Journal 26: 29
103. Mansfield P, Hall D, Rittenhouse E, Sauvage L, Stamm S, Herndon P, Furman E 1979 Cardiac surgery under age two years. A review. Journal of Thoracic and Cardiovascular Surgery 77: 816
104. Mapleson W 1954 Elimination of rebreathing in various semi-closed anaesthetic systems. British Journal of Anaesthesia 26: 323
105. Maruschak G, Potter P, Schauble J, Rogers M 1982 Overestimation of pediatric cardiac output by thermal indicator loss. Circulation 65: 380
106. Mathru M, Rao T, Salem M 1979 Tracheal intubation in pediatric patients. Anesthesiology Review 6: 42
107. Maunuksela E, Gattiker R 1981 Use of pancuronium in children with congenital heart disease. Anesthesia and Analgesia 60: 798
108. Maurer H, McCue C, Robertson L, Haggins J 1975 Correction of platelet dysfunction and bleeding in cyanotic congenital heart disease by simple red cell volume reduction. American Journal of Cardiology 35: 831
109. Mehrizi A, Hirsch M, Taussig H 1964 Congenital heart disease in the neonatal period. Autopsy study of 170 cases. Journal of Pediatrics 65: 721
110. Merin R, Kumazawa T, Luka N 1976 Myocardial function and metabolism in the conscious dog and during halothane anesthesia. Anesthesiology 44: 402
111. Midell A, Hallman G, Bloodwell R, Beall A, Yashar J, Cooley D 1971 Epsilon-aminocaproic acid for bleeding after cardiopulmonary bypass. Annals of Thoracic Surgery 11: 577
112. Miller G 1974 Congenital heart disease in the first week of life. British Heart Journal 36: 1160
113. Mitchell S, Korones S, Berendes H 1971 Congenital heart disease in 56,109 births. Incidence and natural history. Circulation 43: 323
114. Moffitt E, McGoon D, Ritter D 1970 Diagnosis and correction of congenital cardiac defects. Anesthesiology 33: 144
115. Moodie D, Feldt R, Kaye M, Danielson G, Pluth J, D'Fallon M 1979 Measurement of postoperative cardiac output by thermodilution in pediatric and adult patients. Journal of Thoracic and Cardiovascular Surgery 78: 796
116. Moore R 1981 Anesthesia for the pediatric congenital heart patient for noncardiac surgery. Anesthesiology Review 8: 23
117. Moorthy S, Pond W, Rowland R 1980 Severe circulatory shock following protamine (an anaphylactic reaction). Anesthesia and Analgesia 59: 77
118. Mori A, Muraoko R, Yokota V, Okamoto Y, Ando F, Fukumasu H, Oku H, Ikeda M, Shirotani H, Hikasa Y 1972 Deep hypothermia combined with cardiopulmonary bypass for cardiac surgery in neonates and infants. Journal of Thoracic and Cardiovascular Surgery 64: 422
119. Morrison J, Killip T 1973 Serum digitalis and arrhythmia in patients undergoing cardiopulmonary bypass. Circulation 47: 341

120. Moss A 1979 What every primary physician should know about the postoperative cardiac patient. Pediatrics 63: 320
121. Motoyama E, Cook C 1980 Respiratory physiology. In: Smith R (ed) Anesthesia for Infants and Children, 4th edn. C.V. Mosby Company, St. Louis
122. Munson E, Bowers D 1967 Effects of hyperventilation on the rate of cerebral anesthetic equilibrium. Anesthesiology 28: 377
123. Myerowitz PD, Caswell K, Lindsay W, Nicoloff D 1977 Antibiotic prophylaxis for open-heart surgery. Journal of Thoracic and Cardiovascular Surgery 73: 625
124. Nadas A, Hauck A 1960 Pediatric aspects of congestive heart failure. Anesthesia and Analgesia 39: 466
125. Naeye R 1962 Thrombotic state after a hemorrhagic diathesis, a possible complication of therapy with epsilon-aminocaproic acid. Blood 19: 694
126. Nicodemus H, Nassiri-Rahimi C, Bachman L, Smith T 1969 Median effective doses (ED_{50}) of halothane in adults and children. Anesthesiology 31: 344
127. Nightingale D, Glass A, Bachman L 1966 Neuromuscular blockage by succinylcholine in children. Anesthesiology 27: 736
128. Neuman G, Hansen D 1980 The anaesthetic management of preterm infants undergoing ligation of patent ductus arteriosus. Canadian Anaesthetists' Society Journal 27: 248
129. Olinger G, Becker R, Bonchek L 1980 Noncardiogenic pulmonary edema and peripheral vascular collapse following cardiopulmonary bypass: rare protamine reaction? Annals of Thoracic Surgery 29: 20
130. Parr G, Blackstone E, Kirklin J 1975 Cardiac performance and mortality early after intracardiac surgery in infants and young children. Circulation 51: 867
131. Patel K, Venus B, Pratap K, Konchigeri H 1980 Cutaneous PO_2 monitoring during pediatric cardiac surgery. Anesthesiology 53: S343
132. Phornphutkul C, Rosenthal A, Nadas A, Berenberg W 1973 Cerebrovascular accidents in infants and children with cyanotic congenital heart disease. American Journal of Cardiology 32: 329
133. Rackow H, Salanitre E 1969 Modern concepts in pediatric anesthesiology. Anesthesiology 30: 208
134. Radney P, Arai T, Nagashima H 1974 Ketamine-gallamine anesthesia for great-vessel operations in infants. Anesthesia and Analgesia 53: 365
135. Radnay P, Badola R 1973 Generalized extensor spasm in infants following ketamine anesthesia. Anesthesiology 39: 459
136. Ravin M, Drury W, Keitt A, Daicoff G 1973 Red cell 2,3-diphosphoglycerate in surgical correction of cyanotic congenital heart disease. Anesthesia and Analgesia 52: 599
137. Rita L, Seleny F, Levin R 1970 Comparison of pentazocine and morphine for pediatric premedication. Anesthesia and Analgesia 49: 377
138. Roberts J 1978 Cardiovascular conditions of children 6–11 years and youth 12–17 years. National Center for Health Survey, U.S. Department of Health, Education, and Welfare. Publication No. (PHS) 78-1653, series 11, No. 166: 1–47
139. Robinson S, Gregory G 1981 Fentanyl-air-oxygen anesthesia for ligation of patent ductus arteriosus in preterm infants. Anesthesia and Analgesia 60: 331
140. Roe C, Santulli T, Blair C 1966 Heat loss in infants during general anesthesia and operations. Journal of Pediatric Surgery 1: 266
141. Root B, Loveland J 1973 Pediatric premedication with diazepam or hydroxyzine: oral vs. intramuscular route. Anesthesia and Analgesia 52: 717
142. Rosenthal A, Button L, Nathan D, Miettinen O, Nadas A 1971 Blood volume changes in cyanotic congenital heart disease. American Journal of Cardiology 27: 162
143. Rosenthal A, Fyler D 1974 Effect of red cell volume reduction on pulmonary blood flow in polycythemia of cyanotic congenital heart disease. American Journal of Cardiology 33: 410
144. Rosenthal A, Mentzer W, Eisenstein E, Nathan D, Nelson N, Nadas A 1971 Role of red blood cell organic phosphates in adaption to congenital heart disease. Pediatrics 47: 537
145. Ryan J 1975 Use of muscle relaxants in pediatric anesthesia. In: Furman E (ed) Anesthesiologist's Role in Pediatric Acute Care. International Anesthesiology Clinics 13: 1. Little Brown, Boston
146. Salanitre E, Rackow H 1969 Pulmonary exchange of nitrous oxide and halothane in infants and children. Anesthesiology 30: 388
147. Salem M, Bennett E 1980 Anesthetic care of pediatric surgical patients. Critical Care Medicine 8: 541
148. Salem M, Wong A, Mani M, Bennett E, Toyama T 1976 Premedicant drugs and gastric juice pH and volume in pediatric patients. Anesthesiology 44: 216
149. Seelye E 1973 Anaesthesia for children with congenital heart disease. Anaesthetic Intensive Care 1: 512

150. Shahinian L, Malachowski N 1978 Retrolental fibroplasia. Archives of Opthalmology 96: 70
151. Shappell S, Lenfant C 1972 Adaptive, genetic, and iatrogenic alterations of the oxyhemoglobin dissociation curve. Anesthesiology 37: 127
152. Shim W, Halford P 1974 Method for maintaining the neonate's intraoperative core temperature. Surgery 75: 416
153. Stanley T, Webster L 1978 Anesthetic requirements and cardiovascular effects of fentanyl-oxygen and fentanyl-diazepam-oxygen anesthesia in man. Anesthesia and Analgesia 57: 411
154. Stark D, Silvay G 1980 Anesthetic management for cardiac surgery not requiring cardiopulmonary bypass. In: Radney P (ed) Anesthetic Considerations for Pediatric Cardiac Surgery. International Anesthesiology Clinics 18: 71. Little, Brown, Boston
155. Steffey E, Howland D 1977 Isoflurane potency in the dog and cat. American Journal of Veterinary Research 38: 1833
156. Sterns L, Lillehei C 1967 Effect of epsilon aminocaproic acid upon blood loss following open heart surgery: an analysis of 340 patients. Canadian Journal of Surgery 10: 304
157. Stevens W, Cromwell T, Halsey M, Eger E II, Shakespeare T, Bahlman S 1971 Cardiovascular effects of a new inhalation anesthetic, Forane, in human volunteers at constant arterial carbon dioxide tension. Anesthesiology 35: 8
158. Steward D, Sloan I, Johnston A 1974 Anaesthetic management of infants undergoing profound hypothermia for surgical correction of congenital heart defects. Canadian Anaesthetists' Society Journal 21: 15
159. Stoelting R 1972 The hemodynamic effects of pancuronium and d-tubocurarine in anesthetized patients. Anesthesiology 36: 612
160. Stoelting R, Longnecker D 1972 The effect of right-to-left shunt on the rate of increase of arterial anesthetic concentration. Anesthesiology 36: 352
161. Tanner G, Angers D, Barash P, Mulla A, Miller P, Rothstein P 1982 Does a left-to-right shunt speed the induction of inhalational anesthetic in congenital heart disease? Anesthesiology 57: A427
162. Telford J, Keats A 1957 Succinylcholine in cardiovascular surgery of infants and children. Anesthesiology 18: 841
163. Thorburn J, Smith G, Vance J, Brown D 1979 Effect of nitrous oxide on the cardiovascular system and coronary circulation of the dog. British Journal of Anaesthesia 51: 937
164. Todres I, deBros F, Kramer S, Moylan F, Shannon D 1976 Endotracheal tube displacement in the newborn infant. Journal of Pediatrics 89: 126
165. Truccone N, Spotnitz H, Gersony W, Dell R, Bowman F, Malm J 1976 Cardiac output in infants and children after open heart surgery. Journal of Thoracic and Cardiovascular Surgery 71: 410
166. Tweed W, Minuck M, Mymin D 1972 Circulatory responses to ketamine anesthesia. Anesthesiology 37: 613
167. Watkins J 1979 Anaphylactoid reactions to I.V. substances. British Journal of Anaesthesia 51: 51
168. Weintraub H, Heisterkamp D, Cooperman L 1969 Changes in plasma potassium concentration after depolarizing blockers in anaesthetized man. British Journal of Anaesthesia 41: 1048
169. White G 1960 Evolution of endotracheal and endobronchial intubation. British Journal of Anaesthesia 32: 235
170. White R, Moffitt E, Feldt R, Ritter D 1972 Myocardial metabolism in children with heart disease. Anesthesia and Analgesia 51: 6
171. Wong K, Martin W, Hornbein T, Freund F, Everett J 1973 Cardiovascular effects of morhphine sulfate with oxygen and with nitrous oxide in man. Anesthesiology 38: 542
172. Wong K, Mohri H, Dillard D, Martin W, Amory D, Cheney F, Merendino K 1974 Deep hypothermia and diethyl ether anesthesia for open heart surgery in infants: a clinical report of 8 years experience. Anesthesia and Analgesia 53: 765
173. Wong A, Salem M, Mani M, Padillo E, Mehta A 1974 Glycopyrrolate as a substitute for atropine in reversl of curarization in pediatric cardiac patients. Anesthesia and Analgesia 53: 412
174. Woodson R, Torrance J, Shappell S, Lenfant C 1970 Effect of cardiac disease on hemoglobin oxygen binding. Journal of Clinical Investigation 49: 1349
175. Wyse S, Pfitzner J, Rees A, Lincoln J, Branthwaite M 1975 Measurement of cardiac output by thermal dilution in infants and children. Thorax 30: 262
176. Young J, Kisker C, Doty D 1978 Adequate anticoagulation during cardiopulmonary bypass determined by activated clotting time and the appearance of fibrin monomer. Annals of Thoracic Surgery 26: 231
177. Zsigmond E, Matsuki A, Kothary S, Jallad M 1976 Arterial hypoxemia caused by intravenous ketamine. Anesthesia and Analgesia 55: 311

5
The Role of Preload in the Manipulation of the Failing Circulation

Russell C. Raphaely and Richard A. Browning

In his delivery of the Linacre Lecture at Cambridge, England, in 1915, Ernest H. Starling,[41] based upon his own studies[28,29] and those of Otto Frank[13] on isolated heart and heart/lung preparations, concluded that "the energy of contraction, however measured, is a function of the length of the muscle fibre." Many investigators have questioned the validity and significance of the relationship in the presence of an intact circulation. Studies attempting to explore the interaction in vivo have struggled with quantifying energy and fiber length. Acceptably precise estimates of external mechanical work exclude energy liberated during isometric contraction. Therefore, total energy is not measured. Myocardial fiber length in the intact animal has proven to be an elusive variable.

These difficulties prompted Sarnoff to substitute external stroke work, which excludes the energy of contraction during isometric contraction, for energy liberated and atrial pressure for myocardial fiber length to "evaluate more completely the law of the heart and physical determinants of ventricular work in the living animal with a complete circulation."[34]

However, implicit in the pressure-fiber length-volume relationship is the absence of any change in elasticity or tone of the ventricle. Changes in compliance of the ventricles, which occur acutely in critically ill patients, may lead to a misinterpretation of cardiac performance if filling pressures rather than end-diastolic volume (EDV) are utilized.[10] Furthermore, many publications following Sarnoff's work have inappropriately substituted cardiac output or stroke volume for stroke work even though Sarnoff cautions against this.

Echocardiography has been advocated by some as a satisfactory bedside non-invasive method for estimating ventricular volume.[20] Proponents suggest this discipline should be regularly employed and substituted for measurements of filling pressure during manipulation of preload to reverse a failing circulation. Other individuals dispute the accuracy of this method for estimating ventricular volumes.[12] Contrast, or nuclide, cardioangiography has yet to achieve practical use in a critical care unit.

Clinicians overcome the inability to measure end-diastolic volume and assess the variable relationship between end-diastolic volume (fiber length) and filling pressure that acute and chronic diseases produce by examining the pattern of response to a decrease or augmentation of intravascular volume; thereby insight into the existing pressure-volume relationship is gained.

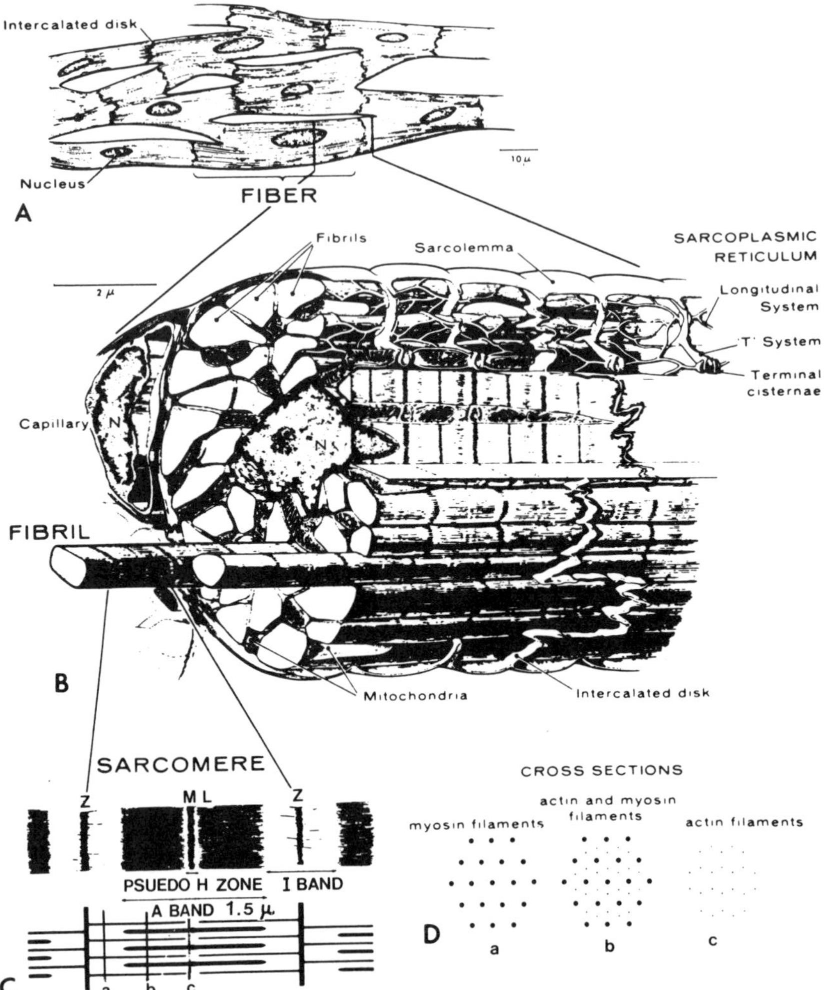

Fig. 5.1. Diagrammatic representation of microscopic features of heart muscle. (A) Branching heart muscle fibers connected at intercalated discs with nuclei located centrally. (B) Illustration of electron micrograph demonstrating parallel fibrils within a fiber that contains mitochondria, nucleus, and sarcoplasmic reticulum and is bordered by an intercalated disc. (C) Illustration of sarcomere showing thick and thin filament relationships resulting in the A and I bands, H zone, Z line. (D) Cross section through the center, distal A band and I band of sarcomere, illustrating thick and thin filament relationship. (Braunwald E, Sonnenblick EH, Ross J, Jr 1984 Contraction of the normal heart. p. 410. In: Braunwald E (ed) Heart Disease: A Textbook of Cardiovascular Medicine. WB Saunders, Philadelphia.)

STRUCTURE OF THE MYOCARDIAL CELL

Knowledge of myocardial cell composition (Fig. 5.1) helps one understand the performance of the heart according to Starling's law. Striated muscle cells or fibers 10 to 20 μm in diameter and 40 to 100 μm in length make up the myocardium. Multiple cross-banded strands, the myofibrils, run the length of the fiber. Serially repeating structures, the sarcomeres, which occupy 50 percent of the cell mass, align themselves so that the ends of each sarcomere in adjacent myofibrils exist next to one another, resulting in the whole fiber possessing a banded or striated appearance under light microscopy.

Strands of contractile protein, the myofilaments, are arranged in a specific manner. Their interaction generates force and causes shorting.

Two adjacent lines, the Z lines, define the boundaries of the sarcomere, the fundamental structure and functional unit of contraction. A distance of 1.6 to 2.2 μm separates the Z lines under physiologic conditions. Alternating light and dark bands within the sarcomere give the myocardium its striated appearance.

At constant length of 1.5 μm, the A band exists as a broad dark structure in the center of the sarcomere. Two I bands flank the A band; these are lighter bands of variable length, depending on sarcomere length. A dark line, the M line, bisects the A band. Immediately adjacent to the M lines are two lighter areas termed the L lines. These collectively constitute the ML complex or pseudo–H zone.

An orderly array of partially overlapping rod-like myofilaments, fixed in length during rest and contraction, constitute the contractile substance. The myofilaments consist of ordered macroaggregates of contractile proteins. The thicker myofila-

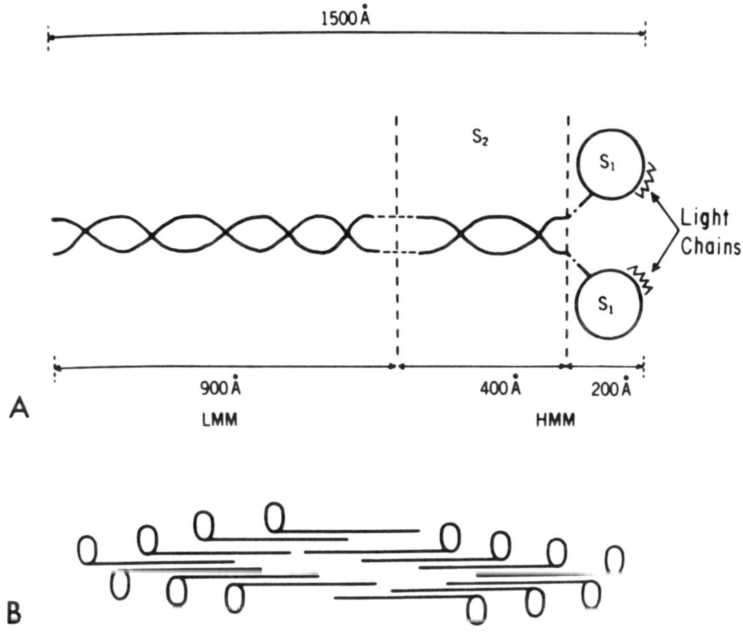

Fig. 5.2. Schematic of individual myosin molecule and collective arrangement in thick filament. (A) Diagrammatic representation of myosin molecule showing two strands and cleavage points separating light and heavy meromyosin elements. Heavy meromyosin contains an S_1 portion where ATPase is located. The S_2 fragment attaches and is similar in shape to the light meromyosin. (Lowey S et al 1969 Substructure of the myosin molecule. I. Subfragments of myosin by enzymatic degradation. J Molec Biol 42: 1.) (B) Illustration of myosin molecules. They are aggregated into a thick filament and arranged such that the long portion faces the center and the active enzymes containing segments occupy the edges of the filament. (Braunwald E, Sonnenblick EH, Ross J, Jr 1984 Contraction of the normal heart. p. 413. In: Braunwald E (ed) Heart Disease: A Textbook of Cardiovascular Medicine. WB Saunders, Philadelphia.)

ments, composed of myosin, 100 nm in diameter and 1.5 to 1.6 μm in length, exist only in the A band. Thinner actin myofilaments, 50 Å in diameter and 1.0 μm in length extend from the Z line through the I band to the A band and terminate at the L line when the sarcomere length equals 2.2 μm. Thick and thin filaments overlap within the A band. The I band contains only thin filaments when sarcomere length is fully extended. The ML complex or, pseudo-H zone, contains only thick filaments.

Contractile Proteins

The thicker myosin filaments with tapered ends consist of molecules which can be broken down into light and heavy meromyosin (Fig. 5.2). Heavy meromyosin 200 Å long contains bilobed globular heads, which are oriented laterally and project from the filament. The bilobed heads appear to be the sights of the formation of cross bridges with the actin filaments. Further cleavage of the heavy meromyosin results in an S_2 fragment 400 Å in length similar to light meromyosin and a 200 Å long portion possessing adenosine triphosphatase (ATPase) activity. This ATPase is inhibited by Mg^{++} but is activated by small amounts of Ca^{++}.

Light meromyosin makes up the rod-like tail lying along the filament for about 1300 nm and oriented toward the center of the filament. This double alpha helix consists of two strands of actin projecting through the Z line, the I band, and into the A band where overlapping of the thin and thick filaments occurs. Thin filaments exists alone in the I band.

Six actin filaments surround one myosin filament in a hexagonal arrangement. Each actin filament may participate in the hexagonal grouping around more than one myosin element.

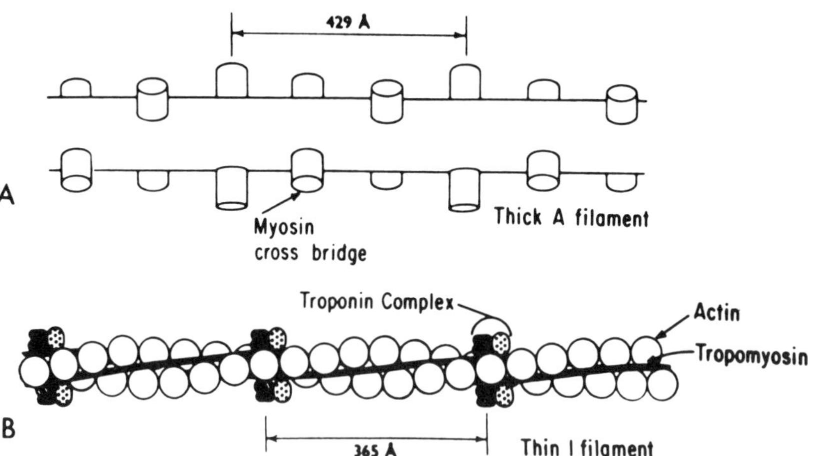

Fig. 5.3. Schematic of thick and thin filaments and their interaction. (A) Spiral configuration of myosin bridges such that a complete revolution of active sites around long axis of filament occurs every 429 Å. (B) Tropinin complex exists at every seventh actin site. Actin molecules align to form a ridge close to which a tropomyosin molecule lies. (Braunwald E, Sonnenblick EH, Ross J, Jr 1984 Contraction of the normal heart. p. 413. In: Braunwald E (ed) Heart Disease: A Textbook of Cardiovascular Medicine. WB Saunders, Philadelphia.)

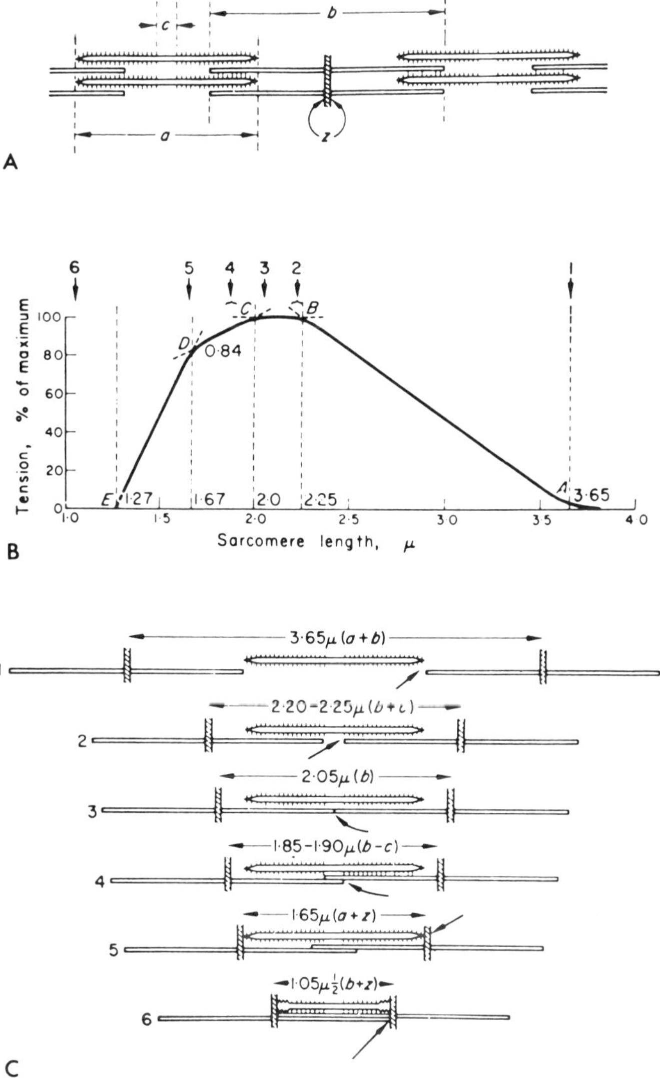

Fig. 5.4. Tension development and myofilament relationships. (A) Diagrammatic scaler representation of 1.0 μm thin and 1.6 μm long thick filaments. (B) Tension development and sarcomere length relationship. Sarcomere length is indicated by numbers with arrows that correspond to filament arrangements in Fig. 5.4C. (C) Myofilament overlap at various sarcomere lengths. (Adapted from Gordon AM et al 1966 The variation in isometric tension with sarcomere length in vertebrate muscle fibers. J Physiol (Lond) 184: 170 by Braunwald E, Sonnenblick EH, Ross J, Jr 1984 Contraction of the normal heart. p. 424. In: Braunwald E (ed) Heart Disease: A Textbook of Cardiovascular Medicine. WB Saunders, Philadelphia.)

Regulatory Protein

The regulatory proteins troponin and tropomyosin constitute 10 percent of the protein content of the myofibril (Fig. 5.3). Both exist as part of the thin filament. The rod-like tropomyosin lies slightly outside the groove created by the actin chains, forming a continuing strand through the center of the thin filament.

Troponin is composed of three components: C, which binds Ca^{++}; I, which possesses an inhibitory function over Mg^{++} stimulation of actinomyosin ATPase activity; and T, which is necessary for the entire complex function and its site of attachment to the tropomyosin and actin. A strand of seven actin molecules exists in association with one troponin complex. One long tropomyosin molecule extends the length of seven actin molecules.

Filament length remains constant at rest and during contraction. Force generation occurs as a result of displacement of the actin filaments by linking them to cross-bridging sites on the myosin filament. The number of cross-bridging sites between actin and myosin determines the tension developed, or magnitude of shortening of the myocardial fiber. Changes in sarcomere length produce a predictable alteration in the overlapping of the thick and thin filaments, which influences the number of cross-bridging sites during contraction. Uncertainty exists as to whether electrostatic forces or physical attachment are responsible for the movements of the myofilaments.

Thick filaments measure 1.5 μm in length with a central portion of approximately 0.2 μm in width possessing no cross-bridging sites. Maximum force development occurs (Fig. 5.4) when sarcomere length is 2.0 to 2.2 μm when optimum overlapping of the 1.0 μm long actin and 1.5-μm long myosin optimally overlap. Force generation decreases when the sarcomere contracts from a length greater than 2.2 μm and ceases at 3.65 μm when no overlapping of the filaments exists.

Double overlapping of the thin filaments and reductions in force generation result when sarcomere length falls below 2.0 μm. Suggested explanations for this include: interference with cross-bridge formation, delayed ability of filaments to bind Ca^{++} required for activation, and diminished sensitivity to calcium ion. Significant internal load may impair shortening at lesser sarcomere dimensions, and repellation of the thin filaments from the opposite half of the A band may also contribute.

STARLING'S LAW OF THE HEART

Length-tension curves describe the influence of myocardial fiber length on force development. Stretching an isolated papillary muscle produces an increase in resting tension and developed tension. Contraction reaches a maximum after which developed tension falls, even though total tension increases as a result of an increase in resting tension. This reflects the incorporation of more interacting sites between the actin and myosin filaments until the optimal overlap is reached. Further lengthening of the myocardial fiber reduces the potential cross-bridging sites, thereby diminishing the force developed with a contraction.

In the intact heart, end-diastolic volume or, more commonly, ventricular end-diastolic pressure (EDP), is usually estimated from mean atrial pressure. It represents length, and stroke work is substituted for developed tension (energy). The product of stroke volume and the difference between mean systolic arterial and mean atrial pressures equals stroke work. A curvilinear line concaved downward results when volume or pressure is located on the X axis and stroke work on the Y axis. Increasing myocardial fiber length increases both developed tension and the rate at which isometric tension develops. Furthermore, integrated systolic isometric tension increases and constitutes the impulse force generated by an isometrically contracting fiber. During isotonic conditions, this force expells blood from the heart.

DIASTOLIC PROPERTIES OF THE INTACT HEART

Myocardial fiber length at end diastole determines tension developed during isometric contraction and magnitude of shortening during isotonic contraction. Volume of the intact ventricle just before systole influences myocardial fiber length. In the absence of readily available volume estimates, clinicians employ more measurable pressure, assuming a known relationship between volume and pressure. This relationship describes the diastolic properties of the intact ventricle. A curvilinear, concave, upward line results when volume is placed on the X axis and pressure is located on the Y axis[19,23] (Fig. 5.5). The instantaneous compliance (dV/dP) can be determined at any point along the curve and changes as a dynamic function of filling. A slowly rising slope exists at low diastolic volumes reflecting the high compliance or easy distensibility of the ventricle during early diastole when filling begins. A steeper exponential relationship occurs near end diastole. On the same curve, therefore, compliance changes as the ventricle fills.[17,19] Though volume is the true determinant of preload, pressure is the most frequent clinically measured entity. The pressure-volume relationship of the ventricle changes under

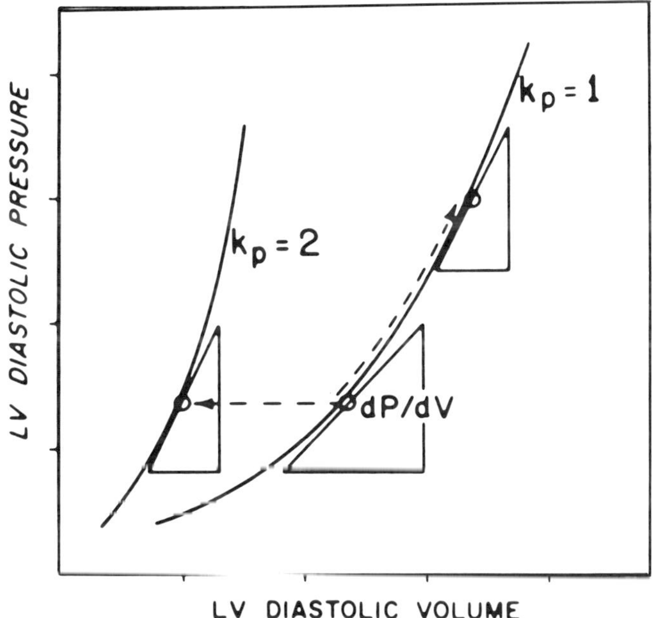

Fig. 5.5. Pressure-volume relationships of the left ventricle (LV). On the Right can be seen the increased operative chamber stiffness (dP/dV) that occurs with normal filling, on the Left, the altered pressure volume relationship that results from a change in the modulus of chamber stiffness (K_p). (Gaasch WH, Levine HJ, Quinonesm MA 1976 Left ventricular compliance: Mechanisms and clinical implications. American Journal of Cardiology 38: 645.)

Table 5.1. Conditions Effecting Modulus of Chamber Stiffness (K_p) in the Left Ventricle

Conditions that shift the pressure-volume curve to the left
Positive end expiratory pressure
Intraventricular septal shift from right ventricular distention
Pericardial disease
Age
Relief of volume overload
Inotropes
Ischemia
Intrinsic increases in myocardial stiffness
Hemorrhagic and septic shock
Ventricular hypertrophy
Conditions that shift the pressure-volume curve to the right
Chronic adaptation to volume overload
Cardiomyopathies
Relief of ischemia
Vasodilators

physiologic and pathophysiologic conditions. For maximal clinical manipulation of preload in any patient, the extent of the alteration must be determined. The pressure-volume curve in Figure 5-5 reveals the decreased compliance or increased stiffness (dP/dV) that occurs with normal filling. Increase in chamber stiffness may also occur by a shift to the left of the pressure-volume curve[16] (Fig. 5.5). This results in a change in the modulus of chamber stiffness (K_p) and defines an altered pressure-volume relationship for that ventricle secondary to a disease process or drug therapy. K_p increases when the ventricle compliance decreases; hence EDP is greater for any given EDV.[23] Leftward shifts (Table 5.1) of the pressure-volume curve result from increases in intrinsic myocardical stiffness (e.g., fibrosis and storage diseases), by a change in ventricular mass and wall thickness, positive end expiratory pressure (PEEP), right ventricular (RV) overload with septal shift, pericardial disease, inotropes, ischemia, hemorrhagic and septic shock, and decreased end diastolic volume due to improved ejection fraction.[1,9,10,18,23,25,33,40,42]

Four important clinical influences on ventricular compliance worthy of further discussion are the effects of PEEP, ventricular interpendence, the elastic limits of the pericardium, and age.

Application of PEEP, accentuates the difference between EDV and wedge pressure (WP)[11], manifested clinically by a decrease in left ventricular (LV) EDV despite no change or even an increase in WP.[9,11] Resultant increases in LV stiffness (dP/dV) may occur from either a shift of the intraventricular septum[22,25] or by an increase in the volume of the surrounding lung causing restricted ventricular relaxation.[38]

Compliance of the left ventricle may decrease as a consequence of changes in the shape of the right ventricle.[43] Increased RV volume may result in a leftward shift of the interventricular septum.[2] The LV volume is thus lowered despite an increase in LVEDP.

Alterations of the pressure-volume curve also result during conditions of volume loading when overall cardiac volume may increase beyond the limits of pericardial distensibility. The pericardium then becomes restrictive, and a functional increase in ventricular stiffness results.[26]

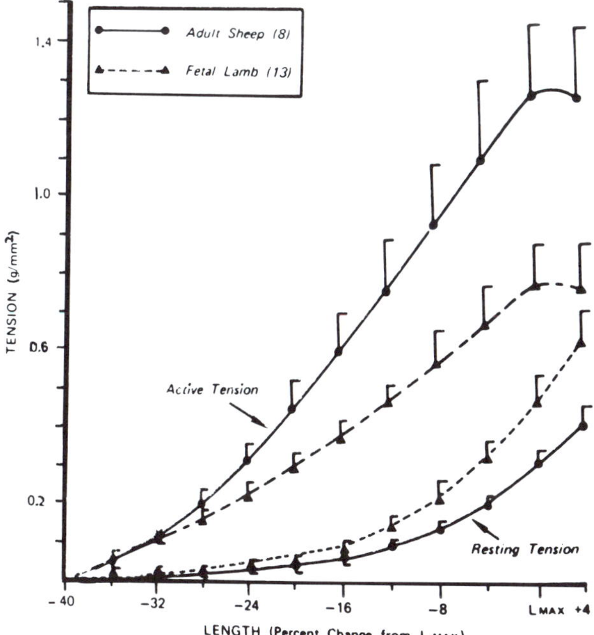

Fig. 5.6. Isometric passive and active length-tension curves from the fetus and adult. Numbers in brackets refer to numbers of animals studied. Each point and the vertical bars represent the mean ± SEM. (Friedman WF 1972 Intrinsic physiologic properties of the developing heart. Progress in Cardiovascular Disease. Grune and Stratton, New York 15: 87–111, by permission.)

The pressure-volume properties of the newborn ventricle differ from those of the adult or older child. Animal studies support the clinical impression that the newborn heart is less compliant than the adult heart.[14,15,31,32] Friedman obtained isometric passive and active length-tension curves from fetal and adult lambs[14] (Fig. 5.6). At all muscle lengths, fetal heart muscle generated significantly less active tension when compared to the adult. A higher resting tension also occurs in the fetus at any muscle length. The left-shifted resting tension curve suggests that a state of reduced compliance exists in fetal heart muscle when compared to the adult and implies an age-dependent difference in the force required to distend the ventricular chambers. Romero et al confirmed this hypothesis by analyzing the pressure-volume characteristics of each ventricle.[31] In the early newborn period (1 to 18 days) the right and left ventricles exhibit reduced compliance when compared to the adult. In the newborn, ventricular filling of one ventricle influences the other ventricle more than in the adult (Fig. 5.7). Newborns easily demonstrate systemic venous congestion in the presence of disorders that primarily increase left ventricular volume or pressure, providing clinical evidence supporting this laboratory observation. These properties of the newborn ventricle limit the benefit obtained from increases in preload observed in the adult ventricle. Less effective augmentation of stroke work by preload results[25] (Fig. 5.8). The explanation for the reduced compliance of the newborn heart remains unclear. However, fetal myocardium contains a significantly greater noncontractile mass than occurs in adult tissue.[14,36]

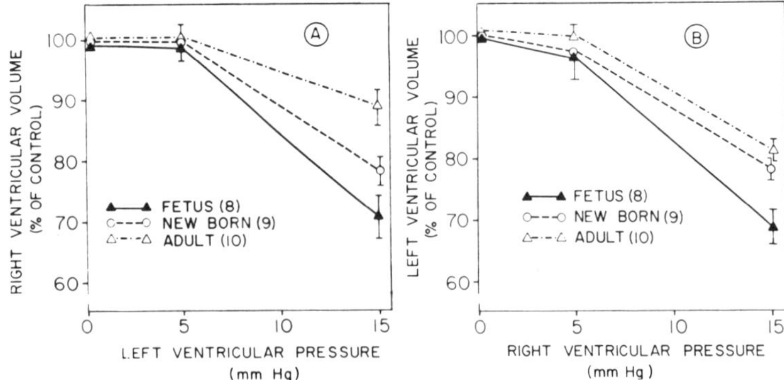

Fig. 5.7. (A) Influence of left ventricular filling on right ventricular volume. At 15 mmHg left ventricular pressure, right ventricular volume is significantly less in both the fetus and newborn when compared to the adult. (B) Influence of right ventricular filling on left ventricular volume. At 15 mmHg right ventricular pressure, left ventricular volume is significantly less in the fetus than either the newborn or the adult. (Romero T, Covell JW, Friedman WF 1972 A comparison of pressure volume relations of the fetal, newborn and adult heart. American Journal of Physiology, 222: 1285.)

Chronic adaptation to volume overload, cardiomyopathy, relief of ischemia, and vasodilator therapy displace the pressure-volume curve to the right.[23]

Parenteral infusion of arterial vasodilators such as sodium nitroprusside and nitroglycerin improve left ventricular compliance.[8] By altering the ventricular mechanical properties, these drugs shift the pressure volume curve to the right. Larger EDV can then be accommodated at constant or lowered wedge pressures, allowing for therapeutic augmentation of LVEDV without a detrimental rise in wedge pressure.

Ventricular compliance determines how the ventricle will respond to fluid manipulations. The compliance allows one to more accurately interpret ventricular volumes from filling pressures—central venous pressure (CVP) or WP—and hence

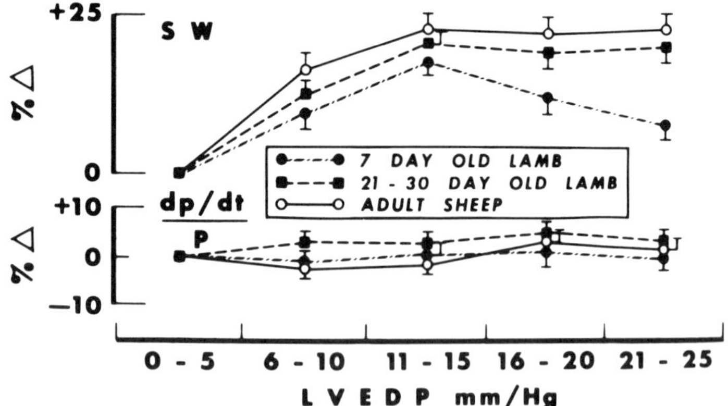

Fig. 5.8. Changes in stroke work induced by saline infusion at constant heart rate. The newborn lamb is unable to increase stroke work in response to increased preload as effectively as the adult sheep. (Romero TE, Friedman WF 1979 Limited left ventricular response to volume overload in the neonatal period: A comparative study with the adult animal. Pediatric Research, 13: 910.)

fiber length. This in turn, permits preload manipulation which will reverse a failing circulation.

PRELOAD

Venous return, total blood volume, distribtuion of blood volume, and atrial function determine preload (ventricular EDV) in the intact animal.[3,7,27]

The return of blood to the heart has a major influence on cardiac output. Peripheral resistance and venous tone determine venous blood flow to the heart.[3] Conditions which decrease peripheral vascular resistance (e.g., fever, pregnancy, exercise, and atrioventricular (AV)-fistula,) markedly augment venous return. Similarly, increases in venous tone (e.g., exercise, drugs, and anxiety)[6,21,37] cause more blood to reach the heart and augment preload.

Total blood volume profoundly effects preload. Hemorrhage decreases EDV, reduces fiber length, and diminishes tension development and shortening.

Distribution of blood has an impact on preload.[3,7] Body position, intrathoracic pressure, and intrapericardial pressure alter the distribution of blood and consequently cardiac filling and preload. Gravitational forces (upright position), intrathoracic pressure elevations (positive pressure ventilation, pneumothorax),[4] and intrapericardial pressure elevations (effusion)[35] all impair blood return to the thorax and decrease cardiac preload.

A vigorous, well-timed atrial contraction augments ventricular filling.[5] The volume of blood ejected during atrial systole at ventricular end-diastole further increases the passively accumulated ventricular EDV. Nodal rhythms or atrioventricular dissociation uncouples this atrial augmentation of ventricular filling. Atrial fibrillation produces ineffective contractions and negates the positive atrial effect on preload. The atrial augmentation of preload effects ventricular filling most significantly in the presence of ventricular hypertrophy or other states of reduced compliance. Absence of the atrial systolic component to filling in these conditions markedly reduces ventricular EDV and, consequently, stroke work falls.[24]

Preload Manipulation

Disease and injury probably effect preload more than any other determinant of cardiac output. Similarly, manipulation of intravascular volume (preload) by expansion or contraction remains the most common therapeutic intervention employed in the care of critically ill patients. The effectiveness of preload volume manipulation is governed by the pressure-volume relationship within the ventricle and by Starling's law of the heart.[41] As described earlier, this law states that "the mechanical energy set free on passage from the resting to the contractile state is a function of the length of the muscle fibre, i.e., of the area of chemically active surfaces." In the intact heart, the end-diastolic volume determines the resting length of the sarcomeres. Alterations in preload, operating through changes in end-diastolic sarcomere length, provide a major determinant of ventricular function. In addition to a plateau being reached on the ventricular performance curve such that no further stroke work occurs, the pressure achieved at a given end-diastolic volume transmitted to the pulmonary capillaries constitutes a practical limit to preload augmentation. As the ventricle moves to the steeper portion of its pressure-volume curve, pulmonary edema results.

Tactics of manipulation

When confronted with evidence supporting the diagnosis of failing circulation (defined as a pressure and flow insufficient to meet tissue requirements) and in the absence of systemic or pulmonary vascular congestion, clinicians infuse a preselected volume of fluids to test the response to preload manipulation. Physicians treating children choose 10 to 20 ml/kg of colloid-containing fluid infused rapidly over 10 to 20 minutes and evaluate the impact on clinical estimates of improving hemodynamics. Variables utilized include systemic arterial pressure, heart rate, skin color and temperature, urine flow, venous caliber, pulse volume, and mentation.

Failing to achieve the desired goal of hemodynamic stability, one proceeds to a titration of fluids to atrial pressure measured by catheter placement discussed in detail in Chapter 3. In our practice, we favor placement of the orifice of a catheter in the superior vena cava just before its entry into the right atrium. Pressure here mirrors right atrial pressure, and blood sampled for gas tensions and content yield mean values that correlate well with those found in mixed venous blood sampled from the pulmonary artery. We insert flow-directed, balloon-tipped pulmonary artery catheters only (1) if we believe the patient possesses an insult suspected of impairing left ventricular performance while sparing or effecting to a lesser magnitude the right ventricle or (2) when guided by right heart pressures one does not achieve hemodynamic stability. In pediatric practice, one most commonly encounters global cardiac dysfunction so that both ventricles are uniformly effected. Patients who have undergone reparative procedures for congenital heart lesions may be exceptions.

We employ a modification of Weil's "5 and 2 Rule"[44] to guide us in the safe augmentation of preload (Fig. 5.9). One observes the CVP for 10 minutes. If that pressure is less than 6 mmHg, we infuse 4 ml/kg over 10 minutes, discontinuing the infusion if the CVP rises at any time more than 4 mmHg. If, following the infusion, the CVP has risen by less than 4 mmHg, but more than 2 mmHg, we observe the patient for an additional 10 minutes. If the CVP remains above 2 mmHg of the starting value, we monitor the patient without administering any additional fluid. If the CVP declines to within 2 mmHg of the initial value, we repeat the maneuvers until systemic arterial pressure reaches a normal value, the patient manifests other signs of circulatory integrity, or a sustained rise of more than 4 mmHg occurs. If the initial CVP lies between 6 and 10 mmHg, we administer 2 ml/kg over 10 minutes and look for the same CVP changes. If the initial CVP exceeds 10 mmHg, we infuse 1 ml/kg over 10 minutes and again observe the CVP change. We emphasize two points. First, we examine the change in CVP measurement in response to the fluid infusion rather than look for an absolute value. Second, because the veins are very distensible vessels and act as a reservoir for fluid, a three-fold increase in the volume of fluid may be necessary before we can see changes in the CVP.

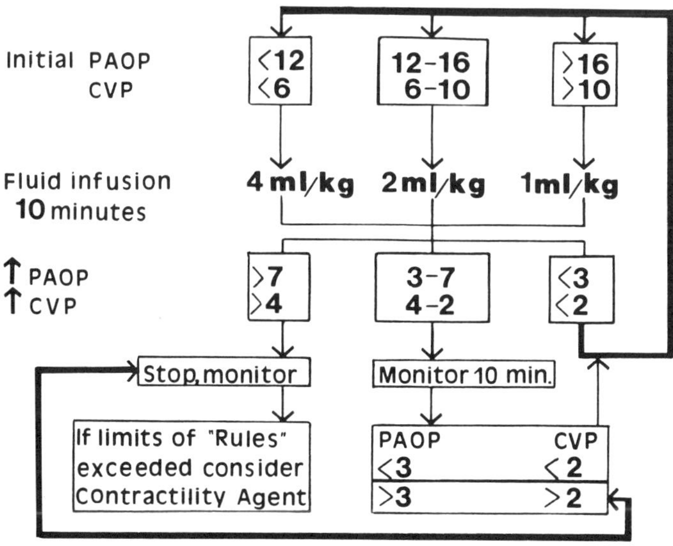

Fig. 5.9. Fluid volumes titrated against central venous (CVP) or pulmonary artery occluded pressures (PAOP) for preload manipulation. (Modified from Weil MH 1980 Patient evaluation, "vital signs," and initial care. pp. 1A–31 In Shoemaker WC, Thompson WL (eds) Critical Care: State of the Art, The Society of Critical Care Medicine, Vol 1, Fullerton, CA.)

Choice of Fluids

If the hemodynamic instability is associated with an insult in which the constituents of the preload deficit are known, we administer fluids which most approximate the lost fluid.

We maintain a hematocrit of 33 percent, preferring to administer packed cells in combination with other blood components, thereby using these scarce resources more efficiently. We employ fresh-frozen plasma and platelets if clotting abnormalities or thrombocytopenia exists. When the hematocrit is greater than 33 percent or blood is not available, we use 5 percent albumin and normal saline solution. Shoemaker[39] examined the effects of colloid-crystalloid fluids containing electrolytes and whole blood on several variables. Overall, he found the synthetic plasma expander dextran with molecular weights of 40,000 to 70,000 as well as albumin, produced the most favorable changes in mean arterial pressure, left ventricular stroke work, pulmonary vascular resistance, and oxygen consumption, if these were used in place of whole blood. Dextrans and hetastarch are widely available and relatively inexpensive, but cause diminished platelet adherence and interfere with clotting. This effect is seldom of clinical significance when less than 20 ml/kg of these solutions are administered.

When circulatory assessment suggests preload should be reduced, vasodilators and potent tubular diuretics find widespread use. Nitroglycerin mostly effects the venous capacitance vessels and seems particularly suitable for diminishing preload and redistributing intravascular volume. By diminishing impedence to ejection, nitroprusside and arterial vasodilators allow more complete emptying of the ventricle, diminish EDV, and thus reduce preload. Ethyacrinic acid and furosemide in doses of 0.5 to 1 mg/kg promptly produce urine flow, which reduces preload by diminishing intravascular volume.

CONCLUSION

Even though disease, injury, and therapy affect preload more than any other determinant of cardiac output, its importance in the management of the failing circulation is often underestimated. Perhaps because of the simplicity of the principle, caretakers often devote little attention to this influence on cardiac output and focus more on manipulation of afterload and contractility.

Ream and Fogdall[30] note in their book *Acute Cardiovascular Management: Anesthesia and Intensive Care*, in an evaluation of the treatment of cardiogenic shock, that mortality rates of 50 to 95 percent existed before the importance of preload augmentation was appreciated. When protocols demanded adequate left ventricular preload, cardiogenic shock unresponsive to this treatment had a uniformly greater than 95 percent mortality. This suggests that with the proper management of preload, only 5 percent of patients who require adjustment of other determinants of cardiac output survive.

Our experience in an active pediatric critical care unit leads us to manipulate preload as the main therapy in management of the failing circulation. An understanding of the principle and a systematic approach to the adjustment of preload will help individuals to achieve a favorable outcome in pediatric patients with a failing circulation.

REFERENCES

1. Alyono D, Ring WS, Anderson RW 1978 The effects of hemorrhagic shock on the diastolic properties of the left ventricle in the conscious dog. Surgery 83: 691
2. Bemis CE, Serur JR, Borkenhagen D, Sonnenblick EH, Urschel CW 1974 Influence of right ventricular filling pressure on left ventricular pressure and dimension. Circulation Research 34: 498
3. Braunwald E 1974 Regulation of the circulation. New England Journal of Medicine 290: 1124
4. Braunwald E, Binion JT, Morgan WL Jr, Sarnoff SJ 1957 Alterations in central blood volume and cardiac output induced by positive pressure breathing and counteracted by metaraminol (Aramine). Circulation Research 5: 670
5. Braunwald E, Frahm CJ 1961 Studies on Starling's law of the heart IV. Observations on hemodynamic functions of left atrium in man. Circulation 24: 633
6. Braunwald E, Ross J Jr, Kahler RL, Gaffney TE, Goldblatt A, Mason DT 1963 Reflex control of the systemic venous bed: Effects on venous tone of vasoactive drugs, and of baroreceptor and chemoreceptor stimulation. Circulation Research 12: 539
7. Braunwald E, Sonnenblick, EH, Ross J Jr 1984 Contraction of the normal heart. p. 409 In: Braunwald E (ed) Heart Disease: A Textbook of Cardiovascular Medicine, WB Saunders, Philadelphia
8. Brodie BR, Grossman W, Mann T, McLaurin LP 1977 Effects of sodium nitroprusside on left ventricular diastolic pressure-volume relations. Journal of Clinical Investigation 59: 59
9. Calvin JE, Driedger AA, Sibbald WJ 1981 Positive end-expiratory pressure (PEEP) does not depress left ventricular function in patients with pulmonary edema. American Review of Respiratory Diseases 124: 121
10. Calvin JE, Driedger AA, Sibbald WJ 1981 Does the pulmonary capillary wedge pressure predict left ventricular preload in critically ill patients? Critical Care Medicine 9: 437
11. Fewell JE, Abendschein DR, Carlson CJ, Rapaport E, Murray JF 1980 Mechanism of decreased

right and left ventricular end-diastolic volume during continuous positive-pressure ventilation in dogs. Circulation Research 47: 467
12. Folland ED, Parisi AF, Moynihan PF, Jones DR, Feldman CL, Tow DE 1979 Assessment of left ventricular ejection fraction and volumes by real-time, two-dimensional echocardiography. Circulation 60: 760
13. Frank O 1959 On the dynamics of cardiac muscle. (Transl. by CB Chapman and E Wasserman) American Heart Journal 58: 282 and 467
14. Friedman WF 1972 Intrinsic physiologic properties of the developing heart. Progress in Cardiovascular Disease 15: 87
15. Friedman WF, George BL 1985 Treatment of congestive heart failure by altering loading conditions of the heart. Journal of Pediatrics 106: 697
16. Gaasch WH, Levine HJ, Quinones MA, Alexander JK 1976 Left ventricular compliance: Mechanisms and clinical implications. American Journal of Cardiology 38: 645
17. Glantz SA, Misbach GA, Moores WY, Mathey DG, Lekven J, Stowe DF, Parmley WW, Tyberg JV 1978 The pericardium substantially affects the left ventricular diastolic pressure-volume relationship in the dog. Circulation Research 42: 433
18. Glantz SA, Parmley WW 1978 Factors which affect the diastolic pressure-volume curve. Circulation Research 42: 171
19. Grossman W, McLaurin LP 1976 Diastolic properties of the left ventricle. Annals of Internal Medicine 84: 316
20. Gueret P, Meerbaum S, Wyatt HL, Uchiyama T, Lang T-W, Corday E 1980 Two-dimensional echocardiographic quantitation of left ventricular volumes and ejection fraction. Circulation 62: 1308
21. Guyton AC, Douglas BH, Langston JB, Richardson TQ 1962 Instantaneous increase in mean circulatory pressure and cardiac output at onset of muscular activity. Circulation Research 11: 431
22. Jardin F, Farcot JC, Boisante L, Curien N, Margairaz A, Bourdarias J-P 1981 Influence of positive end-expiratory pressure on left ventricular performance. New England Journal of Medicine 304: 387
23. Lewis BS, Gotsman MS 1980 Current concepts of left ventricular relaxation and compliance. American Heart Journal 99: 101
24. Linderer T, Chatterjee K, Parmley WW, Sievers RE, Glantz SA, Tyberg JV 1983 Influence of atrial systole on the Frank-Starling relation and the end-diastolic pressure-diameter relation of the left ventricle. Circulation 67: 1045
25. Ludbrook PA, Byrne JD, McKnight RC 1979 Influence of ventricular hemodynamics on left ventricular diastolic sure-volume relations in man. Circulation 59: 21
26. Mirsky I, Rankin JS 1979 The effects of geometry, elasticity, and external pressures on the diastolic pressure-volume and stiffness-stress relations. How important is the pericardium? Circulation Research 44: 601
27. Parker JO, Case RB 1979 Normal left ventricular function. Circulation 60: 4
28. Patterson SW, Starling EH 1914 On the mechanical factors which determine the output of the ventricles. Journal of Physiology 48: 357
29. Piper H, Starling EH 1914 The regulation of the heart beat. Journal of Physiology 48: 465
30. Ream AK, Fogdall RP (eds) 1982 Cardiovascular physiology: Application to clinical problems. p. 9 In: Acute Cardiovascular Management: Anesthesia and Intensive Care. JB Lippincott, Philadelphia
31. Romero T, Covell JW, Friedman WF 1972 A comparison of pressure volume relations of the fetal, newborn and adult heart. American Journal of Physiology, 222: 1285
32. Romero TE, Friedman WF 1979 Limited left ventricular response to volume overload in the neonatal period: A comparative study with the adult animal. Pediatric Research, 13: 910
33. Ross J 1979 Editorial: Acute displacement of the diastolic pressure volume curve of the left ventricle: Role of the pericardium and the right ventricle. Circulation 59: 32
34. Sarnoff SJ 1955 Symposium on regulation of heart: Myocardial contractility as described by ventricular function curves; observations on Starling's Law of the Heart. Physiological Reviews 35: 107
35. Shabetai R, Fowler NO, Guntheroth WG 1970 The hemodynamics of cardiac tamponade and constrictive pericarditis. American Journal of Cardiology 26: 480
36. Sheldon CA, Friedman WF, Sybers HD 1976 Scanning electron microscopy of fetal and neonatal lamb cardiac cells. Journal of Molecular and Cellular Cardiology 8: 853
37. Shepherd JT, Vanhoutte PM 1975 Veins and Their Control. WB Saunders Company, Philadelphia
38. Shirato K, Shabetai R, Bhargava V, Franklin D, Ross J Jr 1978 Alteration of the left ventricular diastolic pressure-segment length relation produced by the pericardium: Effects of cardiac distention and afterload reduction in conscious dogs. Circulation 57: 1191

39. Shoemaker WC 1976 Comparison of the relative effectiveness of whole blood transfusions and various types of fluid therapy in resuscitation. Critical Care Medicine 4: 71
40. Sibbald NJ, Calvin J, Driedger AA 1984 Right and left ventricular preload and diastolic ventricular compliance: Implication for therapy in critically ill patients. In: Shoemaker WC, Thompson WL, Holbrook PR (eds) Textbook of Critical Care Medicine, WB Saunders, Philadelphia
41. Starling EH 1918 The Linacre Lecture on the Law of the Heart. Given at Cambridge in 1915. Longmans, Green & Company, London
42. Suter PM, Fairley HB, Isenberg MD 1975 Optimum end-expiratory airway pressure in patients with acute pulmonary failure. New England Journal of Medicine 292: 284
43. Taylor RR, Covell JW, Sonnenblick EH, Ross J Jr, 1967 The dependence of ventricular distensibility in the filling of the opposite ventricle. American Journal of Physiology 213: 711
44. Weil MH 1980 Patient evaluation, "vital signs," and initial care. p. 31. In: Shoemaker WC, Thompson WL (eds) Critical Care: State of the Art, The Society of Critical Care Medicine, Vol 1, Fullerton, CA

6

Afterload: Nonsurgical Manipulation of the Failing Circulation

David J. Steward

Afterload is the tension in the wall of the ventricle during ejection.[22] It is directly related to the impedance against which the ventricles contract and eject blood. Changes in impedance can significantly affect the volume of blood ejected by the ventricles and the volume of blood that remains in the ventricles at end-systole. These changes also determine the tension required of the ventricular wall. In addition, the aortic impedance is a major determinant of aortic root pressure, and thus may affect coronary blood flow. Factors that comprise the impedance include the aortic or pulmonary artery resistance, the systemic or pulmonary vascular resistance, and the mass and viscosity of blood in the vessels.

In the pediatric patient, drugs may be administered to act upon peripheral vessels, with the objective of lowering left ventricular or right ventricular afterload. Medical techniques such as the intra-aortic balloon pump may be used to reduce afterload. In some circumstances, drugs may be given that increase afterload and affect the distribution of the cardiac output. These various modes of therapy will be discussed here.

DRUG THERAPY TO REDUCE AFTERLOAD

Over the past decade, there has been much interest in the use of vasodilator drugs to reduce afterload and increase the output of the failing heart while having little effect on or even reducing myocardial oxygen requirement.[5,7,10] The principal effect of these drugs is to decrease the resistance of the arterioles and, thereby, to "unload" the heart. A secondary effect is to increase the size of the venous vascular pool. This decreases preload, thus decreasing the ventricular volume.

Reduction of left ventricular afterload in the presence of myocardial failure, may have very little effect on systemic blood pressure. As the impedance to ventricular ejection decreases, provided that the preload is maintained at an optimal level, the stroke volume increases progressively. This augmentation of stroke volume, if the heart rate is stable, results in an increase in cardiac output, which balances the reduction in systemic vascular resistance and tends to maintain the blood pressure. Thus, coronary blood flow may be well maintained, and, in fact, myocardial perfusion may be improved by the fall in ventricular end-diastolic pressure which accompanies afterload reduction.

Reduction of right ventricular afterload in patients with raised pulmonary vascular resistance will similarly decrease the work of the right ventricle, and by reducing the end-diastolic pressure, perfusion of its muscular wall may be improved. In addition, pulmonary blood flow may be increased, and right-to-left shunting through ductus arteriosus or foramen ovale decreased accordingly.

Drugs Used to Reduce Afterload in Pediatric Patients

Sodium nitroprusside

Sodium nitroprusside (SNP) is a direct-acting vasodilator that relaxes both arteriolar and venous smooth muscle.[13] It is a very potent, rapidly acting drug with a short duration of action. Because of these properties, it has become the most commonly used vasodilator for the management of low cardiac output states. Administration of an infusion of SNP at rates of 2.5 to 12 μg/kg/minute in infants following cardiac surgery.[1]

Sodium nitroprusside acts directly on the vascular smooth muscle, causing relaxation independent of autonomic innervation. Arteriolar vascular resistance and venous vascular tone are equally affected.[24] SNP has no direct inotropic effects, and improved ventricular function is due solely to reduced afterload. Venodilation results in venous pooling of blood and reduced venous return; consequently, preload is also diminished. The effect of this reduction in preload is dependant upon the position that the resultant end-diastolic pressure occupies on the ventricular function curve. If the ventricular filling pressure remains near the plateau of a depressed ventricular function curve, afterload reduction with SNP will result in increased stroke volume. However, if the fall in preload reduces the ventricular filling pressure down to the ascending portion of the ventricular function curve, SNP administration may result in a fall in stroke volume. Thus, the intravascular fluid volume must be increased as is necessary to maintain an optimal level of preload if maximum augmentation of stroke volume is to be achieved by the use of SNP.

In infants and children who had recently undergone surgery with cardiopulmonary bypass, SNP infusion and volume expansion to maintain preload (left atrial pressure) at levels of approximately 11 to 12 mmHg was associated with a 41 percent increase in cardiac index.[1] Systemic blood pressure may decrease during SNP infusion, but in the presence of significant ventricular dysfunction, this fall in blood pressure is usually small. SNP infusion in infants and children following cardiac surgery has been reported to decrease mean arterial pressure to 75[1] to 85 percent[30] of pre-infusion values.

The effect of SNP on pulmonary vascular resistance (PVR) has been measured in children following cardiac surgery.[30] PVR decreased 27 percent overall, and by 22 percent in a subgroup of patients with elevated pulmonary vascular resistance.[30] The fall in PVR is greater than that of the systemic vascular resistance, and is greatest in those children with previously increased PVR.

SNP results in little change[1] or a slight increase[30] in heart rate in infants and children. The effect of SNP on myocardial metabolism has not been measured in pediatric patients. In adult patients, SNP has been shown to enhance cardiac output while lowering myocardial oxygen consumption.[26] Reduction in ventricular end-diastolic pressure may improve myocardial perfusion, even in the absence of coronary artery disease.

SNP is metabolized in the body to thiocyanate and cyanide. It has been reported that some children may show tachyphylaxis to SNP, and that if increased infusion rates are employed, dangerous cyanide toxicity may result.[8] In practice, infusion rates should be limited to 8 μg/kg/hr, and during prolonged infusions, the blood thiocyanate level should be checked regularly.[7] Thiocyanate is excreted by the kidneys, but the renal clearance is low due to tubular reabsorption; hence, high blood levels may develop and may persist after SNP is discontinued. Thiocyanate impairs iodine uptake by the thyroid gland, and may lead to hypothyroidism. Toxic blood levels (>10 mg/100 ml) of thiocyanate may result in weakness, nausea, tinnitus, behavioral changes, and psychosis. Tachyphylaxis to SNP should be regarded as an early sign of cyanide toxicity. Serial acid-base determinations should be performed during SNP therapy since progressive metabolic acidosis is another, though later, clue to the development of cyanide toxicity. Sodium thiosulphate (150 mg/kg) is recommended for the treatment of cyanide toxicity.

Nitroglycerin

Nitroglycerin has a greater vasodilating effect on the venous capacitance vessels than on the arterioles.[25] Thus, nitroglycerin has been reported to result in a smaller increase in cardiac index, but a greater fall in ventricular pressure than occurs with SNP.[2]

In infants and children with low cardiac output following intracardiac surgery, the intravenous infusion of nitroglycerin was found to increase the cardiac index significantly.[4] The cardiac index was further increased when the blood volume was expanded to restore the left ventricular (LV) filling pressure to pre-infusion levels. No change occurred in heart rate or mean systemic arterial pressure. Total systemic vascular resistance fell by 22 percent during nitroglycerin infusion. The rate of nitroglycerin infusion required to achieve these hemodynamic effects varied very widely from child to child; doses of 0.4 to 60 μg/kg/min were administered: the mean rate of infusion being 20.8 μg/kg/min.

Nitroglycerin is metabolized in the liver to produce glyceryl dinitrate and nitrite, both of which are weak vasodilators. These metabolites are water-soluble and are excreted in the urine.

Hydrazaline

Hydrazaline is a pthalazine derivative and a long-acting vasodilator which has been used to increase cardiac output in chronic heart failure. The vasodilating effect of hydrazaline is principally directed to the arterioles, where it acts by directly relaxing vascular smooth muscle.[18]

Hydrazaline has no effect on nonvascular smooth muscle, no effect on the heart, and little effect on the venous capacitance vessels. Hydrazoline is metabolized by N-acetylation and ring hydroxylation, plus conjugation with glucuronic acid. Metabolism is significantly delayed in uremic patients, who should be given reduced doses of the drug.

In hypertensive patients, hydrazaline initiates compensatory increases in heart rate and myocardial contractility, effects that are usually blocked with beta-blocking drugs during hydrazaline therapy. In patients with congestive heart failure, this response is diminished, and heart rate usually remains stable.[6]

Hydralazine has been used to treat intractable cardiac failure in childhood.[11] A large increase in stroke volume and cardiac output was observed with no change in heart rate. Systemic and pulmonary vascular resistance were both reduced by hydralazine. This drug has the advantage that it may be taken orally, and thus may allow the patient to resume some normal activities. Oral hydralazine has been successfully used to treat primary pulmonary hypertension[28] in infants with large ventricular septal defects. The decrease in afterload caused by hydralazine results in increased systemic blood flow and a decrease in left to right shunt.[3] It is suggested that this drug may be useful in the management of such infants.

Diazoxide

Diazoxide is a benzothiadizine derivative closely related to the thiazide diuretics.[17] Diazoxide causes arteriolar vasodilation by direct effect on the vascular smooth muscle. There is little effect on capacitance vessels and no direct effect on the heart. It has a prolonged duration of action (8 to 12 hours). Diazoxide has been used primarily to treat severe hypertensive conditions, though it has also been advocated for the treatment of chronic normotensive congestive heart failure in adults.[23] Oral diazoxide has also been demonstrated to be effective in the therapy of primary pulmonary hypertension[16]; pulmonary vascular resistance decreased markedly both during rest and exercise.

Tolazoline

Tolazoline is an alpha-adrenergic blocking agent, which also has a direct effect on vascular smooth muscle. This drug has been used therapeutically, mainly for its effects on pulmonary vascular resistance, though it exerts similar vasodilating effects on systemic arterioles. Tolazoline has been used to reduce right ventricular afterload, and to increase pulmonary blood flow in ventricular septal defect[14], neonatal meconium aspiration,[19] neonatal hypoxia,[12] and congenital diaphragmatic hernia.[20] Doses of 1 to 2 mg/kg of the drug are usually infused via a systemic vein or directly into the pulmonary artery. The response to the drug is very variable from patient to patient.

Phentolamine

Phentolamine is an alpha-adrenergic blocking drug which also has direct vascular smooth muscle relaxing properties.[22] This drug causes less dilation of the venous capacitance vessels than sodium nitroprusside for a given reduction in afterload.[33] Tachycardia may occur with phentolamine, and is due to norepinephrine release, which also results in an indirect positive inotropic effect. Phentolamine has a very transient effect, and long-term infusions of the drug are impractical, due to the high cost of the drug.

Prostaglandins

Prostaglandins affect vascular smooth muscle and may cause contraction or relaxation.[35] Prostaglandin E_1 and prostacyclin appear to have a marked vasodilating effect on the pulmonary vessels and have been administered to achieve this effect.

In patients with pulmonary hypertension, prostaglandin E_1 infused into a peripheral vein decreases pulmonary vascular resistance and pulmonary artery pressure with an accompanying increase in cardiac output.[32] In children after open-heart surgery, prostaglandin E_1 infusion decreased systemic and pulmonary vascular resistance, but with a less consistent pulmonary vascular response than that obtained with sodium nitroprusside.[29] Side effects, including tachycardia, headache, and abdominal cramps necessitated discontinuing the drug in several patients.

Prostacyclin has been used to treat idiopathic pulmonary hypertension,[34] and it is suggested that this substance may offer advantages over other drugs: it is naturally occurring, relaxes vascular smooth muscle, and causes disaggregation of pulmonary microthromboemboli.[34]

THE INTRA-AORTIC BALLOON PUMP

The use of the intra-aortic balloon pump (IABP) in adult patients with left ventricular failure following myocardial infarction or cardiac surgery has become an established method to support the myocardium and improve cardiac output by decreasing afterload.[21] Experience with the IABP in infants and children is limited,[27] but it has been suggested that this technique may be of some value in children over 5 years of age. In younger children, the technical problems of insertion and positioning of the balloon catheter may lead to complications. In addition, the greater elasticity of the aorta in infants and young children impairs the efficiency of the IABP; the pressure generated by the balloon inflating in diastole is diminished, and afterload reduction is less effective. Finally, the cardiac index in pediatric patients with postoperative low output syndrome may be so low that the IABP cannot provide any significant augmentation.[27]

AFTERLOAD REDUCTION: SPECIFIC INDICATIONS

Postoperative Low Cardiac Output Syndrome

Myocardial performance is decreased in the immediate postoperative period and continues to decline over the next few hours. The severity of this myocardial impairment is related to the pre-existing cardiac status, to the length of cardiopulmonary bypass and the duration of ischemic cardiac arrest, and to injury sustained during reperfusion of the heart. The decline in myocardial performance postoperatively is secondary to damage to and edema of the heart muscle, resulting in decreased compliance and contractility of the ventricles. (Remember that even in the normal infant, the heart muscle is less compliant and less contractile than in the adult, due to a lower proportion of contractile elements.) In addition, total systemic vascular resistance is often high in the postoperative period.

In this postoperative state of impaired contractility, afterload reduction offers the opportunity to increase the cardiac index with little change in cardiac work. Cardiac output should be determined, and those patients demonstrated to have a low cardiac index despite adequate preload should be treated by afterload reduction, with or without the addition of inotropic drugs. Sodium nitroprusside has been most commonly used for this purpose. A solution of suitable concentration should be prepared and infusion commenced at a rate of 1 μg/kg/min, and increased as is required to achieve the desired effect. Systemic blood pressure and atrial loading pressures should be carefully monitored, and the preload augmented by additional fluid infusions as is necessary to maintain it at optimal level. Serial repeat determinations of cardiac index will be required to assess the effect of afterload reduction and to determine when this therapy can be discontinued.

CONTROL OF PULMONARY HYPTERTENSION

Pulmonary hypertension in pediatric patients is most commonly seen in the immediate newborn period, or in later infancy and childhood of the patient with congenital heart disease.

In the neonate, the pulmonary vasculature is highly reactive. Hypoxemia and acidemia result in a large increase in pulmonary vascular resistance. Some infants may have additional abnormalities of the pulmonary blood vessels. For example, in those with congenital diaphragmatic hernia, hypoplasia of the lungs is accompanied by a contracted vascular bed. Increased pulmonary vascular resistance in the neonate will lead to pulmonary hypoperfusion, impaired gas exchange in the lungs, and consequent hypoxemia. The ductus arteriosus will then remain open or reopen and a fetal pattern of the circulation will persist. High right-sided pressures in the heart also result in continued shunting via the foramen ovale. Drug therapy to decrease pulmonary vascular resistance is indicated if this resistance remains high despite adequate oxygenation, hyperventilation, and correction of acidosis.

Pediatric patients with congenital heart disease (e.g., ventricular septal defect, VSD) may develop pulmonary vascular disease as a result of pulmonary hyperperfusion. Though surgical treatment is aimed to protect the pulmonary vasculature, for example, by early total repair or by pulmonary artery banding, some patients cannot or do not receive optimal treatment, and hence may develop pulmonary hypertension; other patients may develop pulmonary hypertension in spite of apparently optimal treatment. Such patients face the risk of a high operative mortality due to postoperative right ventricular failure with consequent low cardiac output. Episodic acute pulmonary hypertension may occur following repair of congenital heart defects (e.g., VSD or truncus arteriosus), and may be a cause of early mortality.

It has been demonstrated that the use of vasodilators may permit survival through the period of postoperative myocardial impairment. Of course, it is essential that the pulmonary vasculature is still reactive and will respond to vasodilators, a fact which may be demonstrated at the time of cardiac catheterization. The drug used most commonly to induce pulmonary vasodilation has been sodium nitroprusside. The drug can be administered into a systemic vein, and at infusion rates similar to those used to reduce left ventricular afterload. Sodium nitroprusside infusion should be commenced intraoperatively prior to weaning the patient from cardiopulmonary bypass.[9] Pulmonary artery pressure and cardiac output should be measured to assess the effect of the infusion.

Though the pulmonary vascular resistance may return to preoperative elevated levels after sodium nitroprusside is discontinued, the use of this drug for a period may enable the patient to survive the period of postoperative right ventricular dysfunction.

Fentanyl has been demonstrated to cause little alteration in pulmonary or systemic hemodynamics of infants,[14a] but does prevent increases of pulmonary vascular resistance associated with airway manipulations or suctioning.[14b] The use of fentanyl in infants who have hyper-reactive pulmonary vasculature and require extended postoperative intubation and ventilation is recommended.[14b]

It is vitally important to control pulmonary vascular resistance, and hence right ventricular impedance, in patients who may have postoperative pulmonary hypertension. All such patients should have the pulmonary artery pressure monitored continuously. Elevation of the pulmonary artery pressure above the normal must be treated promptly: inspired oxygen concentrations must be increased to insure the best possible oxygenation of arterial blood. Metabolic acidosis must be corrected and a degree of respiratory alkalosis produced by moderate hyperventilation. Sodium nitroprusside infusion should be initiated or continued. Fentanyl should be administered to prevent increases in pulmonary vascular resistance resulting from airway manipulations or other stimuli.

DRUG THERAPY TO INCREASE AFTERLOAD

Measures to increase afterload are very rarely indicated, except during cardiopulmonary resuscitation (CPR) and occasionally during cardiopulmonary bypass. At these times, drugs that increase left ventricular afterload may have a beneficial effect on the distribution of blood flow.

During CPR, the administration of epinephrine (0.1 ml/kg of a 1:10,000 solution) has been demonstrated to increase blood flow to the brain and heart.[15] Epinephrine is more effective than the pure vasoconstrictor, phenylephrine, in increasing regional blood flow to the heart during CPR. This is due to the combined alpha- and beta-adrenergic effects of epinephrine, which result in systemic vasoconstriction but coronary vasodilation.[15]

Low perfusion pressures during cardiopulmonary bypass may result in uneven transmural perfusion of the myocardium. In such instances, increasing afterload by infusion of methoxamine has been demonstrated to improve myocardial perfusion, especially to the subendocardium.[31]

REFERENCES

1. Appelbaum A, Blackstone AH, Kouchoukos NT, Kirklin JW 1977 Afterload reduction and cardiac output in infants early after intracardiac surgery. American Journal of Cardiology 39: 445
2. Armstrong PW, Walker DC, Burton JR, et al 1975 Vasodilator therapy in acute myocardial infarction: a comparison of sodium nitroprusside and nitroglycerin. Circulation 52: 1118
3. Beekman RH, Rocchini AP, Rosenthal A 1982 Hemodynamic effects of hydralazine in infants with a large ventricular septal defect. Circulation 65: 523
4. Benson LN, Bohn D, Edmonds JF, Fortune RL, Price SA, Williams WG, Rowe RD 1979 Nitroglycerin therapy in children with low cardiac index after heart surgery. Cardiovascular Medicine 4: 207
5. Chatterjee K, Parmley WW 1977 The role of vasodilator therapy in heart failure. Progress in Cardiovascular Disease 21: 301
6. Chatterjee K, Parmley W, Massre B, Greenberg B, Werner J, Klausner S, Norman A 1976 Oral hydralazine therapy for chronic refractory heart failure. Circulation 54: 879
7. Cohn JN, Franciosa JA 1977 Vasodilator therapy of cardiac failure. New Eng J Med 297: 27
8. Davies DW, Greiss L, Kadar D, et al 1975 Sodium nitroprusside in children: Observations on

metabolism during normal and abnormal responses. Canadian Anaesthesiology Society Journal 22: 553

9. Faraci PA, Rheinlander HF, Cleveland RJ 1980 Use of nitroprusside for control of pulmonary hypertension in repair of ventricular septal defect. Annals of Thoracic Surgery 29: 70
10. Franciosa JA, Akhtar N, Notargiacomo AV, Cohn JN 1973 Hemodynamic and metabolic response to nitroprusside infusion in experimental acute myocardial infarction. Circulation 48: 165
11. Fried R, Steinherz LJ, Levin AR, Linday L, Tan CTC, Miller D 1980 Use of hydralazine for intractable cardiac failure in childhood. Journal of Pediatrics 97: 1009
12. Goetzman BW, Sunshine P, Johnson JD, Wennberg RP, Hackel A, Merten DF, Bartoletti AL, Silverman NH 1976 Neonatal hypoxia and pulmonary vasospasm: response to tolazaline. Journal of Pediatrics 89: 617
13. Goodman LS, Gilman A 1980 The Pharmacological Basis of Therapeutics, 6th edn. McMillan, New York,
14. Grover RF, Reeves JT, Blount SG 1961 Tolazoline hydrochloride (priscoline), an effective pulmonary vasodilator. American Heart Journal 61: 5

14a. Hickey PR, Hansen DD, Wessel DL, Lang P, Jonas RA 1985 Pulmonary and systemic responses to fentanyl in infants. Anesth Analg. 64: 483

14b. Hickey PR, Hansen DD, Wessel DL, Lang P, Jonas RA, Elixon EM 1985 Blunting of stress responses in the pulmonary circulation of infants by fentanyl. Anesth Analg. 64: 1137

15. Holmes HR, Babbs CF, Vorhees WD, Tacker WA, De Garavilla B 1980 Influence of adrenergic drugs upon vital organ perfusion during CPR. Critical Care Medicine 8: 137
16. Klinke WP, Gilbert JAL 1980 Diazoxide in primary pulmonary hypertension. New England Journal of Medicine 302: 91
17. Koch-Weser J 1976 Diazoxide. New England Journal of Medicine 294: 1271
18. Koch-Weser J 1976 Hydrazoline. New England Journal of Medicine 295: 320
19. Levin DL, Gregory GA 1976 The effect of tolazoline on right to left shunting via a patent ductus arteriosus in meconium aspiration syndrome. Critical Care Medicine 4: 304
20. Levy RJ, Rosenthal A, Freed MD 1977 Persistent pulmonary hypertension in a newborn with congenital diaphragmatic hernia: successful management with tolazoline. Pediatrics 60: 740
21. McEnany MT, Kay HR, Buckley MJ, et al 1978 Clinical experience with intraaortic balloon pump support in 728 patients. Circulation 58: 124
22. Mason DT 1978 Afterload reduction and cardiac performance. American Journal of Medicine 65: 106
23. Massie BM, Stern R, Hanlon JT, Haughom RN 1982 Beneficial hemodynamic effects of diazozide in refractory congestive heart failure. American Heart Journal 104: 581
24. Miller RR, Mason DT, Zelis R et al 1975 Clinical use of sodium nitroprusside in chronic ischemic heart disease: effects on peripheral vascular resistance and venous tone and on ventricular volume, pump and mechanical function. Circulation 57: 328
25. Miller RR, Vismara LA, Williams DO et al 1976 Pharmacological mechanism for left ventricular unloading in clinical congestive heart failure: differential effects of nitroprusside, phentolamine, and nitroglycerine on cardiac function and peripheral circulation. Circulation Research 39: 127
26. Miller RR, Williams DO, Mason DT et al 1976 Pharmacologic mechanisms for left ventricular unloading in clinical congestive heart failure: differential effects of nitroprusside, phentolamine, and nitroglycerine on cardiac function and peripheral circulation. Circulation Research 39: 127
27. Pollock JC, Charlton MC, Williams WG, Edmonds JF, Trusler GA 1980 Intraaortic balloon pumping in children. Annals of Thoracic Surgery 29: 522
28. Rubin LJ, Peter RH 1980 Oral hydralazine therapy for primary pulmonary hypertension. New England Journal of Medicine 302: 69
29. Rubis LJ, Stephenson LW, Johnston MR, Nagaraj S, Edmunds LH 1981 Comparison of the effects of prostaglandin E_1 and nitroprusside on pulmonary vascular resistance in children after open heart surgery. Annals of Thoracic Surgery 32: 563
30. Stephenson LW, Edmunds H, Raphaely R, Morrison DF, Hoffman WS, Rubis LJ 1979 Effects of nitroprusside and dopamine on pulmonary arterial vasculature in children after cardiac surgery. Circulation 60 (Supp I): 104
31. Symmonds JB, Kleinman LH, Wechsler AS 1977 Effects of methoxamine on the coronary circulation during cardiopulmonary bypass. Journal of Thoracic Cardiovascular Surgery 74: 577
32. Szczeklik J, Dubiel JS, Mysik M, Pyzik Z, Krol R, Horzela T 1978 Effects of prostaglandin E_1 on pulmonary circulation in patients with pulmonary hypertension. British Heart Journal 40: 1397
33. Taylor SH, Sutherland GR, Mackenzie MB et al 1968 The circulatory effects of intravenous phentolamine in man. Circulation 31: 741
34. Watkins WD, Peterson MB, Crone RK 1980 Prostacyclin and prostaglandin E_1 for severe idiopathic pulmonary artery hypertension. Lancet 1: 1083
35. Weir EK, Grover RF 1978 The role of endogenous prostaglandins in the pulmonary circulation. Anesthesiology 48: 201

7
Nonsurgical Contractility Manipulation of the Failing Circulation

Ronald M. Perkin and Nick G. Anas

The critically ill patient often presents a well-defined need to support or augment the cardiovascular response to an acute illness. Circulatory failure is a general term that refers to an inadequacy of the cardiovascular system to maintain oxygen delivery to match the metabolic demands of the cells, both in the central and peripheral circulations.[72] Reduction in myocardial contractility, resulting in an absolute decrease in cardiac output and a state of acute cellular oxygen deficiency, is a contributing factor in many different types of circulatory failure.[72] In addition, the stress of trauma, surgery, sepsis, or fever induces a requirement for increased oxygen delivery because of greater cellular metabolic demand.[82] Failure to provide the oxygen substrate for cellular oxidative phosphorylation will eventually result in circulatory failure. Therefore, heart failure is defined as the inability to pump blood at the flow rate (cardiac output) needed to provide for the oxygen demand and cellular metabolic requirements of the critically ill patient, for whatever reason.[82] All shock states tend to merge into a common path.[37,81] That common path is myocardial failure, initially due to inadequate oxygen supply, and excessive demand.[81]

Delivery of oxygen is a direct function of the cardiac output and the arterial oxygen content.[43] Therefore, therapeutic efforts, in addition to treatment of the primary underlying process, involve optimizing cardiac output and arterial oxygen content. A reduced arterial oxygen content, existing with anemia, poor arterial oxygen saturation, or both, will result in greater dependency upon cardiac output to maintain oxygen delivery.[82] If for any reason the necessary increase in cardiac output to satisfy the patient's oxygen demands does not occur, even though it may be significantly increased above normal, cellular anoxic damage ensues, thus establishing an irreversible cycle.[72,82]

In some severely ill patients, adequate oxygen delivery may not be possible even after efforts are made to optimize preload, afterload, heart rate, and arterial oxygen content. In these situations, depression of myocardial contractility probably exists, whether it be due to the presence of myocardial disease or damage, continuing hypoxemia and acidosis, or the presence of a circulating myocardial depressant factor.[82] Therapy, then, must focus on enhancing contractility of the myocardium using both pharmacologic and nonpharmacologic methods.

To understand the disturbances in cardiac contraction and the rational treatment of depressed myocardial contractility, it is necessary to review the structure and function of the normal cardiac cell and of the normal contractile function.

NORMAL MYOCARDIAL CELL STRUCTURE AND FUNCTION

The sarcolemma is a surface membrane that surrounds the myocardial cells. In diastole, it maintains a high intracellular potassium concentration and low sodium and calcium concentrations. The sarcolemma possesses an enzyme system that utilizes adenosine triphosphate (ATP) for energy in order to maintain these differences in cation concentrations.[69] This sodium-potassium stimulated ATPase is responsible for the active transport of sodium and possibly calcium out of the cardiac cell and for the uptake of potassium.[1,45] A crucial factor in the generation of the cardiac action potential is the remarkable ability of the sarcolemma to alter its permeability to allow for a complex sequence of changes in ion conductance during different phases of the cardiac cycle.[47] In most regions of the myocardium, the action potential consists of at least five morphologically defined phases (Fig. 7.1).[4,47] The upstroke of the action potential (phase 0), corresponding to depolarization, is followed by a brief phase of early repolarization (phase 1), and then by a plateau (phase 2), which is largely responsible for the long duration of the cardiac action potential. Repolarization (phase 3) and the resting potential (phase 4) are similar to that in other excitable cells.[45]

The ionic basis of the cardiac action potential is now reasonably well understood.[45] At rest, the sarcolemma is highly permeable to potassium but relatively impermeable to sodium and calcium. In the upstroke phase, opening of a "fast channel" allows sodium ions to enter the cell, carrying a rapid inward (depolarizing) flow of current.[4] At the same time, potassium conductance decreases. The plateau

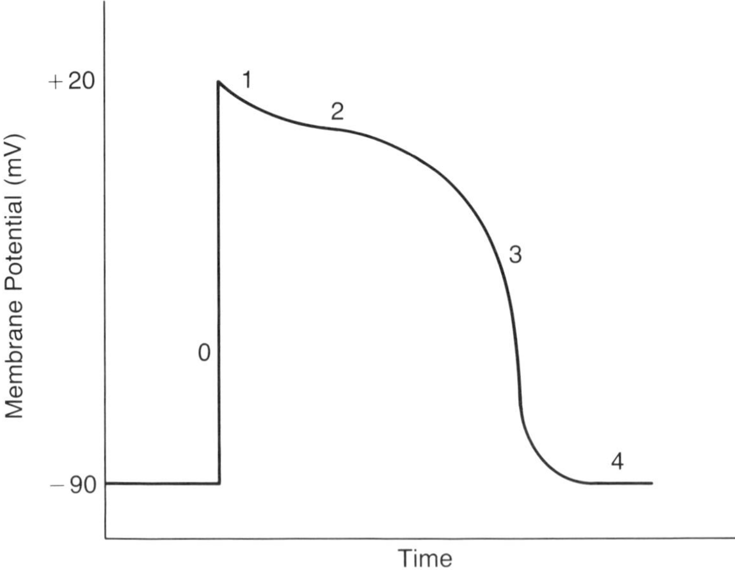

Fig. 7.1. The cardiac action potential.

of the action potential results from opening of a "slow channel," which allows calcium ions to enter the cell, carrying a slow inward (depolarizing) current.[4] Because the slow channels are normally 100 times more selective for calcium than for sodium or potassium, the slow inward current is propagated primarily by calcium ions.[15,47] These slow calcium channels, which require metabolic energy, are blocked by verapamil and its analogs, manganese ion, and acidosis, but are activated by catecholamines and the xanthines.[47,97] The slow inward current is subsequently overcome by an outward current that is carried by potassium ions, which are present in high concentration inside the cell. The closing of the slow channels and the progressive opening of potassium channels shift the balance of these opposing currents to favor the outward (repolarizing) potassium current. The resulting return to normal resting potential completes the cardiac action potential.

Once the electrical cells initiate and propagate the wave of depolarization, the myocardial working cells are stimulated to initiate muscle contraction. The sequence of events that links the electrical activation to mechanical activity is termed excitation-contraction coupling.[45]

The muscle cells of the heart are composed of functioning units called *sarcomeres*. Contained within and filling the sarcomere are several structures, which include (1) myofibrils, (2) mitochondria, (3) centrally located nuclei, and (4) an extensive internal tubular network called the *sarcoplasmic reticulum*.[45,69] The myofibrils of the cell perform the contraction process. Each sarcomere is constructed of numerous thin, longitudinal strands (actin proteins) interdigitating with thicker strands (myosin proteins).[63] Actin and myosin have great attraction, and, left together, they form crossbridges that fuse the two strands together into a conglomerate, actomyosin.[69] In heart muscle, there is some overlap of the actin and myosin strands. When actin and myosin form crossbridges, they slide together to maximize their overlap.[63] This sliding together is what shortens the sarcomere length and thus, if all sarcomeres shorten together, contracts the cell.

There are two additional proteins, however, intermingled with the actin and myosin strands: tropomyosin and a complex known as troponin.[63] Tropomyosin inhibits the crossbridge formation between actin and myosin. Troponin, which is attached to tropomyosin, can prevent this inhibition if—and only if—calcium ions are bound to a certain part of the troponin complex.[69] If calcium ions are freely available to the myofibrils, they bind to troponin, which in turn releases the inhibition that tropomyosin has been imposing on actin to prevent crossbridge formation with myosin.[47] With this inhibition gone, crossbridges are formed and contraction occurs. Removal of the calcium from the troponin causes relaxation.[35,56]

In addition to calcium, crossbridge formation requires energy.[47] On the end of the myosin crossbridge is an ATPase that splits ATP to provide the energy. This enzyme requires magnesium.[69] Thus, both ATP and magnesium must be present for contraction. Because sarcomeres are like links in a chain, all must contract in order for the chain to contract. If only some contract, they will pull out to full extension those others in the chain that are still relaxed; as a result, little or no overall chain contraction will occur.[69] A similar argument holds for cells. All the cells must contract together in order for the heart muscle as a whole to contract.

The sarcoplasmic reticulum forms a fine filamentous network of tubules and functions to retrieve calcium from the myofibrils, thereby facilitating relaxation.[56] The retrieval process is energy dependent and involves activation of a calcium sensitive ATPase located on the sarcolemma.[15] When activated, calcium is pumped from the sarcoplasma up an extreme gradient to the internal storage in the sarcoplasmic reticulum. This pump consumes enormous amounts of energy because of the high concentration gradient against which it must work.[35,56] Since the transition from systole to diastole requires a reduction in intracellular calcium, it follows that an inadequate supply of ATP must result in incomplete relaxation.[35] At the same time, intracellular calcium will remain at abnormally high levels. Calcium can also be taken up and released by other intracellular structures, particularly the mitochondria.[69] When intracellular calcium rises, ATP generated by the mitochondria is involved in the uptake of calcium by these organelles.[15] However, excessive uptake of calcium by the mitochondria interferes with its function.[68]

With this review of ultrastructure, the excitation-contraction coupling can be described. In recent years, there has been increased understanding of the mechanics by which the action potential initiates the contractile process. All studies have emphasized a central role of calcium.[45] As the wave of depolarization spreads throughout the heart muscle, calcium enters the cell through the slow channels. The absolute quantity of calcium that crosses the sarcolemma during the plateau (phase 2) of the action potential is relatively small and incapable of bringing about complete activation of the contractile apparatus.[15,45] However, this influx of calcium appears to release a much larger quantity of calcium from its storage sites in the sarcoplasmic reticulum.[63,69,97] This calcium diffuses toward the myofibrils and binds to troponin, allowing activation of the contractile system. The number of contractile sites activated—and, therefore, the resultant force generated—are directly related to the quantity of calcium present in the area of the myofibrils. This, in turn, is ultimately dependent on the influx of calcium that accompanies the action potential.[15,97] This influx is a function of the extracellular calcium concentration, the duration of the action potential, and the number of action potentials per unit time.[63]

Relaxation results from a cessation of the slow inward calcium current coupled with the uptake and storage of intracellular calcium primarily by the sarcoplasmic reticulum. As the intracellular calcium concentration falls, calcium dissociates from the troponin, resulting in inhibition of the interaction between actin and myosin.[56]

The rates at which the muscle contracts and relaxes are dependent, respectively, on the *rates* at which calcium is delivered to and removed from the myofibrils. The *extent* of activation and inactivation, which is represented in the myocardium as the isometric systolic and diastolic tensions, respectively, depends on the intracellular calcium concentration achieved during systole and diastole.[15]

Therefore, normal cardiac contraction and relaxation are critically dependent on precisely timed modulations of the intracellular calcium concentration.[15] For these reasons, it is important to carefully outline and, in some cases, reiterate some of the more important mechanisms which control the intracellular calcium concentration. Abnormalities in any of these mechanisms can affect myocardial performance. Several mechanisms that control intracellular calcium concentration have been identified.[15,97]

1. Slow calcium channels allow inward movement of calcium along its concentration gradient and across the sarcolemma.

2. Total calcium within the cell is also affected by a sodium-calcium exchange across the sarcolemma.[29,56] This is a bidirectional exchange system: the direction is dependent upon the relative concentration of sodium and calcium.[4] The sodium-calcium exchange mechanism operates by utilizing the energy of the concentration gradient of sodium to transport calcium, while the sodium concentration gradient is maintained by the activity of the energy requiring sodium-potassium pump of the sarcolemma.[15]

3. A calcium-stimulated magnesium ATPase in the membrane of the sarcoplasmic reticulum transports calcium into the lumen of the sarcoplasmic reticulum and sequesters it there in an energy dependent process.[35,56]

4. Calcium can also be taken up and released by other intracellular structures. These include the inner layer of the cell membrane (sarcolemma) and its invaginations (transverse tubular system) and particularly the mitochondria.[97]

5. The sarcolemma possess a calcium-stimulated ATPase that extrudes calcium from the cell in an energy-requiring process.[15,97]

6. Finally, a variety of inophores can effect the movement of calcium along its concentration gradient directly across the sarcolemma.[75]

FACTORS INFLUENCING CONTRACTILITY

Change in contractility (inotropic state) of the heart is an alteration in cardiac performance that is independent of changes resulting from variations in preload or afterload.[45,103] When loading conditions remain constant, an improvement in contractility will augment cardiac performance (positive inotropic effect) while a depression in contractility will lower cardiac performance (negative inotropic effect).[45] Cardiac function can be assessed by examining the performance characteristics of individual muscle fibers or of the overall pumping characteristics of the ventricle.[77] In patients it is often difficult to obtain the parameters that assess cardiac muscle directly, and this is particularly true in the acutely ill patient. Instead, ventricular function has usually been examined on the basis of the Frank-Starling principle, which relates the force of ventricular contraction to the myocardial fiber length immediately before the onset of ventricular systole.[77] Since neither of these is easy to measure, cardiac index, stroke index, and stroke work index have been used as indices of the force of contraction, and end-diastolic volume and end-diastolic pressure have been used as indices of fiber length.[77] The relationships are typically presented using Frank-Starling (ventricular performance) type curves (Fig. 7.2).[90]

Contractility itself cannot presently be assessed directly; only changes in ventricular performance can be observed. From these observations, inferences can be drawn regarding change in contractility. Changes in ventricular performance after alterations in preload or afterload may be difficult to ascribe to changes in contractility unless the changes in ventricular performance are in the same direction as changes in afterload and opposite to the changes in preload. It may be inferred

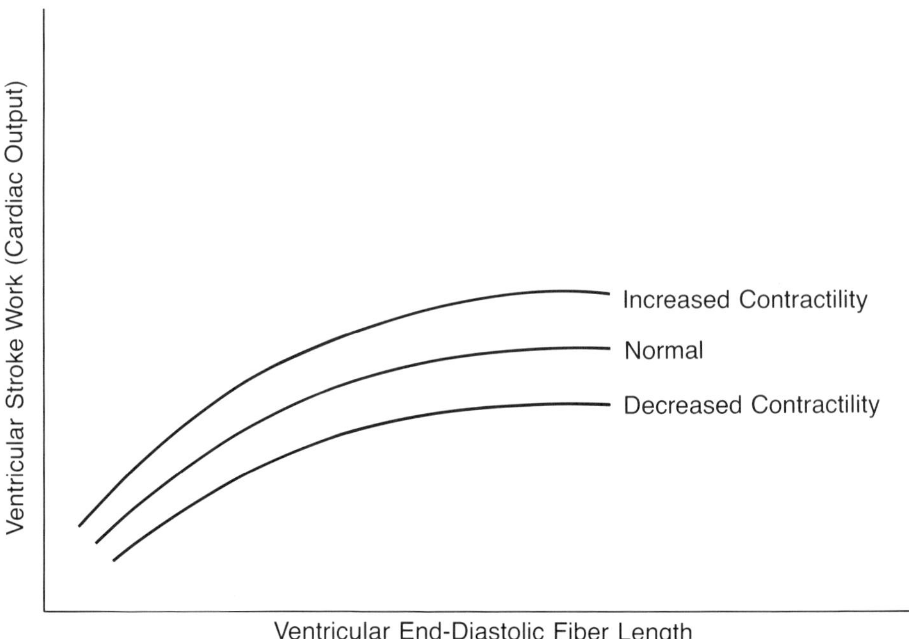

Fig. 7.2. Ventricular function curves.

that changes in ventricular performance that are disproportionate to changes in preload or afterload, even in the same direction, indicate changes in contractility. Additionally, there are several factors that could affect the ventricular end-diastolic pressure. These include heart rate, preload, afterload, pericardial or pleural pressure, diastolic properties of the ventricle, and the ventricular inotropic state.[35,44] Recognition of these factors is important when considering the ventricular end-diastolic pressure as an index of ventricular function.[44]

In summary, abnormal contractility cannot be diagnosed with confidence in the intensive care patient, but trends can often be detected. Fortunately, contractility need not be accurately assessed to adequately evaluate cardiovascular status and plan treatment. It is sufficient to achieve a characterization of ventricular performance along with and in relation to circulatory factors affecting venous return. There are important potentially reversible factors which depress contractility.

Myocardial Blood Flow and Oxygen Delivery

The contractility of the heart depends on the adequacy of myocardial blood flow and oxygen delivery.[40] There is rarely an anatomic impairment to coronary flow in the pediatric patient unless a coronary artery has an anomalous origin or is injured surgically. Myocardial oxygen delivery, therefore, depends on the maintenance of adequate coronary arterial perfusion pressure, oxygenation, and oxygen-carrying capacity of the blood.[90]

The heart is an aerobic organ.[68] It therefore requires a continuous supply of oxygen to generate the energy required for the maintenance of its cellular structure and function. This energy is made available as ATP, which is produced in the mitochondria.[68] In addition, creatinine phosphate serves as a reserve energy supply when the rate of oxidative phosphorylation falls to such an extent that adenosine diphosphate (ADP) is rephosphorylated slowly and begins to accumulate in the cytosol.[68] The phosphate moiety of creatinine phosphate can be transferred to ADP via creatinine phosphokinase activity to generate ATP.[63,98] It has been demonstrated during conditions of reduced oxygen availability and ischemia, creatinine phosphate depletion precedes ATP depletion.[68] Nevertheless, when heart muscle becomes hypoxic, ischemic, or both, it is the depletion of the tissue stores of ATP which triggers the deterioration in structure and function that, if left uncorrected, will result in cell death.[95,97]

Hypoxemia is a common accompaniment of circulatory failure.[72] Hypoxemia causes vasodilatation in the heart and brain and reflex vasoconstriction in the vessels of skeletal muscle, skin, and splanchnic beds.[39,52] The combination of a direct dilator effect and an indirect vasoconstrictor effect redistributes blood flow to organs that depend on aerobic metabolism.[39] Despite these and other compensatory mechanisms which permit delivery of oxygen to the vital organs, myocardial contractility and relaxation may be impaired as arterial oxygen tension declines.[52,56]

Although myocardial oxygen extraction can be increased, the margin for increase is small.[42] As a result, the increased oxygen delivery needed by the heart when its work increases is obtained mainly by an increase coronary blood flow. Therefore, myocardial oxygen supply is principally related to coronary blood flow, which in turn, is governed by mechanical, neural, humoral, and metabolic factors.[42] These factors are integrated by autoregulatory mechanisms which modulate coronary vascular resistance and thereby coronary blood flow.[42,74] Coronary perfusion pressure can be expressed as the difference between systemic diastolic pressure and ventricular end-diastolic pressure.[74] The range of perfusion pressures over which coronary blood flow remains constant while perfusion pressure is varied is the autoregulatory range.[42] The fall in flow at low perfusing pressures (the low end of the autoregulatory range) suggests that vasodilatation can no longer compensate for any further fall in perfusing pressure. At this point, coronary blood flow becomes dependent on the perfusion pressure.[42] When coronary perfusion pressure is lowered progressively, maximal vasodilatation is reached first in the subendocardial vessels.[95] This is one reason why subendocardial muscle (the innermost or deepest quarter of the thickness of the free wall of the left or right ventricle) is exceptionally vulnerable to necrosis and fibrosis, even when the coronary arteries are normal. Subendocardial ischemic damage is due to marked underperfusion even in patients with normal coronary arteries.[42] Left ventricular subendocardial damage has been noted when there is severe aortic stenosis or incompetence, profound shock of diverse etiologies, prolonged hypothermia after cardiopulmonary bypass, and congestive cardiomyopathies. It has also been noted in some types of cyanotic heart disease.[42,95] Similar damage to right ventricular subendocardial muscle has been found in patients with right ventricular hypertrophy, especially if they also have cyanotic heart disease.[42,83,101] The right ventricle is inordinately susceptible to the effects of the afterload imposed on it by the pulmonary circulation.[83] Being a thin-walled structure with little active reserve to increase the force of contraction, progressive increments in pulmonary artery pressures cause right ventricular dilatation and may even induce ischemia in a previously normal right ventricle.[76,83] Recent studies have begun to question whether there may not be a depression in right ventricular contractility with severe pulmonary artery hypertension.[76,83,101]

Coronary blood flow also depends on the diastolic time.[95] Subendocardial muscle of the left ventricle, and in some circumstances the right ventricle, can be perfused only in diastole.[83] The dependence of subendocardial blood flow on diastolic perfusion is why so many studies have shown that reduced coronary perfusing pressures cause profound subendocardial ischemia.[37,76,95] Prolonged hypotension produces ischemia and greater depression of ventricular function.[40] Thus, there is further decline of cardiac output and more profound lowering of arterial pressure, which leads to additional reduction of coronary blood flow, continued deterioration of cardiac function, and an ultimately fatal outcome.[81] Patients with shock from noncardiogenic events may develop impaired myocardial performance from prolonged increases in cardiac work associated with tachycardia, limited coronary blood flow, and reduced myocardial oxygenation.[81,95]

The overall effect of ATP depletion on myocardial function can be most easily understood in terms of the consequences of failure of the various ATP-dependent systems (Fig. 7.3).[15,68] First, at the level of the sarcolemma ATP provides the energy for two enzymes, the sodium-potassium ATPase and a calcium-sensitive ATPase.[1,63] Failure of these two enzymes will result in a net gain in intracellular calcium, sodium, and water and in a net loss of intracellular potassium.[68] Second, contraction depends upon the available energy generated by the hydrolysis of ATP, the important ATPase enzyme being located in the terminal heads of the myosin subunits.[69] Therefore, energy in the form of ATP is needed if the mechanical activity of the heart is to be maintained. Third, the retrieval of calcium by the sarcoplasmic reticulum is ATP-dependent and involves the activation of a calcium-sensitive ATPase.[40] Since the transition from systole to diastole requires a reduction in intracellular calcium, it follows that an inadequate supply of ATP must result in imperfect relaxation followed by arrest in systole.[35,40] If the inadequate supply of ATP is due to an impaired delivery of oxygen associated with reduced coronary blood flow, then the failure of the myocardium to relax during diastole can only further impair coronary blood flow.[40,81] There are other adverse consequences of the raised intracellular calcium concentration, apart from imperfect relaxation. The most important of these relates to mitochondrial function.[68] Since the mitochondria are avid accumulators of calcium, they will begin to become overloaded with calcium. Under these conditions, the mitochondria eventually become incapable of producing ATP even when placed in an ideal environment.[68,97]

Therefore, reduction of ATP will cause progressive loss of structure and function. The rate at which this loss of structure and function develops will, according to this hypothesis, depend upon the rate of depletion of ATP, the availability of calcium, and the avidity of the mitochondria for calcium.[68] The rate of depletion of ATP and the availability of calcium will, in turn, depend upon other factors. The neonatal heart has enhanced ability to maintain glycolysis and normal levels of ATP during hypoxia.[52] The duration of inadequate oxygenation can be prolonged by the administration of exogenous substrate, such as glucose,[52] while inotropic agents may exacerbate ischemic damage because of their enhancement

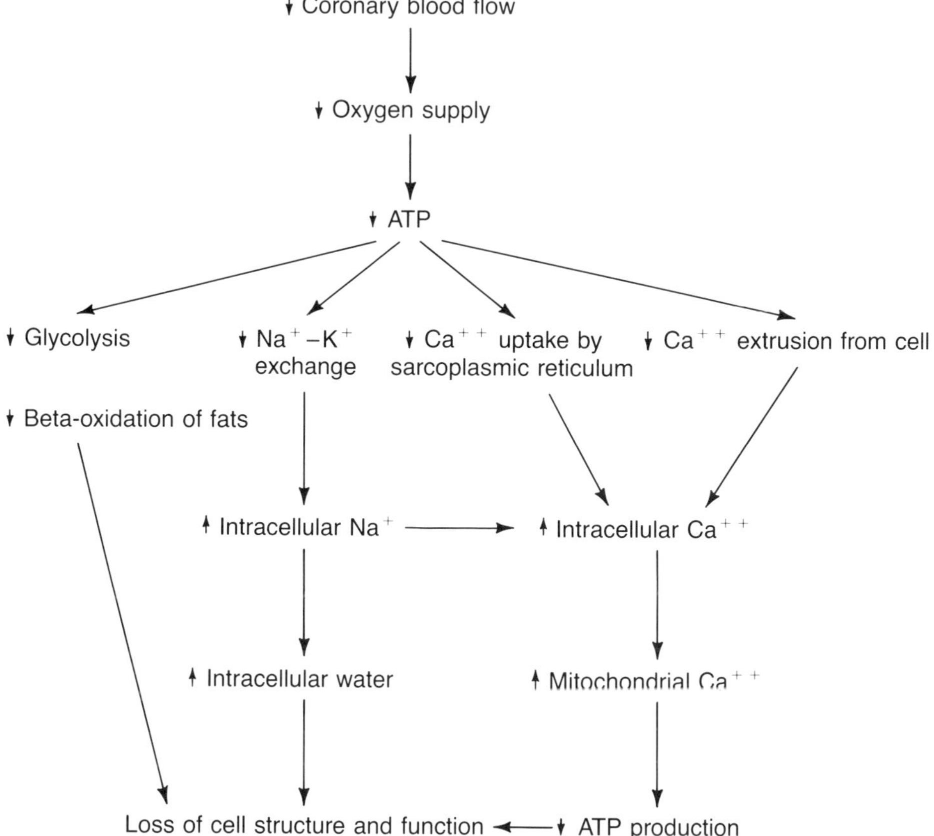

Fig. 7.3. Sequence of events involved in myocardial ischemic damage.

of ATP utilization and because they promote the entry of calcium into the myocardium.[68] Heart rate, contractile state, and peripheral vascular resistance are also of importance, since these are the main determinants of myocardial oxygen consumption and ATP utilization.[89]

The metabolic alterations which occur during ischemia and oxygen deficiency are numerous and contribute to the cascade of structural and functional abnormalities. In hearts where mitochondrial oxidation is reduced, failure to remove lactate from the cells results in high levels of nicotinamide adenine dehydrogenase (NADH), which inhibits glycolysis and fatty acid oxidation.[40,98] Inhibition of beta-oxidation of fatty acids will result in increased levels of acyl coenzyme A (CoA) and acyl carnitine. The rise in acyl CoA, acyl carnitine and free fatty acids may have secondary effects that contribute to cell damage.[10,98] These compounds are active detergents and bind extensively to cell membranes resulting in disruption and distortion of these membranes.[98] In addition to the detergent action, these products may have effects on specific enzymatic processes. In vitro studies reveal inhibition of sodium-potassium ATPase and alteration of calcium metabolism by the sarcoplasmic reticulum.[98] The presence of excess fatty acids in hypoxic or ischemic hearts depresses cardiac function.[48]

Acid-Base Balance

Acidosis (pH 6.8 to 7.2) causes depression of the contractile state.[9,65] Isolated cardiac muscle and heart preparations in vitro invariably exhibit decreased contractile force during either metabolic or respiratory acidosis.[65] In some patients, the direct myocardial effect of acidosis may be masked by the action of the sympathoadrenal system. Beta-receptor stimulation during acidosis results from increased release of norepinephrine from cardiac nerve endings and epinephrine and norepinephrine from the adrenal medulla.[65] In addition to its effects on cardiac function through direct action and through release of catecholamines, acidosis influences the heart by a third mechanism: depression of myocardial responsiveness to catecholamines.[9,65] Catecholamine binding to beta-receptors is influenced significantly by the pH of the environment. Maximum binding occurs at a pH between 7.4 and 7.5. The amount of catecholamines bound decreases considerably when the pH falls below 7.4.[65] This observation may explain the decreased myocardial response to catecholamines during acidosis, and the return to normal response when the acidosis is corrected.[9] In contrast, the effects of vagal stimulation are markedly enhanced at pH levels below 7.1, probably as a consequence of inhibition of acetylcholinesterase.[65] The resulting tendency for a given quantity of acetylcholine to have a protected duration of action leads to an increased danger of vagally mediated bradycardia and arrest during acidosis.[65]

The exact mechanisms by which the pH influences the inotropic state of the heart remains uncertain, but several mechanisms may play important roles. First, hydrogen ions compete with calcium for binding to the myocardial protein troponin.[40,65] In the presence of elevated concentration of intracellular hydrogen ion, a smaller percentage of the available calcium is able to react with troponin, fewer actin-myosin interactions occur, and the strength of contraction is reduced.[45] A second mechanism by which contractile force may be lowered during acidosis involves the binding and release of calcium to sarcoplasmic reticulum. Intracellular acidosis is thought to inhibit the release of calcium from the sarcoplasmic reticulum.[40,65] The ability of the sarcoplasmic reticulum to readily release calcium can affect the strength of contraction by controlling the amount of calcium that is potentially available for binding to troponin. Third, opening of the slow channel is reduced by acidosis. Therefore, acidosis appears to limit movement of calcium ions from the extracellular space into the cell, which also would interfere with excitation-contraction coupling. Finally, acidosis causes a rise in extracellular potassium, and hyperkalemia may influence the contractility as well as the rhythm of the heart.[45,65]

The effect of alkalosis on ventricular function has received less attention, and the existing data are controversial.[9,65] Most information does not substantiate any change in ventricular performance with induced alkalosis.[9] There are reports suggesting alkalosis has a depressant effect on the myocardium.[102,106] Respiratory alkalosis can increase coronary vascular resistance which in some patients, may result in decreased contractility. Also, in hemorrhagic shock, elevation in plasma epinephrine parallels the onset of acidosis; if acidosis is prevented by the intravenous administration of sodium bicarbonate, then the plasma epinephrine response to hemorrhage is blunted.

Hormonal and Metabolic Factors

Hypoglycemia

Glucose is a necessary energy substrate for metabolism in the myocardium.[40] Severe hypoglycemia may result in myocardial depression and circulatory failure.[72] Hypoglycemia is a common metabolic problem in the intensive care unit and may complicate shock of diverse etiologies, renal failure, sepsis, pancreatitis, and hypothermia, as well as the administration of many commonly prescribed medications.

Electrolyte and mineral imbalances

Abnormalities in calcium, potassium, sodium, phosphorus, and magnesium metabolism impair normal myocardial function.[71]

Calcium is essential to several vital cardiovascular processes, including (1) electrical activation of cardiac cells, (2) excitation-contraction coupling, (3) smooth muscle contraction in coronary and peripheral arteries, and (4) intracellular energy storage and utilization.[7,15,49] An adequately ionized calcium concentration is necessary for normal excitation, conduction, and contractile function of the myocardium.[97] Several clinical reports have provided evidence of a relation between hypocalcemia and heart failure.[8,24,32] A rise in the intracellular calcium level, derived from extracellular fluid and intracellular stores, is the immediate trigger for cardiac contraction. Thus, cardiac contractility can be impaired during hypocalcemia and improved after restoration of serum calcium levels.[28] In addition, the inotropic action of many drugs is also dependent on extracellular calcium, and ineffectiveness of these drugs during hypocalcemia can contribute to decreased cardiac function.[22,24]

The critically ill patient is vulnerable to the development of hypocalcemia by a variety of mechanisms. Because many hypocalcemic patients are either hypoalbuminemic or alkalotic, measuring ionized calcium levels is preferable.[49,50] Although the optimal level of ionized calcium has not been documented in normal or ill patients, a minimal level appears to be about 1.7 mEq/L.[49]

An increased extracellular potassium ion concentration can reduce myocardial contractility.[45] This does not appear to be a direct effect of potassium ion on the contractile process. Rather, high extracellular potassium probably exerts a negative inotropic action by accelerating repolarization of the cardiac action potential; in turn, this shortens the plateau phase during which time calcium is able to enter the cell.[45] Rapid accumulation of potassium ion in the extracellular space surrounding ischemic cells may thus contribute to pump failure.

Altered extracellular concentrations of sodium influence myocardial contractility. Whereas calcium is essential for myocardial contraction, it has been shown that sodium has the ability to depress this contractile response.[45] The net effect of the opposing actions of these cations on myocardial contractility depends not on the absolute concentrations of sodium or calcium but on the ratio between these two cations.[15] These cations compete for transport into the cell, and the ion transported is determined by their relative concentrations in the extracellular fluid.[45]

Magnesium deficiency has been associated with a number of cardiac disorders.[17,21] Although dysrhythmias are most commonly mentioned, magnesium plays an essential role in cardiac contractility, and hypomagnesemia may result in heart failure and circulatory shock.[21,99] The reason magnesium seems to be so important in cardiac disorders is that it is necessary for the generation of membrane sodium-potassium dependent ATPase as well as the ATPase that splits ATP to provide the energy for muscle contraction.[17] Additionally, magnesium depletion, by impairing parathyroid gland function, may cause hypocalcemia which would depress myocardial contractility.[71]

Hypophosphatemia impairs myocardial performance.[70,71] Numerous studies have shown that myocardial contractility may be affected by a fall in the phosphate stores of the body. ATP depletion is the most likely mechanism of the myocardial depression observed.[70]

Thyroid function

Alterations in thyroid physiology and thyroid function tests occur in some patients with serious nonthyroidal illness.[100] Low concentrations of serum triiodothyronine (T_3) occur in these patients and are attributable largely to reduced extrathyroidal conversion of thyroxine (T_4) to T_3.[23] Concentrations of serum total T_4 may be low, normal, or high; alterations in serum binding of T_4 explain the abnormality in most cases.[23] Concentrations of serum reverse T_3 are usually high because metabolic clearance is reduced.[23] The degree of impairment in thyroid hormone metabolism that occurs may correlate with the severity of illness. Hypothyroxinemia has been correlated with mortality in critically ill patients.[85] The most striking thyroid hormone response to shock and trauma is a profound decrease in plasma T_3 levels.[100] These findings of severe chemical hypothyroidism in circulatory failure suggest that therapy with T_3 might be beneficial for these patients.[100] However, the use of thyroid hormone in such patients to improve cardiac output, heart rate, and systemic blood pressure is controversial.[23,66,97] Most evidence suggests that despite the low serum concentration of T_3, sick patients with nonthyroidial illness are clinically euthyroid ("sick-euthyroid" syndrome), and therefore should not be treated with thyroid hormone.[23]

Adrenal function

Although the usual physiologic response that occurs in circulatory failure is increased secretion of adrenocortical hormones, not all patients in shock have increased blood cortisol levels.[72,84] Acute adrenal insufficiency has been reported following cardiac surgical procedures and during severe bacterial infections.[3,84] Although the main effect of adrenal insufficiency occurs in the vascular bed, the electrolyte imbalance may have profound effects in the myocardium.

Temperature

Myocardial performance is temperature dependent. Hypothermia depresses myocardial contractility resulting in depressed cardiac output.[41,69] In addition, hypothermia will result in peripheral vasoconstriction and metabolic acidosis, which will further impair tissue perfusion and hemodynamic stability.[41] When the infant is subjected to cold stress, it attempts to maintain body temperature by increased heat production from the metabolism of free fatty acids released from brown fat stores. This may be effective in maintaining body temperature, but at the expense of a marked increase in metabolic rate and oxygen consumption.[90] This places a great stress on the cardiorespiratory system, perhaps exceeding the ability of the infant to compensate. In the older child, the primary intrinsic mechanism to reverse hypothermia is shivering. This rigorous muscle activity increases oxygen consumption and therefore cardiac work. Similarly, hyperthermia increases metabolic rate, oxygen consumption, and cardiac work.[90]

The Effect of Positive End-Expiratory Pressure

Some investigators have suggested that positive end-expiratory pressure (PEEP) decreases myocardial contractility.[26] The mechanisms of impaired contractility include (1) reflex cardiac depression mediated by the stimulation of lung stretch receptors, (2) depressed contractility mediated by the release of vasoactive substances resulting from lung distention, and (3) myocardial ischemia secondary to reduced coronary arterial blood flow.[86] However, the vast majority of researchers have not shown that PEEP impairs ventricular contractility.[26,86] It is therefore unlikely that impaired ventricular contractility contributes to the decrease in cardiac output often seen as a result of PEEP. The effects of PEEP are primarily mechanical and are mediated through a combination of right ventricular preload limitation and outflow obstruction; both effects are additive in limiting left ventricular preload.[76,86]

Pharmacologic Agents That Decrease Contractility

Drugs known to have negative inotropic actions are inhalation anesthetic agents, barbiturates, calcium-channel blockers, and beta-adrenergic receptor antagonists.[69] In addition to these exogenous compounds, various endogenous factors have been postulated to be mediators of circulatory failure.[2,53] One of the more prominent of these is a myocardial depressant factor found in a variety of types of shock.[53] A number of other endogenous substances are being identified which have negative inotropic action and may contribute to circulatory failure.[2,53,64] Treatment of circulatory shock must consider the presence of these toxic factors.[2,54] Therapeutic efforts to counteract these factors may be useful in the pharmacologic approach to circulatory failure.[54]

THERAPEUTIC MEASURES TO IMPROVE MYOCARDIAL CONTRACTILITY

This section describes the management of acute, life-threatening circulatory failure, with emphasis on measures designed to improve myocardial contractility. Although heart failure may be the final common pathway of many acute illnesses and is responsive to certain therapeutic interventions regardless of the cause, optimal therapy requires identification of both primary and secondary causes of decompensation. This goal can only be achieved by a detailed history, frequent physical examination, and laboratory evaluation since some primary or secondary causes may not be apparent.

Therapeutic measures to improve myocardial contractility include (1) improvement in myocardial oxygen delivery, (2) reduction of myocardial oxygen demands,

(3) correction of extramyocardial factors, (4) appropriate utilization of inotropic drugs, and (5) avoidance of cardiac depressant drugs.

Measures to Improve Myocardial Oxygen Delivery

Myocardial oxygen delivery depends on the maintenance of coronary blood flow and adequate oxygen content of the coronary perfusate.[90] As previously discussed, in many cases of heart failure and circulatory shock, coronary blood flow becomes dependent on aortic diastolic pressure, ventricular end-diastolic pressure, and diastolic time. Any compromise of coronary blood flow leads to subendocardial ischemia, which results in a self-perpetuating process eventually leading to terminal heart failure.[81] Decreasing ventricular size, increasing coronary perfusion pressure, lowering ventricular end-diastolic pressure, or decreasing heart rate may improve subendocardial perfusion, correct the imbalance of energy supply and demand, and therefore improve myocardial contractility.

Perhaps the most important consideration is the maintenance of adequate coronary perfusion pressure by increasing aortic diastolic pressure, decreasing ventricular end-diastolic pressure, or both.[89] However, an excessive rise in pressure is to be avoided since increased afterload on the ventricle necessitates additional oxygen requirements.[89] The minimal acceptable coronary perfusion pressure is unknown and will depend on disease state, myocardial oxygen demand, and arterial oxygen content. Estimation of subendocardial perfusion by using a ratio of diastolic pressure time index to systolic pressure time index is thought to be helpful in the management of these patients.[42,90]

The administration of inotropic agents, such as catecholamines, will increase myocardial oxygen requirements unless there is concomitant decrease in ventricular volume and tension.[89] Dobutamine, an agent which improves cardiac output and coronary blood flow while lowering left ventricular end-diastolic pressure, has improved the histology and biochemistry of endomyocardial biopsies in cardiomyopathic patients.[95] These studies provide evidence that improved coronary blood flow is associated with improved function, morphology, and biochemistry of the myopathic ventricle.[95] Further evidence emphasizing the importance of maintaining coronary perfusion pressure comes from studies of acute right ventricular pressure overload and failure; a common problem following repair of certain congenital heart defects.[101] Ischemia of the right ventricular free wall is the mechanism by which failure occurs in right ventricular pressure overload.[83,101] Without decreasing right ventricular afterload, increasing aortic pressure and hence myocardial perfusion pressure increases myocardial blood flow, reverses ischemia, and consequently improves right ventricular function.[101] These findings suggest that maintaining systemic pressure is an important factor in the clinical management of right ventricular overload and failure. Some inotropic agents may increase myocardial oxygen consumption to a greater extent than they improve coronary blood flow.[74] Thus, the discrepancy between oxygen requirements and supply is widened, possibly contributing to further ischemic.[74] In addition to the better known effects pharmacologic agents (inotropic drugs, vasopressors, or both) have on myocardial oxygen consumption and coronary blood flow, the effect of such drugs on diastolic time, with consequent implications for coronary perfusion, should be considered.[14]

Occasionally, the judicious use of vasopressors, for example norepinephrine, is required in such desperate situations as cardiogenic shock.[101] In some patients, naloxone may act as a vasopressor while reversing some of the pathophysiologic changes seen in shock.[2,34] Naloxone has no significant side-effects in clinical use and may prove to be a first line drug in profound shock, for temporary stabilization of hemodynamic factors while specific therapy is instituted.[34]

Efforts to decrease myocardial wall stress and ventricular end-diastolic pressure may be helpful in improving coronary blood flow and, therefore myocardial contractility. When contemplating such therapy, the various factors that can affect ventricular end-diastolic pressure must be considered. Extramyocardial factors such as hypothermia, acidosis, pain, excessive mean airway pressure, and pericardial effusion can all increase end-diastolic pressure and should be corrected prior to initiating other therapy.[44] Myocardial ischemia will impair ventricular relaxation (by impairing function of the sarcoplasmic reticulum) and therefore, decrease ventricular distensibility resulting in a higher intraventricular diastolic pressure for any given ventricular volume.[18,35,83] This may further impair the gradient for subendocardial flow.[83] Therefore, measures taken to improve the function of the sarcoplasmic reticulum (e.g., normothermia, adequate coronary perfusion, and ample oxygen and metabolic substrates) will improve ventricular relaxation, increase ventricular compliance, decrease ventricular end-diastolic pressure, and improve myocardial contractility.[69] Treatment with diuretics and vasodilators may favorably affect end-diastolic pressure but may adversely affect coronary blood flow.[18,90]

Finally, measures to increase the arterial oxygen content should be instituted; as hypoxemia is a common accompaniment of circulatory shock.[51,72] In approaching the problem of hypoxemia, one must consider all factors that determine the partial pressure of oxygen in arterial blood (P_aO_2). These determinants include ventilatory, circulatory, and metabolic factors as well as the quantity and quality of hemoglobin present.[43] Therapeutic interventions that change circulatory (e.g., cardiac output and pulmonary vascular resistance) and metabolic (e.g., oxygen consumption) determinants of the P_aO_2 may result in dramatic change in P_aO_2 without altering underlying lung function.[43] Sudden changes in P_aO_2 are usually circulatory or metabolic in origin if gross ventilatory changes have been excluded (e.g., pneumothorax, malpositioned or obstructed endotracheal tube, and change in inspired oxygen tension).

Oxygen delivery to the heart (as well as the entire body) can be improved by increasing the P_aO_2, increasing the hemoglobin, and correcting those conditions that cause a leftward shift of the oxyhemoglobin dissociation curve making it more difficult for the hemoglobin to release the oxygen to the tissues. Those conditions which cause a leftward shift are alkalosis, hypothermia, hypophosphatemia, and a decreased red cell 2, 3-diphosphoglycerate.[43] Although increasing the inspired concentration of oxygen (F_IO_2) is one means of increasing P_aO_2 and therefore improving oxygen delivery; the risks of oxygen toxicity also increase. In some patients, improvement of P_aO_2 may require positive pressure ventilation. However, the P_aO_2 is not the only indicator of tissue oxygenation. For example, increasing PEEP may improve P_aO_2 but decrease cardiac output.[43,86] The result may decrease tissue oxygen delivery, which is the product of cardiac output and arterial oxygen content.

Measures to Decrease Myocardial Oxygen Consumption

The major determinants of myocardial oxygen consumption include myocardial tension (determined by ventricular pressure, intraventricular volume, and myocardial mass), contractile state of the heart, and heart rate.[89] Of lesser importance quantitatively, but contributing to oxygen requirements are the external work performed by the heart; the energy required for activation and relaxation; and the basal, or resting, metabolism of the myocardium.[89] Optimizing preload, afterload, and heart rate may decrease myocardial oxygen consumption and therefore improve myocardial performance. These therapeutic modalities are discussed in Chapters 5, 6 and 8. Because inotropic drugs may adversely affect myocardial oxygen consumption, their use should be reserved for situations in which these other modes of therapy are ineffective or contraindicated.[81] An increasing myocardial oxygen consumption, however, does not always occur when inotropic agents are administered. Instead, the change in myocardial oxygen consumption after an inotropic stimulus depends upon the degree to which myocardial tension is reduced in relation to the extent to which contractile state is augmented.[89]

Devices and techniques have been developed to assist the failing circulation by reducing work load and oxygen requirements of a failing heart. They include the intra-aortic balloon pump and long term cardiopulmonary bypass using membrane oxygenators. Intra-aortic balloon diastolic augmentation and counterpulsation is an effective means of increasing coronary blood flow and decreasing left ventricular work, thereby improving the balance between myocardial oxygen supply and demand.[90]

One effective means of reducing myocardial oxygen requirements is to reduce total body oxygen consumption. Measures to reduce oxygen consumption include mechanical ventilation of the lungs, prevention of hyperpyrexia, control of pain or anxiety, and muscle paralysis.[90] In patients with circulatory failure, the work of breathing is substantially increased. This can be caused by hyperventilation elicited by acidemia, hypoxemia, or other neural factors; or it can also be due to alterations in pulmonary mechanics secondary to either pulmonary vascular congestion or increased resistance to flow (pulmonary hypertension).[60,72] However, in low cardiac output states, the oxygen supply to the inspiratory muscles, which is dependent on blood flow, may not meet the energy demanded by the increased work of breathing.[30,79] As a result, either other body tissues (possibly including the brain, heart, and liver[58]) are deprived of much needed oxygen or the inspiratory muscles are deprived, resulting in an inability to maintain adequate ventilation.[30] Thus, in the presence of circulatory shock, artificial ventilation should be considered in order to diminish inspiratory muscle oxygen demands.[60] Instituting artificial ventilation in this situation will markedly decrease the oxygen consumption of the respiratory muscles liberating what limited oxygen supplies are available for the rest of the body.[30,60] It will also decrease lactate production, decrease the myocardial oxygen consumption by decreasing cardiac work, and prevent respiratory failure due to inspiratory muscle fatigue.[6,82]

The effect of intubation and positive-pressure ventilation may extend beyond these considerations. Positive mean airway pressure will decrease left ventricular afterload, which should increase stroke volume and hence decrease end-diastolic volume and myocardial oxygen.[82]

Correction of Extramyocardial Factors Which Directly Affect Myocardial Contractility

In order to improve contractility, attention must be directed to some of the cellular and biochemical aspects of myocardial failure. Acid-base and electrolyte disorders accompanying many major physiologic disturbances may contribute to myocardial dysfunction. Thus, an appropriate cellular milieu must exist before relying on inotropic agonists.

Metabolic acidosis may result from anaerobic metabolism and decreased tissue perfusion with release of lactate, or from accumulation of organic acids because of renal failure. Severe hypoventilation may contribute to both hypoxemia and respiratory acidosis. The reduction in arterial and intracellular pH causes depression of myocardial contractility, decreased responsiveness to catecholamines, inhibition of glycolysis and other key metabolic pathways, and increased pulmonary vascular resistance.[9,65] Correction of acidosis may restore cardiac output and eliminate the need for more aggressive therapy.[40] Correction with sodium bicarbonate is indicated when marked metabolic acidosis exists (arterial blood pH < 7.20).[72] Doses of sodium bicarbonate are based on body weight and base deficit (mEq = bodyweight in kilograms $\times$ base deficit $\times$ 0.3). Bicarbonate should be used to partially correct the pH to levels which do not pose an immediate threat to life (7.25 to 7.30). Metabolic alkalosis may be detrimental. Electrolyte abnormalities, fluid overload, and hypertonicity are recognized complications of bicarbonate therapy. In some patients use of another buffer, tris-hydroxymethyl-amino-methane (THAM), may be preferable, though it has the disadvantages of causing respiratory depression, hypoglycemia, and hyperkalemia.[96] Recent reports demonstrate that dichloroacetate can have positive metabolic and hemodynamic effects in patients with lactic acidosis of various causes.[91] Dichloroacetate reduces circulating lactate concentrations by stimulating the activity of pyruvate dehydrogenase, the enzyme that catalyzes the rate-limiting step in the oxidation of lactate to pyruvate.[91] Of equal importance, dichloroacetate improved cardiac performance before any change in arterial pH was achieved.[91] Dichloroacetate is known to stimulate aerobic oxidative metabolism in cardiac tissue and to improve cardiac function in animals with experimentally induced myocardial ischemia or lactic acidosis.[91] Such a drug would be very beneficial in the management of circulatory failure, and further investigation is warranted.

Abnormalities in electrolyte concentrations may also adversely affect myocardial contractility and should be corrected. The most important of these, calcium, is discussed in the section on inotropic agents. Discussion of other electrolyte abnormalities is beyond the scope of this text and the reader is referred to recent reviews of this subject.[71]

The human heart normally derives its contractile energy from oxidative phosphorylation, primarily using free fatty acids and oxygen.[25,40] Under usual conditions, increased energy needs are met by regulating coronary artery blood flow, thereby increasing oxygen and substrate delivery to myocardial muscle. The inability to increase coronary blood flow in such conditions as circulatory failure with profound hypotension may result in insufficient delivery of oxygen to myocardial energy requirements. Substrate availability may also be inadequate with high cardiac work loads, such as in patients with hyperdynamic septic shock or extensive burns.[25] As previously discussed, the oxygen-deprived ventricle undergoes a series of self-perpetuating functional, metabolic, and structural alterations.[40]

In patients in whom oxygen availability represents a critical limitation, the myocardium is capable of metabolizing glucose by anaerobic glycolysis to produce lactate and energy.[40] Because myocardial glycogen stores are limited, glucose must be provided to preserve the myocardium and enhance its performance. Unfortunately, this anaerobic pathway is inefficient and can probably supply only a portion of myocardial needs.[25,57] Insulin and potassium may be added to facilitate muscle uptake of glucose and to prevent hypokalemia.[51] Administration of solutions consisting of glucose, insulin, and potassium (GIK) have been used in patients with circulatory failure of multiple etiologies, and it is well-documented that the GIK administration improves cardiac performance in these patients.[5,25,48] Such infusions improve contractility, restore cell membrane potentials, and lower the concentration of plasma free fatty acids, even under conditions of marked hypoxia.[48,51,57] In addition to increasing glycolysis and decreasing total free fatty acids, GIK infusion changes plasma free fatty acid composition, which may contribute to beneficial effects on electrical and mechanical stability of the ischemic myocardium.[62]

Inotropic Drugs

A number of classes of drugs are currently available to stimulate myocardial contractility. Each class has its own basic mechanism of action. The final common step, however, is an increase in intracellular calcium, which increases contraction.[59]

When using pharmacologic means to support the failing myocardium, it is important to understand the pathophysiology of the many causes of heart failure.[59] There are numerous ways in which myocardial dysfunction or excessive demands can lead to failure.[59] Often, heart failure is produced by an increased load superimposed upon an already poorly functioning myocardium. Another situation, seen frequently in the intensive care unit, is the increased demand of sepsis added to myocardial dysfunction produced by hypotension, acidosis, and hypoxemia.

Inotropic drugs are used as an adjunct to other measures directed at the primary disease. Often their use is temporary, designed to assist the failing myocardium through a critical period of the disease process. In other situations, inotropic agents may be used on a long-term basis as the primary mode of therapy. In yet other circumstances, an inotropic agent may be contraindicated. Thus, the pathophysiologic process first must be considered before deciding to use inotropic drugs. In acute situations, it is desirable to use short-acting, titratable drugs because the situation may rapidly change. The list of inotropic drugs is not very long (Table 7.1) and the basic mechanisms of action are relatively few (Fig. 7.4).[59,88]

Calcium

Ionized calcium is the physiologic stimulus for myocardial contraction and, when administered intravenously, can increase the serum level resulting in increased myocardial contractility.[13,88] Therefore, when the serum ionized calcium level is low, administration of calcium has a positive inotropic action.[27] The effect is transient, lasting approximately 10 to 15 minutes.[38] However, when the ionized calcium

Table 7.1. Inotropic Agents

Agent
Calcium
Catecholamines
Cardiac glycosides (digitalis)
Glucagon and the phosphodiesterase inhibitors
Glucagon
Xanthines (including theophylline and aminophilline)
Agents under investigation
Amrinone
Inophores

concentration is normal or high, administration of calcium may increase systemic vascular resistance and blood pressure without increasing cardiac output.[28]

The advantages of the use of calcium salts as inotropic agents, especially the highly ionized calcium chloride, is subject to some controversy.[7] This issue is complicated by the fact that although calcium plays an essential role in cardiovascular function, the in vivo concentration of ionized calcium required for these functions has not been determined.[7] Levels of ionized calcium can change precipitously after albumin administration, blood transfusion, or rapid changes in acid-base status.[7,49] Whether any of these changes also alter cardiovascular function

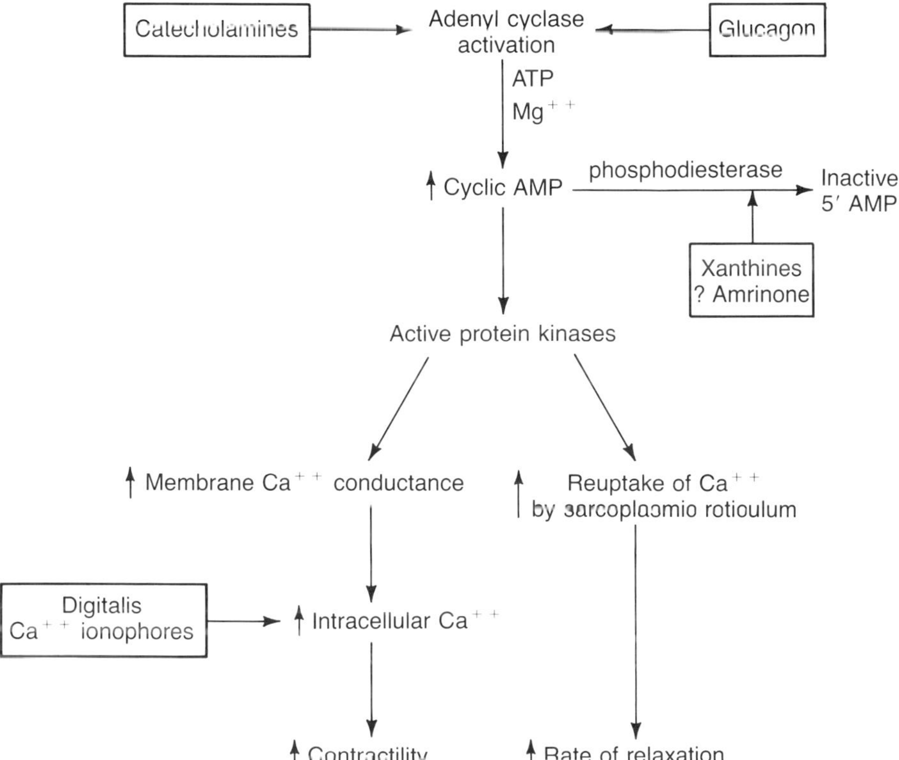

Fig. 7.4. Proposed mechanisms by which the inotropic agents increase contractility of the myocardium.

has not been well delineated.[7] Currently, there is no clear indication when supplemental calcium is required in the management of shock. Further studies are needed to determine the optimal level of ionized calcium during and after resuscitation from circulatory shock in order to offer recommendations.[38,49]

Special attention must be paid to the potential adverse effects of calcium, especially to the ischemic myocardium. Recent data implicate the calcium ion as a triggering element in a number of adverse reactions in a wide variety of tissues after shock, sepsis, trauma, and anoxia.[104] Reports have also linked ionic calcium shifts to abnormalities in cellular metabolism, intracellular release of free fatty acids, and production of oxidative free radicals.[104]

As discussed earlier, the interaction between myocardial ischemia and intracellular calcium concentration is complex. During ischemia, several factors contribute to an increased intracellular calcium concentration. Activation of slow calcium channels, impaired uptake of calcium by the sarcoplasmic reticulum, and impaired extrusion of calcium from the cell all contribute.[40,68] Hypocalcemia—seen so frequently in patients with circulatory shock—may be explained, at least in part, by this intracellular pooling of calcium.[94] The increased intracellular calcium concentration results in uptake of calcium by the mitochondria. The energy of oxidation is directly used by the mitochondria to take up calcium without the intermediate production of ATP.[68] This calcium pumping by the mitochondria is obligatory, energy consuming, and uncouples the use of oxidation-derived energy from the production of ATP.[97,104] Myocardial ischemia, therefore, is characterized by a reduction of myocardial ATP stores. This raises intracellular calcium which, in turn, triggers a vicious cycle by further depleting ATP stores.[15,69,97] In such instances, one should beware of administering calcium[92]; in fact, use of calcium blockers may be more appropriate therapy.[36,78] Preventing the accumulation of intracellular calcium might lessen the decrease in contractility and impaired relaxation which are characteristic of myocardial ischemia.[13,36,78,104] Therefore, when a cell is well-supplied with oxygen and nutrients, raising intracellular calcium slightly by using intravenous calcium chloride results in stronger cellular contraction and thus increased cardiac output.

Dysrhythmias may complicate calcium administration. Calcium, with its cellular membrane effects, can slow depolarization of cardiac cells, especially in the presence of digitalis or low serum potassium levels.[19] Calcium replacement therapy is appropriate in patients with circulatory failure to correct a state of sustained hypocalcemia.[28] A precise definition of the optimal dosage of replacement calcium is not available; however, 5 to 10 mg/kg of 10 percent calcium chloride solution by slow intravenous infusion through a centrally placed catheter is the usual dose.[69] For more sustained effect, continuous infusion of calcium chloride may be required.[27] Additional doses or regulation of the calcium infusion should be based on serum calcium measurements.[27]

Catecholamines

The catecholamines increase contractility by stimulating $beta_1$-adrenergic receptors located on the surface of cardiac cells.[103] $Beta_1$ stimulation activates adenyl cyclase in the cell surface membrane which subsequently converts ATP to adenosine 3′,5′ monophosphate (cyclic AMP or cAMP). Cyclic AMP then activates protein kinases which catalyze phosphorylation reactions of multiple membrane systems.[88] One protein kinase appears to catalyze a critical phosphorylation reaction at the inner gate of the slow channel, which increases calcium influx by means of the slow inward current.[4] The increased calcium transport thereby enhances contractility, frequency, and conduction velocity in the heart.[63] Phospholamban is a protein associated with the sarcoplasmic reticulum, which when phosphorylated by cyclic AMP increases the uptake of calcium by the sarcoplasmic reticulum accounting for the more rapid relaxation of cardiac muscle exposed to catecholamines.[15] Therefore, by increasing cyclic AMP, catecholamines augment calcium availability to the contractile system and enhance calcium removal, which produces more rapid relaxation.[88]

The catecholamines are the most potent positive inotropic agents available; however, effects are not limited to inotropy.[72] They also possess chronotropic properties and complex effects on vascular beds of the various organs of the body.[59] Consequently, the choice of an agent may depend as much on the state of the circulation as it does on the myocardium. Manipulation of the side chain of the catecholamine molecule has yielded synthetic catecholamines with greater propensity to activate one receptor or another.[88] The available catecholamines are norepinephrine, epinephrine, isoproterenol, dopamine, and dobutamine (Table 7.2).[20,33,46,61,72,80]

Although cardiac muscle contraction is under the regulatory control of the adrenergic nervous system, some patients with myocardial failure are refractory to pharmacologic stimulation by beta-agonists.[16] Mechanisms for a reduced adrenergic response in some patients include (1) an alteration in the number of $beta_1$-adrenergic receptors on the myocardial cell membrane or (2) a change in the affinity of these receptors for circulating catecholamines.[16,55,67,93] Regardless of the mechanism, the adrenergic support, which is vital to the heart under stress, may be undermined by extreme beta-adrenergic subsensitivity in the failing human heart.[93] Although the cause of beta-receptor down-regulation induced by heart failure is not known, it is possible that it is a result of exposure to an increased concentration of circulating or tissue catecholamines followed by further down-regulation due to therapeutic doses of beta-agonists.[16,32] Beta-receptor down-regulation may be so pronounced as to make the adrenergic pathway incapable of providing the necessary inotropic support.[16,67] In this situation, it may be necessary to use inotropic agents that act either beyond the level of membrane-bound receptors, or through distinctly different receptor-effector pathways.[32]

The catecholamines listed in Table 7.2 have been used extensively in infants and children, but the dose-response relationships have not been investigated fully.[73,105] Older children seem to respond in a manner quite similar to adults, however, markedly different responses may be seen in newborns.[12,31,73] Age related differences in receptor population and sensitivity may partially explain the observed discrepancies. The importance of careful observation of the effects of catecholamines in children, with special emphasis on the response of neonates and infants, must be emphasized.[73]

The available catecholamines must be given by continuous intravenous infusion which should be administered into centrally placed catheters. A constant-infusion pump should be used, and the infusions should never be interrupted as the half-

Table 7.2. Catecholamines

Drug	Recommended Dose	Comment
Norepinephrine	0.05–1.0 μg/kg/min (alpha, beta)	Predominant alpha adrenergic stimulation overshadows the $beta_1$ effects on the myocardium. Used only in situations in which arterial pressure has decreased to levels which acutely jeopardize coronary and cerebral perfusion. May cause hypocalcemia, hypoglycemia, ischemic dysrhythmias and ischemia of renal and splanchnic beds.
Epinephrine	0.005–0.02 μg/kg/min (beta) 0.02–1.0 μg/kg/min (alpha, beta)	Vasodilation of splanchnic bed and skeletal muscle at low doses. Major metabolic effects: increases free fatty acids, and increases glucose. Higher doses may lead to renal and mesenteric ischemia. Reserved for those situations where the failing myocardium is unresponsive to other inotropic drugs.
Isoproterenol	0.01–0.5 μg/kg/min (beta)	Synthetic catecholamine which acts almost exclusively on beta-adrenergic receptors as an agonist. Positive inotropic and chronotropic effects while decreasing systemic and pulmonary vascular resistances. Not generally useful in shock because it increases cutaneous and muscular vasodilation, thus redistributing blood to nonessential areas. Indicated in the therapy of cardiac failure complicated by bradycardia or asthma, and perhaps pulmonary hypertension.
Dopamine	0.05–2.0 μg/kg/min (dopaminergic) 2.0–10.0 μg/kg/min (beta, dopaminergic) 10.0–20.0 μg/kg/min (alpha, beta) >20.0 μg/kg/min (alpha)	Stimulates cardiac beta receptors by direct and indirect mechanisms. Has unique vasodilating effects on certain vascular beds, especially the renal vasculature, but also on the mesenteric coronary and intracerebral vascular beds. The specific peripheral effects of dopamine make this catecholamine particularly useful when low dose infusions can restore cardiovascular stability and also augment renal function.
Dobutamine	1.0–10.0 μg/kg/min (alpha, beta)	Relatively new synthetic catecholamine with a biochemical structure similar to isoproterenol. Racemic mixture—overall activity is due to the sum of the activation of individual stereoisomers. Positive inotropic effect with minimal chronotropic or peripheral vascular effects.

life of the drugs may be only 1 or 2 minutes. The catheter should never be flushed because rapid administration of these drugs can be fatal. All drug infusions should be carefully labeled with the drug name, concentration, and diluent. A secondary catheter should be used for all other drugs, blood products, and fluids. Although dose recommendations are made, there is no usual drug or dose in shock; therapy must be continually tailored to the patient's response. Newer, orally active, $beta_1$-receptor stimulating catecholamines (e.g., prenalterol) are now being studied.[103]

Cardiac glycosides (digitalis)

Digitalis glycosides have been used for 200 years and remain the prime orally active inotropic agent currently available for use in humans.[88] Their action occurs by binding a partial inhibition of the sodium-potassium stimulated ATPase of the sarcolemma, and therefore, reduces the transmembrane exchange of sodium and potassium.[1,103] As a result, intracellular sodium is increased. The increase in intracellular sodium augments an influx of calcium, presumably by triggering a sodium-calcium exchange reaction.[1,103] The resultant rise in intracellular calcium concentration produces a positive inotropic effect.

The efficacy of the glycosides is limited by a low toxic-to-therapeutic ratio. The direct actions of digitalis include a dose-related increased force of contraction. Thus, increasing levels of digitalis produce linear increases in myocardial contractility.[10] Recent studies suggest that low serum levels of digoxin are as effective as high levels in improving heart function in children.[70a] The inotropic effect may be opposed by a direct and reflex peripheral vasoconstrictor effect.[87] Digitalis may, therefore, produce an increase in an inotropic state, which is offset by increased afterload, resulting in no change in cardiac output.[87]

Toxic manifestations of digitalis include conduction disturbances in both atrial and ventricular muscles. Digitalis may produce virtually all cardiac dysrhythmias, including frequent premature beats and atrial tachycardia with atrioventricular (AV) block, nodal tachycardia, and other degrees of AV block. Factors which may increase the sensitivity of the myocardium to digitalis include hypokalemia, hypercalcemia, hypomagnesemia, thyroid status, hypoxia, myocardial ischemia, and alkalosis.[10] This situation is complicated by the fact pharmacokinetic variables of digitalis vary among the different age groups.[10,12] Different rates of metabolism and excretion of the drug account for part of this variability.[10] Neonates and infants need more digoxin than adults on a body weight basis because of a larger volume of distribution, but this excess must be matched against their capacity to eliminate the drug.[10]

For these reasons and because its effect on contractility is not as great as the catecholamines, digitalis is not the inotropic drug of choice in shock.[103] If a sustained inotropic effect is needed after the patient has stabilized, initiation of digitalis therapy at low doses may be indicated.[87]

Glucagon and the phosphodiesterase inhibitors

It has long been known that glucagon, an endogenous pancreatic hormone, could increase contractility without affecting either beta-receptors or the receptor for digitalis glycosides.[88] Glucagon increases cAMP by direct activation of adenyl cyclase. Whereas glucagon intravenously may be used to stimulate contractility acutely or as an antidote for beta-blockade toxicity, it should not be used repeatedly.[88] Moreover, its action to increase contractility may be variable.[59,88] The modest increment in heart function following glucagon administration, together with troublesome gastrointestinal symptoms, have removed it from current therapeutic recommendations.[103]

Phosphodiesterase inhibitors, such as the xanthines, raise cAMP by inhibiting the cAMP-degrading enzyme phosphodiesterase.[103] Xanthines, especially theophylline and aminophylline, increase cardiac output as a direct result of positive inotropic and chronotropic effects.[59] Such effects potentiate the mechanical and biochemical actions of catecholamines. Xanthines may also have an effect on myocardial uptake of calcium ion.[59] More recently, a number of other phosphodiesterase inhibitors with positive inotropic properties have been developed. The ultimate efficacy and safety of these compounds is currently under investigation.[103]

Other inotropic agents under investigation

Recent interest has focused on a new class of inotropic drugs, the prototype of which is amrinone.[11,23a] This dipyridine ring, which is neither a catecholamine nor a digitalis glycoside, augments myocardial contractility in animals and humans, while producing peripheral vasodilation.[11] The mode of action of amrinone is unknown, although it does enhance calcium movements in the red cell. In the heart, it does not affect the sodium-potassium simulated ATPase or enzymes associated with $beta_1$-receptor stimulation.[11] It may inhibit phosphodiesterase, leading to increased cAMP.[88] This would explain both augmented myocardial contractility and reduced peripheral vascular resistance.[88] Moreover, phosphodiesterase inhibition does not depend on a cell surface receptor and may be a way to alter myocardial contractility in the presence of down-regulation.[88] The elucidation of amrinone's mechanism of action will prove most interesting and perhaps lead to a new understanding of the contractile process, as well as to the development of other potent cardiotonic agents.[23a]

Inophores are naturally occurring compounds that modify the permeability of biologic membranes.[75,103] Positive inotropic effects of investigational inophores have been reported in isolated cardiac muscle and intact heart preparations.[103] The mechanism of action by which contractility is increased and calcium influx altered by these compounds is unclear.[59] The available data indicate the positive inotropic effect occurs at least in part, as a result of catecholamine release.[59,75]

SUMMARY

Many interventions that augment or depress the contractile state of heart muscle are the result of alterations in calcium exchange. An understanding of the concepts of cellular ionic flows must be the basis for interpreting myocardial performance and initiating therapy.

REFERENCES

1. Akera T, Brody TM 1982 Myocardial membranes: regulation and function of the sodium pump. Annual Review of Physiology 44: 375
2. Albert SA, Shire GT, Illner H 1982 Effects of Naloxone in hemorrhagic shock. Surgery, Gynecology and Obstetrics 155: 326
3. Alford WC, Meador CK, Mihalevich J, Burrus GR, Glassford DM, Stoney WS, Thomas CS 1979 Acute adrenal insufficiency following cardiac surgical procedures. Journal of Thoracic and Cardiovascular Surgery 78: 489
4. Antman EM, Stone PH, Muller JE, Braunwald E 1980 Calcium channel blocking agents in the treatment of cardiovascular disorders. Part I: Basic and clinical electrophysiologic effects. Annals of Internal Medicine 93: 875
5. Archer LT, Beller BK, Drake JK, Whitsett TL, Hinshaw LB 1978 Reversal of myocardial dysfunction in endotoxin shock with insulin. Canadian Journal of Physiology and Pharmacology 56: 132

6. Aubier M, Trippenbach T, Roussos C 1981 Respiratory muscle fatigue during cardiogenic shock. Journal of Applied Physiology 51: 499
7. Auffant RA, Downs JB, Amick R 1981 Ionized calcium concentration and cardiovascular function after cardiopulmonary bypass. Archives of Surgery 116: 1072
8. Bashour T, Basha HS, Cheny TO 1980 Hypocalcemia cardiomyopathy. Chest 78: 663
9. Beierholm EA, Grantham RN, O'Keefe DD, Laver MB, Daggett WM 1975 Effects of acid-base changes, hypoxia, and catecholamines on ventricular performance. American Journal of Physiology 228: 1555
10. Bendayan R, McKenzie MW 1983 Digoxin pharmacokinetics and dosage requirements in pediatric patients. Clinical Pharmacology 2: 224
11. Benotti JR, Grossman W, Braunwald E, Duvolos DD, Alousi AA 1978 Hemodynamic assessment of amrinone. New England Journal of Medicine 299: 1373
12. Berman W, Yabek SM, Dillon T, Niland C, Corlew S, Christensen D 1983 Effects of digoxin in infants with congested circulatory state due to a ventricular septal defect. New England Journal of Medicine 308: 363
13. Bixler TJ, Flaherty JT, Gardner TJ, Bulkley BH, Schaft HV, Gott VL 1978 Effects of calcium administration during postischemic reperfusion on myocardial contractility, stiffness, edema and ultrastructure. Circulation (Suppl 1) 58: 186
14. Boudoulas H, Rittgers SE, Lewis RP, Leier CV, Weissler AM 1979 Changes in diastolic time with various pharmacologic agents. Circulation 60: 164
15. Braunwald E 1982 Mechanism of action of calcium channel blocking agents. New England Journal of Medicine 307: 1618
16. Bristow MR, Ginsburg R, Minobe W, Cubicciotti RS, Sageman WS, Lurie K, Billingham ME, Harrison DC, Stinson EB 1982 Decreased catecholamine sensitivity and beta-adrenergic-receptor density in failing human hearts. New England Journal of Medicine 307: 205
17. Burch GE, Giles TD 1977 The importance of magnesium deficiency in cardiovascular disease. American Heart Journal 94: 649
18. Calvin JE, Driedger AA, Sibbald WJ 1981 Does the pulmonary capillary wedge pressure predict left ventricular preload in critically ill patients? Critical Care Medicine 9: 437
19. Carlon GC, Howland WS, Goldiner P, Kahn RC, Bertoni G, Turnball AD 1978 Adverse effects of calcium administration. Archives of Surgery 113: 882
20. Chernow B, Rainey TG, Lake R 1982 Endogenous and exogenous catecholamines in critical care medicine. Critical Care Medicine 10: 409
21. Chernow B, Smith J, Rainey TG, Finton C 1982 Hypomagnesemia, implications for the critical care specialist. Critical Care Medicine 10: 193
22. Chopa D, Janson P, Sawin CT 1977 Insensitivity to digoxin associated with hypocalcemia. New England Journal of Medicine 296: 917
23. Chopra IJ, Hershman JM, Pardridge W, Nicoloff JT 1983 Thyroid function in nonthyroidal illnesses. Annals of Internal Medicine 98: 946
23a. Colucci WS, Wright RF, Braunwald E 1986 New positive inotropic agents in the treatment of congestive heart failure. Parts I–II. New England Journal of Medicine 314: 290, 349
24. Connor TB, Rosen BL, Blaustein MP, Applefeld MM, Doyle LA 1982 Hypocalcemia precipitating congestive heart failure. New England Journal of Medicine 307: 869
25. Dennis RC, Harlow C, Egdahl RH 1980 Enhancement of myocardial function with glucose, insulin and potassium. Surgery, Gynecology and Obstetrics 151: 185
26. Dorinsky PM, Whitcomb ME 1983 The effect of PEEP on cardiac output. Chest 84: 210
27. Drop LJ, Laver MB 1975 Low plasma ionized calcium and response to calcium therapy in critically ill man. Anesthesiology 43: 300
28. Drop LJ, Scheidegger D 1980 Plasma ionized calcium concentration. Journal of Thoracic and Cardiovascular Surgery 79: 425
29. Fabiato A, Fabiato F 1979 Calcium and cardiac excitation-contraction coupling. Annual Review of Physiology 41: 473
30. Field S, Kelly SM, Macklem PT 1982 The oxygen cost of breathing in patients with cardiorespiratory disease. American Review of Respiratory Diseases 126: 9
31. Friedman WF 1972 The intrinsic physiologic properties of the developing heart. Progress in Cardiovascular Diseases 15: 87
32. Ginsburg R, Esserman LJ, Bristow MR 1983 Myocardial performance and extracellular ionized calcium in a severely failing human heart. Annals of Internal Medicine 98: 603
33. Glass DD 1980 Cardiovascular drugs. In: Civetta JM (ed) Intensive Care Therapeutics. Appleton-Century-Crofts, New York
34. Groeger JS, Carlon GC, Howland WS 1983 Naloxone in septic shock. Critical Care Medicine 11: 650

35. Grossman W, McLaurin LP 1976 Diastolic properties of the left ventricle. Annals of Internal Medicine 84: 316
36. Hackel DB, Mikat EM, Whalen G, Reimer K, Rochlani SP 1979 Treatment of hemorrhagic shock in dogs with verapamil-effects on survival and on cardiovascular lesions. Laboratory Investigation 41: 356
37. Hackel DB, Ratliff NB, Mikat E 1974 The heart in shock. Circulation Research 35: 805
38. Harrigan C, Lucas CE, Ledgerwood AM 1983 Significance of hypocalcemia following hypovolemic shock. Journal of Trauma 23: 488
39. Heistad DD, Abboud FM 1980 Circulatory adjustments to hypoxia. Circulation 61: 463
40. Hillis LD, Braunwald E 1977 Myocardial ischemia. New England Journal of Medicine 296: 971, 1034, 1093
41. Hoff BH 1979 Multisystem failure: a review with special reference to drowning. Critical Care Medicine 7: 310
42. Hoffman JIE 1978 Determinants of transmural myocardial perfusion. Circulation 58: 381
43. Hotchkiss RS, Wilson RS 1983 Mechanical ventilatory support. Surgical Clinics of North America 63: 417
44. Iskandrian AS, Segal BL, Hakki AH 1981 Left ventricular end-diastolic pressure in evaluating left ventricular function. Clinical Cardiology 4: 28
45. Katz AM 1977 Physiology of the Heart. Raven Press, New York
46. Kehler CH, Fogdall RP 1982 Inotropic agonists and antagonists. In: Ream AK, Fogdall RP (eds) Acute Cardiovascular Management—Anesthesia and Intensive Care. JB Lippincott, Philadelphia
47. Keung ECH, Aronson RS 1983 Physiology of calcium current in cardiac muscle. Progress in Cardiovascular Disease 25: 279
48. Kobayashi H, Yoshioka T, Maemura K, Ohashi N, Sawada Y, Sugimoto T 1983 Hemodynamic and diuretic effects of GIK treatment on extensive burn patients. Journal of Trauma 23: 116
49. Kovalik SG, Ledgerwood AM, Lucas CE, Higgins RF 1981 The cardiac effect of altered calcium homeostasis after albumin resuscitation. Journal of Trauma 21: 275
50. Ladenson JH, Lewis JW, Boyd JC 1978 Failure of total calcium corrected for protein, albumin, and pH to correctly assess free calcium status. Journal of Clinical Endocrinology and Metabolism 46: 986
51. Lange LG, Sobel BE 1982 Pharmacological salvage of myocardium. Annual Review of Pharmacology and Toxicology 22: 115
52. Lees MH 1980 Perinatal asphyxia and the myocardium. Journal of Pediatrics 96: 675
53. Lefer AM 1978 Properties of cardioinhibitory factors produced in shock. Federation Proceedings 37: 2724
54. Lefer AM, Spath JA 1977 Pharmacologic basis of the treatment of circulatory shock. In: Antonaccio MJ (ed) Cardiovascular Pharmacology. Raven Press, New York
55. Lefkowitz RJ 1979 Direct binding studies of adrenergic receptors: biochemical, physiologic, and clinical implications. Annals of Internal Medicine 91: 450
56. Lewis BS, Gotsman MS 1980 Current concepts of left ventricular relaxation and compliance. American Heart Journal 99: 101
57. Liedtke AJ 1981 Alterations of carbohydrate and lipid metabolism in the acutely ischemic heart. Progress in Cardiovascular Disease 23: 321
58. Lockhat D, Magder SA, Luo BJ, Ducas D, Roussos C 1983 Blood flow distribution during inspiratory elastic load with and without hypotension in dog. American Review of Respiratory Diseases 127: 232
59. Lucchesi BR 1977 Inotropic agents and drugs used to support the failing heart. In: Antonaccio MJ (ed) Cardiovascular Pharmacology. Raven Press, New York
60. Macklem PT 1980 Respiratory muscles: The vital pump. Chest 78: 753
61. Mayock DE, Standaert TA, Guthrie RD, Woodrum DE 1983 Dopamine and carotid body function in the newborn lamb. Journal of Applied Physiology 54: 814
62. McDaniel HG, Papapietro SE, Rogers WJ, Mantle JA, Smith LR, Russell RO, Rackley CE 1981 Glucose-insulin-potassium induced alterations in individual plasma free fatty acids in patients with acute myocardial infarction. American Heart Journal 102: 10
63. Meerson FZ, Katz AM 1983 The Failing Heart: Adaptation and Deadaptation. Raven Press, New York
64. Michelassi F, Castorena G, Hill RD, Lowenstein E, Watkins WD, Petkan J, Zapol WM 1983 Effects of leukotrienes B_4 and C_4 on coronary circulation and myocardial contractility. Surgery 94: 267
65. Mitchell JH, Wildenthal K, Johnson RL 1972 The effects of acid-base disturbances on cardiovascular and pulmonary function. Kidney International 1: 375

66. Morkin E, Flink IL, Goldman S 1983 Biochemical and physiologic effects of thyroid hormone on cardiac performance. Progress in Cardiovascular Disease 25: 435
67. Motulsky HJ, Insel PA 1982 Adrenergic receptors in man-direct identification, physiologic regulation, and clinical alterations. New England Journal of Medicine 307: 18
68. Nayler WG 1981 Preservation of the myocardium: some biochemical considerations. In: Longmore DB (ed) Towards Safer Cardiac Surgery. GK Hall Medical, Boston
69. New W 1982 Cellular mechanisms: a clinical view. In: Ream AK, Fogdall RP (eds) Acute Cardiovascular Management-Anesthesia and Intensive Care. JB Lippincott, Philadelphia
70. O'Connor LR, Wheeler WS, Bethune JE 1977 Effect of hypophosphatemia on myocardial performance in man. New England Journal of Medicine 297: 901
70a. Park MK 1986 Use of digoxin in infants and children, with specific emphasis on dosage. Journal of Pediatrics 108: 871
71. Perkin RM, Levin DL 1980 Common fluid and electrolyte problems in the pediatric intensive care unit. Pediatric Clinics of North America 27: 567
72. Perkin RM, Levin DL 1982 Shock in the pediatric patient. Parts I–II. Journal of Pediatrics 101: 163, 319
73. Perkin RM, Levin DL, Webb R, Aquino A, Reedy J 1982 Dobutamine: A hemodynamic evaluation in children with shock. Journal of Pediatrics 100: 977
74. Poole-Wilson PA 1981 Is inotropic stimulation outdated? In: Longmore DB (ed) Towards Safer Cardiac Surgery. GK Hall Medical, Boston
75. Pressman BC, Fahim M 1982 Pharmacology and toxicity of the monovalent carboxylic inophores. Annual Review of Pharmacology and Toxicology 22: 465
76. Prewitt RM, Ghignone M 1983 Treatment of right ventricular dysfunction in acute respiratory failure. Critical Care Medicine 11: 346
77. Rahimtoola SH 1973 Left ventricular end-diastolic and filling pressures in assessment of ventricular function. Chest 63: 858
78. Resnekov L 1981 Calcium antagonist drugs-myocardial preservation and reduced vulnerability to ventricular fibrillation during CPR. Critical Care Medicine 9: 360
79. Robertson CH, Foster GH, Johnson RL 1977 The relationship of respiratory failure to the oxygen consumption of, lactate production by, and distribution of blood flow among respiratory muscles during increased inspiratory resistance. The Journal of Clinical Investigation 59: 31
80. Ruffolo RR, Spradlin TA, Pollock GD, Waddell JE, Murphy PJ 1981 Alpha and beta adrenergic effects of the stereoisomers of dobutamine. Journal of Pharmacology and Experimental Therapeutics 219: 447
81. Shine KI, Kuhn M, Young LS, Tillisch JH 1980 Aspects of the management of shock. Annals of Internal Medicine 93: 723
82. Sibbald WJ, Calvin JE, Holliday RL, Driedger AA 1983 Concepts in the pharmacologic and nonpharmacologic support of cardiovascular function in critically ill surgical patients. Surgical Clinics of North America 63: 455
83. Sibbald WJ, Driedger AA 1983 Right ventricular function in acute disease states: pathophysiologic considerations. Critical Care Medicine 11: 339
84. Sibbald WJ, Short A, Cohen MP, Wilson RF 1977 Variations in adrenocortical responsiveness during severe bacterial infections. Annals of Surgery 186: 29
85. Slag MF, Morley JE, Elson MK, Crowson TW, Nuttall FQ, Shafer RB 1981 Hypothyroxinemia in critically ill patients as a predictor of high mortality. Journal of the American Medical Association 245: 43
86. Smith PK, Tyson GS, Hammon JW, Olsen CO, Hopkins RA, Maier GW, Sabiston DC, Rankin JS 1982 Cardiovascular effects of ventilation with positive expiratory airway pressure. Annals of Surgery 195: 121
87. Sodums MT, Walsh RA, O'Rourke RA 1981 Digitalis in heart failure-farewell to the foxglove? Journal of the American Medical Association 246: 158
88. Sonnenblick EH, Le Jemtel TH 1982 Newer inotropic agents In: Braunwald E, Mock MB, Watson JT (eds) Congestive Heart Failure—Current Research and Clinical Applications. Grune and Stratton, New York
89. Sonnenblick EH, Skelton CL 1971 Myocardial energetics: basic principles and clinical implications. The New England Journal of Medicine 285: 668
90. Southorn PA, Marsh HM 1982 Postoperative management of the cardiac surgical patient: cardiovascular care. In: Tarhan S (ed) Cardiovascular Anesthesia and Postoperative Care. Year Book Medical Publishers, Chicago
91. Stacpoole PW, Harmon EM, Curry SH, Baumgartner TG, Misbin RI 1983 Treatment of lactic acidosis with dichloroacetate. New England Journal of Medicine 309: 390

92. Stueven H, Thompson BM, Aprahamian C, Darin JC 1983 Use of calcium in prehospital cardiac arrest. Annals of Emergency Medicine 12: 136
93. Tarazi RC 1983 The progression from hypertrophy to heart failure. Hospital Practice 18: 101
94. Trunkey D, Carpenter MA, Holcroft J 1978 Ionized calcium and magnesium: The effect of septic shock in the baboon. Journal of Trauma 18: 166
95. Unverferth DV, Magorien RD, Lewis RP, Leier CV 1983 The role of subendocardial ischemia in perpetuating myocardial failure in patients with nonischemic congestive cardiomyopathy. American Heart Journal 105: 176
96. VanVliet PKJ, Gupta JM 1973 THAM versus sodium bicarbonate in idiopathic respiratory distress syndrome. Archives of Diseases in Childhood 48: 249
97. VanWinkle WB, Schwartz A 1976 Ions and inotropy. Annual Review of Physiology 38: 247
98. Vary TC, Reibel DK, Neely JR 1981 Control of energy metabolism of heart muscle. Annual Review of Physiology 43: 419
99. Vicent JL, Buset M, Dufage P, Berre J, Degaute JP, Kahn RJ 1982 Circulatory shock associated with magnesium depletion. Intensive Care Medicine 8: 149
100. Vitek V, Shatney CH, Lang DJ, Cowley RA 1983 Thyroid hormone responses in hemorrhagic shock: study in dogs and preliminary findings in humans. Surgery 93: 768
101. Vlahakes GJ, Turley K, Hoffman JIE 1981 The pathophysiology of failure in acute right ventricular hypertension: hemodynamic and biochemical correlations. Circulation 63: 87
102. Wagner CW, Nesbit RR, Mansberger AR 1979 Treatment of metabolic alkalosis with intravenous hydrochloric acid. Southern Medical Journal 72: 1241
103. Weber KT 1982 New Hope for the failing heart. American Journal of Medicine 72: 665
104. White BC, Winegar CD, Wilson RF, Hoehner PJ, Trombley JH 1983 Possible role of calcium blockers in cerebral resuscitation: a review of the literature and synthesis for future studies. Critical Care Medicine 11: 202
105. Yeager SB, Horbar J, Lucey JF 1980 Sympathomimetic drugs in the neonate. New England Journal of Medicine 303: 1122
106. Zwillich CW, Pierson DJ, Creagh EM, Weil JV 1976 Effects of hypocapnia and hypocapnic alkalosis on cardiovascular function. Journal of Applied Physiology 40: 333

8
Heart Rate and Rhythm as Determinants of Cardiac Output

Randall C. Wetzel, Judith L. Stiff, and Mark C. Rogers

Although disorders of rate and rhythm in critically ill children are common, they often go unrecognized until the child presents dramatically with either cardiac failure or central nervous system hypoperfusion leading to syncope. Therefore, the rapid recognition of abnormal rates and rhythms is an essential part of the pediatric critical care physician's knowledge. Furthermore, since heart rate is relatively more important than stroke volume in regulating cardiac output in the fetus, neonate, and young child, than it is in adults, alterations in heart rate and rhythm may have different physiologic consequences in this age group than in adults.

As is clear from other chapters in this book, cardiac output is dependent on heart rate and stroke volume. Stroke volume, in turn, is determined by the inotropic state of the heart, the end diastolic volume of the heart (preload), and myocardial afterload. These factors are not independent. In certain circumstances, the timing and sequencing of electrical depolarization of the ventricular muscle affects contractility and preload. It is also obvious that alterations in myocardial preload and afterload may alter heart rate and rhythm. Clearly, adrenergic stimulation will affect the heart rate and rhythm as well as the inotropic state of the heart. These interrelationships of heart rate and rhythm with the determinants of stroke volume should be borne in mind during the following discussion. As the determinants of stroke volume are discussed elsewhere in this book, this chapter is limited to the effects of heart rate and rhythm on cardiac output.

The normal range of heart rate in children is wide (Fig. 8.1). Heart rate decreases with age. Whereas a heart rate of less than 100 beats/minute is considered a bradycardia in the newborn, the same heart rate in the older child is considered a tachycardia. Furthermore, the younger the child, the greater the range for normal (Fig. 8.1). For example, a newborn heart rate may vary between 100 and 200 beats/minute and still be considered normal. These physiologically normal rapid heart rates in young children often lead to confusion in treating critically ill children, and are sometimes confused with abnormal supraventricular tachydysrhythmias.

The dependence of cardiac output on heart rate in infants and small children is due to several reasons.[4,11,22] First, the fetal and neonatal myocardium has less muscle mass per unit volume, and this muscle mass is poorly organized compared to the adult myocardium.[5] Secondly, the sympathetic innervation of the myocardium is also deficient when compared with adults. Finally, the fetal myocardium

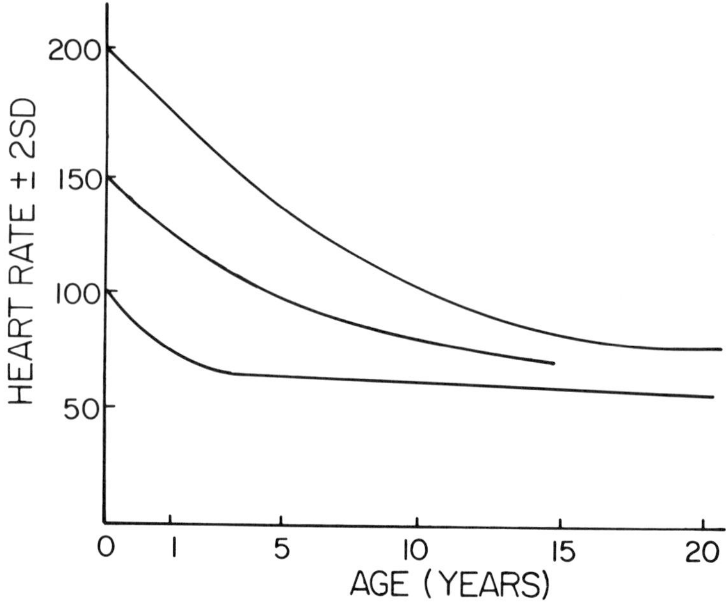

Fig. 8.1. Heart rate ± two standard deviations versus age. There is wide normal variation in the first year of life. (Wetzel RC, Rogers MC 1981 Pediatric Hemodynamic Monitoring. In Critical Care: State of the Art. Shoemaker WC, Thompson WL (eds) The Society of Critical Care Medicine, Vol. 2.)

appears to be resistant to catecholamines and, therefore, the inotropic effects of catecholamine stimulation.[18] These facts lead to a decreased response in stroke volume to any given level of physiologic stress.

On the other hand, increasing heart rate within the normal range can readily increase cardiac output. With increasing age, stroke volume increases while there is a concurrent decrease in heart rate (Fig. 8.2). Furthermore, the acceptable range of normal heart rates narrows with advancing age. This would lead one to expect that the maximal cardiac index achievable in younger children would occur at higher heart rates than in adults (Fig. 8.3). In dealing with critically ill children, the maintenance of near maximal heart rates for age is an efficacious way of providing maximal cardiac output. For this reason, augmentation of cardiac output by either pharmacologically or electrically increasing heart rate should be considered in the management of low output states in children. Conversely, one would expect that in the younger child, whose myocardium has limited ability to increase stroke volume, the abnormalities in heart rate or rhythm would have more seriously detrimental effects on cardiac output than adults.

In children, as in adults, heart rate is a major determinant of myocardial oxygen consumption. In children the oxygen consumption cost of increasing cardiac output by increasing heart rate can be met by increased myocardial oxygen delivery, whereas in adults, this may be limited by cardiovascular disease. Even so, it should be noted that it is possible for children to demonstrate signs of myocardial ischemia during rapid heart rates, and it is therefore wise to consider myocardial oxygen consumption when dealing with tachydysrhythmias in children.

This chapter is not intended to be a discussion of the complex abnormalities in

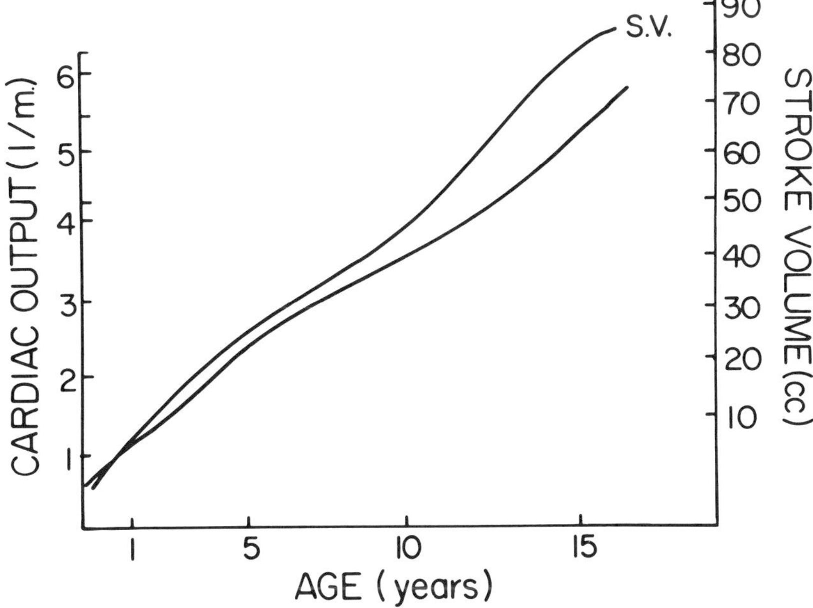

Fig. 8.2. Stroke volume and cardiac output versus age, derived from normative data. (Wetzel RC, Rogers MC 1981 Pediatric Hemodynamic Monitoring. In Critical Care: State of the Art. Shoemaker WC, Thompson WL (eds), The Society of Critical Care Medicine, Vol. 2.)

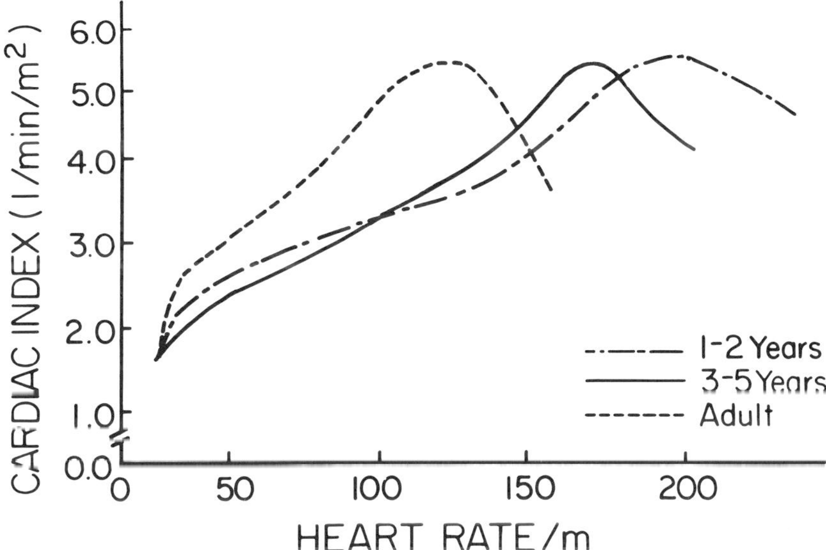

Fig. 8.3. This graph demonstrates changes in cardiac index with heart rate for three different age groups. It is derived from normative data and illustrates the increased dependence of cardiac output on heart rate in young children. (Wetzel RC, Rogers MC 1981 Pediatric Hemodynamic Monitoring. In Critical Care: State of the Art. Shoemaker WC, Thompson WL (eds), The Society for Critical Care Medicine, Vol. 2.)

rate and rhythm which have been increasingly described in children; however, it should serve as a guideline for the critical care physician's management and stabilization of acute life-threatening arrhythmias. This chapter first reviews the physiology and then discusses the symptomatology and diagnosis of children with abnormalities in rate and rhythm. This is followed by a discussion of specific abnormalities in rate and rhythm and their therapy.

PHYSIOLOGY

In order to understand disorders of rate and rhythm, one must know the physiology that underlies the generation and conduction of the cardiac impulse. It is not the purpose of this chapter to exhaustively describe and define the electrophysiology of the child's myocardium; however, a brief precis of the generation of the action potential and the depolarization of the conduction pathways of the myocardium is worthwhile, and will serve as a refresher for the understanding of disorders of rate and rhythm in the myocardium.

The characteristic feature of all myocardial tissue is a spontaneously depolarizing action potential during diastole (phase 4). Myocardial cells depolarize at different rates, depending on their position in the heart. The most rapidly depolarizing cells are in the sinoatrial node. The order of rapidity of depolarization descends from the sinoatrial (SA) node, atrial conducting tissue, atrioventricular (AV) node through the bundle of His conducting tissue, and, finally, the ventricular myocardium. This descending array of automaticity explains why, under normal circumstances, the SA node is the generator of the electrical impulse which determines normal heart rate. This normally generated sinoatrial activity spreads through the atria to the AV node, along the bundle of His through both right and left bundle branches and into the Purkinje fibers distributed throughout the ventricular myocardium. Finally, depolarization of the myocardium, in an orderly fashion, causes myocardial contraction. Abnormalities in myocardial rate and rhythm may arise from (1) abnormal impulse formation at any of these levels or (2) abnormal conduction of this impulse formation. In the absence of the more rapidly depolarizing SA node, pacemaker function may be taken over by successively lower areas such as the AV node or a ventricular pacemaker site, which gives rise to an "escape rhythm." If any of these areas have an increase in their automaticity, they may be responsible for tachydysrhythmias which can thus be generated from any level of the myocardium (sinus tachycardia, nodal tachycardia, ventricular tachycardia). On the other hand, interference with the regular pacemaker beat can lead to bradydysrhythmias, which can be due to the lack of impulse generation (as in sick sinus syndrome) or a conduction delay or blockade. Finally, escape rhythms may arise below the sinus node in the absence of sinus node impulse formation or conduction.

PATHOPHYSIOLOGY

Abnormalities in rate and rhythm in the child's heart are due to numerous congenital or acquired conditions. Certain congenital heart diseases are particularly prone to disorders in heart rate. For example, children with Wolff-Parkinson-

White syndrome have a propensity for developing supraventricular tachydysrhythmias. Congenital complete heart block can occur in association with structural abnormalities associated with congenital heart disease such as Ebstein's anomaly, mitral stenosis, and transposition of the great vessels. Congenital complete heart block also occurs in association with maternal systemic illnesses such as systemic lupus erythematosus.[25] It may also occur at birth idiopathically and familially.[12] Complete heart block may also follow cardiac surgery in children; however, this is frequently reversible.[2]

Systemic diseases also give rise to secondary abnormalities in myocardial rate and rhythm. One of the most obvious of these is disordered serum electrolytes, which may give rise to superventricular bradycardias, bradydysrhythmias, or tachydysrhythmias. Central nervous sytem abnormalities such as increased intracranial pressure may cause abnormally slow cardiac rates and compromised cardiac output.[21] Neuromuscular disorders such as Friedreich's ataxia and the muscular dystrophies have adverse effects on myocardial rate and rhythm. Glycogen storage diseases, endocrine disorders, and collagen-vascular diseases have also been associated with disorders in rate and rhythm. Another cause of abnormal rates and rhythms seen in the pediatric intensive care unit is drug toxicity. Digitalis, aminophylline, sympathomimetic drugs administered for asthma, barbiturates, and many other pharmacologic substances can lead to profound disturbances in cardiac rate and rhythm.

Critical care physicians see cardiac dysrhythmias associated with acute illness that is not primarily cardiac in origin. Myocardial contusion accompanying thoracic trauma can lead to ventricular dysrhythmias, abnormalities in conduction, and most commonly, sinus tachycardia. Severe systemic infections are frequently associated with cardiac dysrhythmias, sinus tachycardia being the most frequent. Apart from the above-mentioned drug intoxications which frequently lead children to present to the intensive care unit, abnormalities in myocardial rate and rhythm may arise in the post-anesthetic state, secondary to chemotherapy, and, as mentioned above, from central nervous system abnormalities such as elevated intracranial pressure, encephalitides, and meningitis.

DIAGNOSIS

Children may present to the pediatric critical care area with bizarre symptoms which may be primarily caused by cardiac dysrhythmia. The most common symptoms of cardiac dysrhythmias in children result from a decrease in cardiac output, either acutely or subacutely. Acute decreases in cardiac output cause sudden decreases in cerebral blood flow and lead to symptoms which include syncope, abnormal and inappropriate behavior, vertigo, and occasionally delerium. More subacute changes in cardic output caused by dysrhythmias can present with symptoms due to cardiac failure such as decreased peripheral perfusion, vomiting, dyspnea, diaphoresis, and pallor. Two less frequent presentations of myocardial rhythm disturbances in children include angina, which may be manifested in infants by uncontrollable screaming and unexplained irritability, or the complaint of consciously sensed abnormalities in heart rhythm such as skipped beats or racing hearts as described by older children.

Routine electrocardiographic monitoring in the pediatric intensive care unit may be the first indication that a child's symptoms are due to an underlying cardiac dysrhythmia. All children who present with loss of consciousness or an abnormal mental status require thorough and urgent evaluation of their cardiac rate and rhythm. Obviously, heart rate and rhythm require intensive evaluation in all children who present with signs and symptoms compatible with heart failure.

The primary diagnostic tool in evaluating abnormalities in rate and rhythm is the electrocardiogram (ECG). Although there are developmental alterations in the heart rate, QRS duration, PR interval, and QT interval, there are well-defined standards for these presented in pediatric cardiac textbooks. A 12 lead ECG should be obtained in all children with suspected disturbances in rate and rhythm and a rhythm strip of 1 to 2 minutes' duration should also be obtained. This rhythm strip is traditionally obtained by recording lead two; however, the morphology of all leads should be investigated to determine which lead best delineates the relationship of the P wave, QRS complex, and T wave. This is frequently found in one of the anterior chest leads such as V_1 or V_2.

The diagnosis of life-threatening abnormalities in cardiac rate and rhythm requires familiarity with the normal ECG for the appropriate developmental stage in the critically ill child.[7,9] Identification of all components of the ECG, from the P wave to the end of the T wave—and their relationship to each other—is the basis for diagnosing all cardiac abnormalities in rate and rhythm. Occasionally, it will be necessary to obtain prolonged ECG monitoring with a Holter-type monitor or to obtain tracings from unorthodox positions such as an esophageal electrode or intracardiac ECG recordings to absolutely delineate abnormalities in rhythm. However, these techniques will rarely be necessary in the critical care situation.

The remainder of this chapter considers the diagnosis and management of acute disturbances in cardiac rate and rhythm from a pragmatic, clinical point of view in all children who present with a suspicion of a myocardial rhythm or rate disturbance. The following schema is meant to be clinically applicable and is based on the initial ECG findings.

SPECIFIC DISTURBANCES

Tachydysrhythmias

In newborns, sinus rates of up to 200 may be considered normal. With age, sinus rate decreases. Although sinus tachycardia is normally defined as a heart rate greater than 100 beats per minute, this definition is not as appropriate for children, and the normal age-appropriate range must be considered before determining if a rapid sinus rhythm is pathologic. Sinus tachycardia occurs in children after exercise; with fever; after volume contraction such as in hemorrhagic shock; with certain drug ingestions; in children with anemia, hyperthyroidism, anxiety, or hypoxemia; and also usually accompanies heart failure of any cause. Sinus tachycardia is often normal and is seen in children frequently not associated with any hemodynamic defect. Indeed, it generally indicates a physiologic response to an underlying pathologic abnormality, which requires an increase in cardiac output. Treatment of sinus tachycardia, which is a normal physiologic compensation for a pathologic state, is not indicated and can be disastrous. Sinus tachycardia is

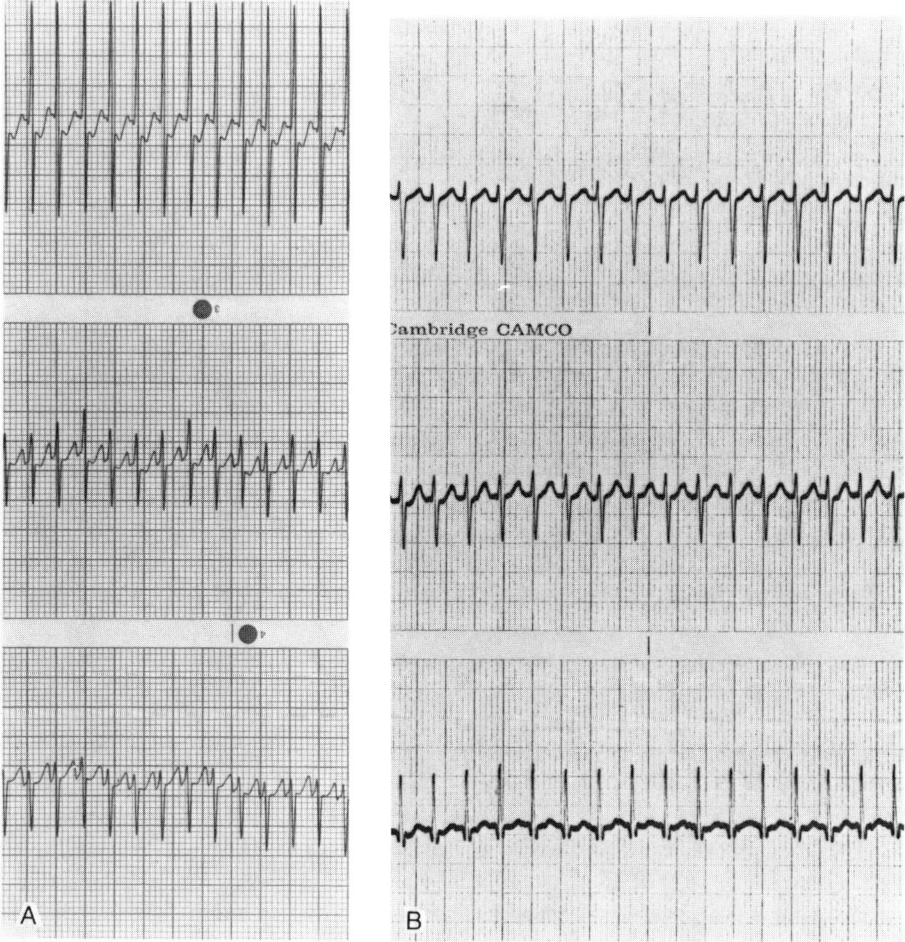

Fig. 8.4. Two examples of neonatal supraventricular tachycardia. Note narrow, regular QRS complexes, regular RR intervals, and a heart rate of 300 bpm. Regular P waves in Fig. A are not as clearly defined in Fig. B.

recognized by the regular relationship of the P wave with the QRS complex, a one-to-one AV conduction of the P wave, a regular RR interval, and a regular QRS morphology.

Supraventricular Tachydysrhythmias

Paroxysmal supraventricular tachycardia (SVT; paroxysmal atrial tachycardia, PAT) is the most frequently observed serious dysrhythmia in pediatric practice (Fig. 8.4). The ECG shows a narrow QRS complex with regular RR intervals. The P waves may be abnormal in morphology, there may be a prolonged PR interval, and the P wave may be difficult to define. In neonates and infants, heart rates of 200 to 300 beats/minute may occur. In older children, heart rates of 150 to 250 beats/minute are more common. SVT is characteristically paroxysmal; that is, it shows a rapid, beat-to-beat onset and offset. Although in neonates and children, the QRS morphology is almost always normal; when aberrant conduction complicates SVT, the ECG may demonstrate wide QRS complexes that most commonly are morphologically similar to the QRS pattern seen with right bundle branch block. Although widened QRS complexes may make it difficult to differentiate SVT from ventricular tachycardia, the latter generally has a left bundle branch block pattern.

Supraventricular tachycardia may occur in utero (leading to the birth of an hydropic infant), in the neonatal period, and throughout all age groups. Most commonly, it occurs in children under 6 months of age and the condition is slightly more common in males than in females. Although it frequently reflects underlying Wolff-Parkinson-White (WPW) syndrome, it may be associated with metabolic abnormalities, Ebstein's anomaly, infection, fever, or drugs. Most commonly, however, no cause can be identified.

Although it was previously thought that the underlying cause of supraventricular tachycardia was a rapidly depolarizing focus in the atrium or AV node, more recent understanding of the underlying mechanism indicates that SVT is caused by a re-entry phenomena.[19] These re-entry phenomena may occur through the AV node or via an aberrant conducting tissue pathway, forming a complete circle of conducting tissue. This leads to depolarization of a pacemaker focus by retrograde conduction of the original impulse to the atrium, the so-called circus movement. The ability of atrial muscle to rapidly repolarize explains why this re-entry phenomena can be effective. Anterograde conduction via an aberrant pathway may also lead to initiation of a circus rhythm. Wolff-Parkinson-White syndrome was the earliest recognized pattern of re-entry phenomena. These patients characteristically have a short PR interval with a widened QRS complex and a slurred upstroke (delta wave). This delta wave represents early depolarization of the ventricular musculature by an anomalous bundle of conduction tissue (bundle of Kent). Frequently, the SVT is triggered by a premature ventricular contraction, which through the aberrant conducting tissue, leads to recurrent atrial depolarization and triggers the consequent supraventricular tachycardia.

In a smaller number of patients with SVT, there is a short PR interval and a normal QRS complex. This Lown Ganong-Levine syndrome can also give rise to paroxysmal supraventricular tachycardia. Characteristically, the PR interval in children under 3 years old is less than 80 msec. Between the ages of 3 and 16 years, the PR interval is less than 100 msec and in adults, it is less than 120 msec. However, the majority of children with supraventricular tachycardia will demonstrate a normal PR interval and normal QRS complex. Although the re-entry pathways in these children have not been demonstrated, they are assumed to exist and involve either normal nodal tissue or an aberrant bypass of bundle tissue.

Patients with supraventricular tachycardia generally present with congestive heart failure. As mentioned above, this may appear as hydrops in the newborn infant with fetal supraventricular tachycardia. However, in older age groups, classical findings of heart failure are present. Frequently, the picture of supraventricular tachyarrhythmia may be confused with other causes of low output states associated with tachycardia such as septic shock, fever, sepsis, and even volume contraction secondary to hemorrhagic shock or excessive fluid loss. Presentation with symptoms of chest pain may occur in older age groups, although screaming and irritability in infants may also be a manifestation of supraventricular tachyarrhythmias. Supraventricular tachyarrhythmia may occur with a conduction blockade, most often with a two-to-one block. Presence of an isoelectric baseline between P waves usually helps differentiate these from atrial flutter and atrial fibrillation.

Two other forms of supraventricular tachycardia occur. They are non–re-entry atrial tachycardia and junctional tachycardias. Both of these occur due to rapid depolarization of an ectopic focus in either the atrium or in the nodal tissue. They are nonparoxysmal and are often quite recalcitrant to therapy. They almost always indicate underlying organic heart disease, such as ischemia or myocarditis, and can occur as a symptom of digitalis toxicity.

Atrial Fibrillation and Atrial Flutter

Although the presence of atrial fibrillation and atrial flutter is infrequently life-threatening, the differentiation from other, more serious, supraventricular tachycardias in the pediatric intensive care unit makes their recognition important.

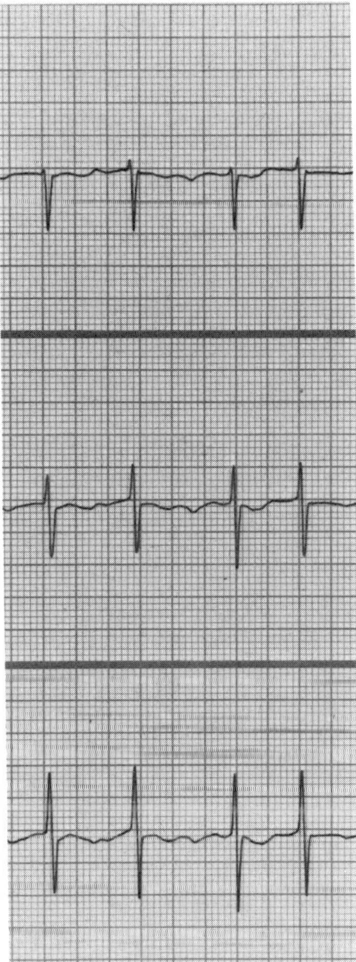

Fig. 8.5. Atrial fibrillation. Note absence of P waves and irregular RR interval with normal QRS morphology (V_4-6).

Atrial fibrillation is due to the rapid and chaotic depolarization of multiple atrial foci and a variable ventricular response. The ECG manifestations of atrial fibrillation are those of a rapid ventricular response which is irregular, with irregular RR intervals and an isoelectric baseline with no clearly defined P waves (Fig. 8.5). Frequently, aberrant conduction may distort the shape of the ventricular complexes. The most common underlying causes of atrial fibrillation in the pediatric age group are rheumatic heart disease, congenital mitral valve disease, and hyperthyroidism. Occasionally, these arrhythmias are noted in cardiomyopathies, pericarditis, atrial septal defects and with Ebstein's anomaly. In adults, atrial fibrillation decreases the component of atrial filling of the ventricles and therefore decreases myocardial preload. In children, however, the physiologic relevance of this is not quite so clear, and atrial fibrillation in younger age groups is often better tolerated than in the elderly.

Atrial flutter is a less common pediatric atrial tachydysrhythmia which is characterized by rapid uniform flutter waves that can occur 250 to 500 times a minute, and may give rise to a characteristic saw-tooth configuration of the ECG (Fig. 8.6). AV conduction is almost always partially blocked, leading to an irregular ventric-

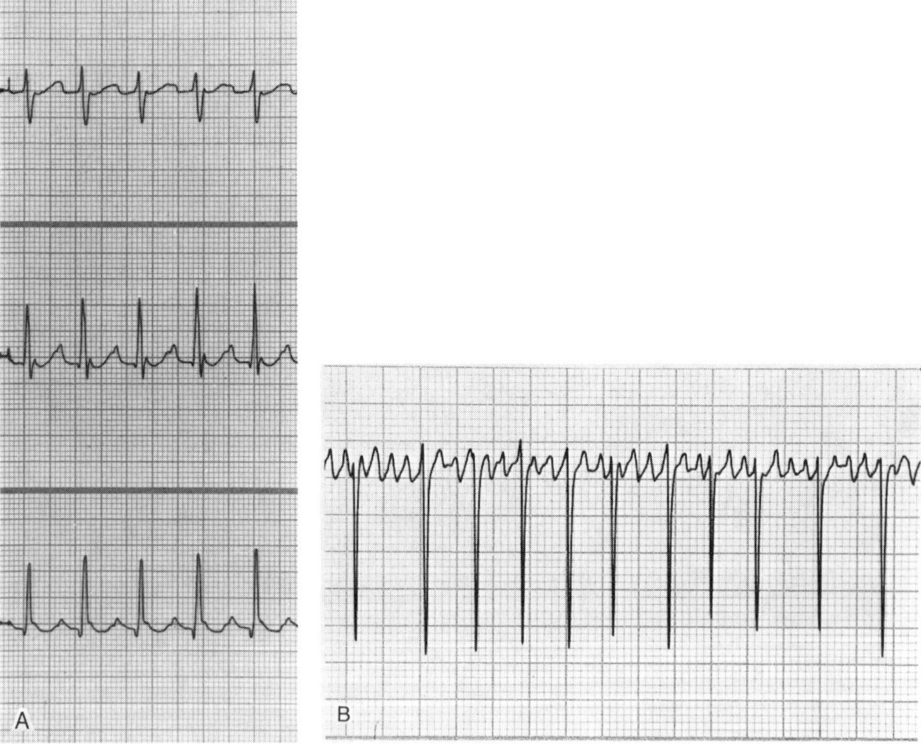

Fig. 8.6. Two examples of atrial flutter. (A) Flutter with a regular 2:1 AV conduction block and regular RR intervals, with a rate of 140 (leads I through III). (B) (lead V_1) Flutter in another patient showing characteristic sawtooth pattern with variable RR intervals. The example of flutter in (A) is more subtle than that in (B).

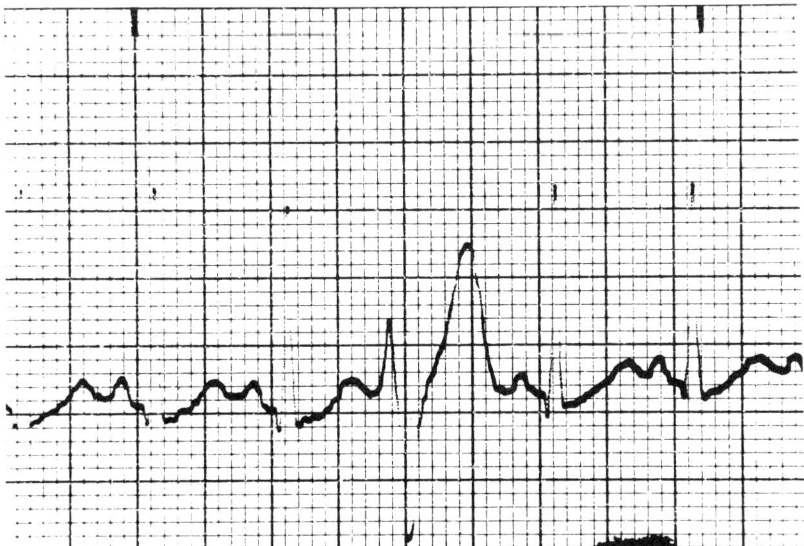

Fig. 8.7. A single ventricular extrasystole. Note wide QRS with opposite vector from sinus QRS, abnormal T morphology and fully compensatory pause.

ular response. Frequently, atrial flutter may be quite difficult to diagnose and may be confused with SVT, or sinus tachycardia with AV conduction blockade. The underlying causes are similar to those for atrial fibrillation.

Ventricular Dysrhythmias

Ventricular tachydysrhythmias in children often present dramatically and require as urgent treatment as they do in adults. As an understanding of ventricular ectopy is crucial to understanding ventricular tachydysrhythmias, ectopic premature ventricular beats will be discussed first. Premature ventricular beats are recognized by abnormal, wide, slurred QRS complexes, usually followed by inverted T waves and the absence of a preceding P wave (Fig. 8.7). They are generated from ectopic ventricular foci. Frequently, the differentiation of premature ventricular beats from premature atrial beats with conduction aberrancy is difficult; however, the presence of a compensatory pause between QRS complexes is a good indicator of a ventricular ectopic beat. In addition, PACs usually have the same initial vector as sinus beats, whereas PVCs generally demonstrate a different initial vector. The significance of individual PVCs, or PVCs occurring in couplets or triplets (ventricular tachycardia) is that they indicate underlying myocardial irritability caused either by ischemia, drugs, or an irritative focus set up after myocardial trauma or surgery. The threat is a constant risk of deterioration to a full-blown, sustained ventricular tachycardia or ventricular fibrillation with severe hemodynamic compromise.

Ventricular tachycardia is defined as the occurrence of three or more premature ventricular contractions in a row (Fig. 8.8). The occurrence of ventricular tachycardia with heart rates of 150 to 200 beats per minute always requires therapy. The etiology of VT may be an electrolyte or metabolic imbalance, a cardiac tumor,

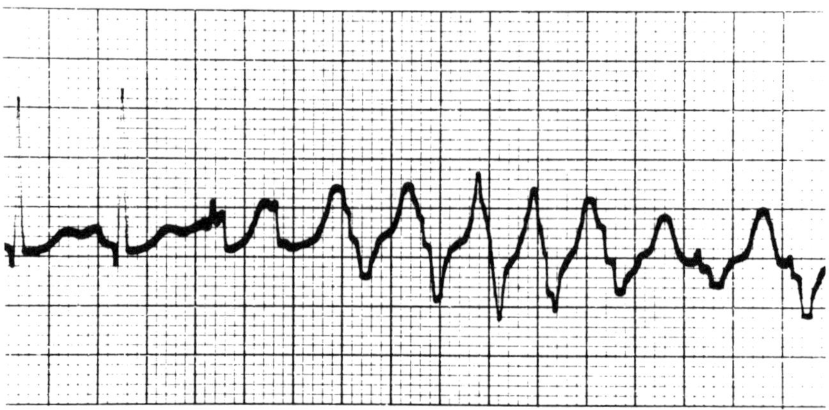

Fig. 8.8. Sinus rhythm degenerating into ventricular tachycardia.

an effect of cardiac surgery, a myocarditis, a cardiomyopathy or a prolonged QT syndrome.[14] However, most frequently, VT arises idiopathically. Hemodynamic compromise is the rule and may lead to syncope or even sudden death. Ventricular fibrillation is manifest by chaotic, irregular ventricular depolarization and is recognized by the absence of a recognizable, regular pattern of QRS complexes (Fig. 8.9). Ventricular fibrillation requires therapy similar to that for cardiac arrest.

The differentiation of ventricular tachycardia from supraventricular tachycardia can frequently be difficult. Rapid rates of over 150, inadequate circulation and a wide QRS complex occur in both SVT and VT. Determination of the preceding rhythm and differentiation of PVCs from PACs can guide the differentiation be-

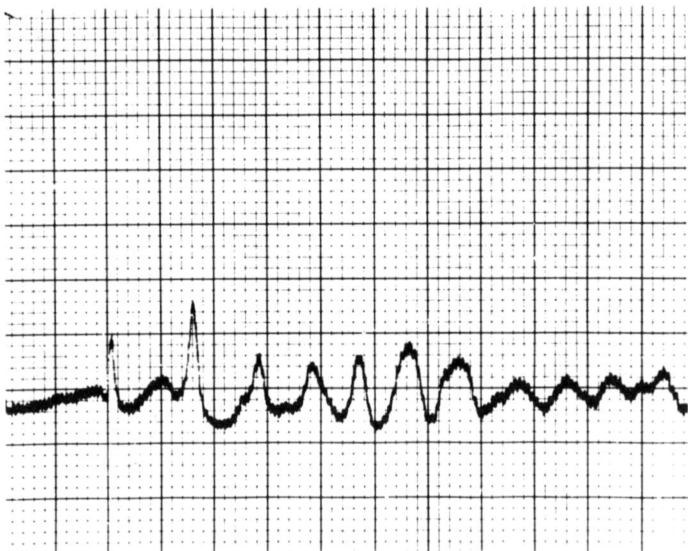

Fig. 8.9. Bradycardia with a ventricular ectopic (R on T) initiating course ventricular fibrillation. Note disorganized, rapid chaotic electrical activity.

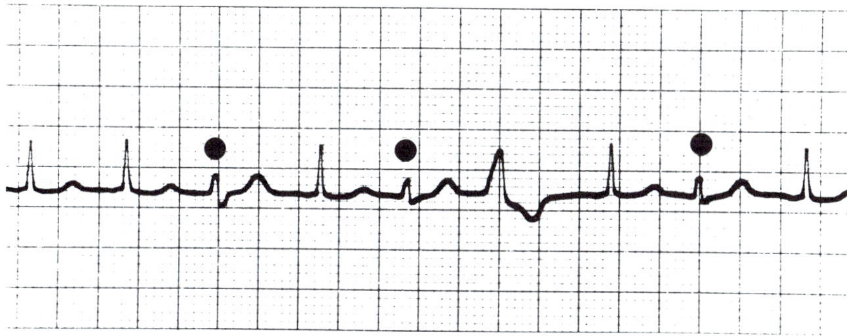

Fig. 8.10. This rhythm strip shows an example of fusion beats, marked with dots. There is also a ventricular ectopic beat. A fusion beat represents a combination of a ventricular ectopic beat with a supraventricular beat and is intermediate in form between the two. Their significance is the same as for ventricular ectopic beats.

tween the two arrhythmias. Preexisting atrioventricular dissociation suggests ventricular tachycardia. The presence of fusion beats (Fig. 8.10), whose etiology and morphology is an amalgamation of a supraventricular with a ventricular beat, indicates the presence of an ectopic ventricular focus and may help differentiate SVT from VT. The generation of a fusion beat requires a ventricular ectopic beat and, therefore, their significance is the same as that of PVCs. Frequently, a trial of therapy is required to differentiate the two arrhythmias. Vagal stimulation such as Valsalva maneuver, occular pressure, or carotid massage rarely affects ventricular tachycardias but frequently slows or aborts supraventricular tachycardias.

Bradydysrhythmias

Sinus bradycardia is a sinus rhythm occurring at a rate of less than 60 beats per minute. This may be normal in athletic adolescents and may occur in states of increased vagal stimulation. Sinus bradycardia may be associated with hyperkalemia, hyperthyroidism, hypothermia, and elevated intracranial pressure, as well as with certain drugs. The crucial fact that differentiates pathologic sinus bradycardia from nonthreatening sinus bradycardia is the presence of perfusion compromise due either to a decreased cardiac output or an irregular and potentially life-threatening escape rhythm. These should certainly be looked for in the face of heart rates less than 60 beats per minute.

Bradycardia refers to the ventricular rate, and bradydysrhythmias other than sinus bradycardia are due to either incomplete conduction of a normal sinus pacemaker beat or failure to generate a sinus beat. Generally, failure of generation of a sinus beat results in an idioventricular rhythm or a nodal rhythm. Nodal bradycardias originate from the AV node and are differentiated into high, medium, or low by the timing of the P wave with respect to the QRS complex. Frequently, the P waves may be inverted. Idioventricular rhythms show regular complexes which are morphologically identical with PVCs. However, failure of a lower pacemaker site to generate any electrical activity in the heart by an escape rhythm leads to asystole, the most profound bradydysrhythmia.

Conduction interference may occur in a spectrum including first, second, or third degree AV block. The consequence of these patterns of bradydysrhythmia are decreased cardiac output caused by an inordinately slow ventricular rate, or a hemodynamically unstable escape rhythm. Recognizing these types of AV conduction delay and complete conduction block is important; they may indicate an underlying source of syncopal episodes, and more importantly, they may indicate that the impending deterioration of the cardiac rhythm toward the total loss of ventricular contractions may occur.

First degree AV block is recognized by a prolonged PR interval indicating delayed atrial to ventricular conduction. Second degree AV block indicates the interruption of conduction of some, but not all, atrial beats to the ventricle. It can occur following a progressive prolongation in the PR interval followed by a blocked beat as in the Wenckebach phenomenon (Mobitz type I) or without a prolongation in the PR interval prior to the blocked beat (Mobitz type II). Mobitz type II block usually demonstrates a regular block of every second, third, or fourth beat. The Wenckebach phenomenon is generally due to interference of AV nodal conduction, whereas Mobitz type II block is usually due to abnormal conduction delay in the His bundle or its branches. Mobitz type II blockade frequently progresses to complete AV blockade and is, therefore, a more ominous rhythm than the Wenckebach phenomenon. Third degree, or complete, AV block occurs when no atrial beats are conducted to the ventricles. If an escape rhythm does not develop, cardiac arrest or Stokes-Adams attacks may follow. Complete AV block, either congenital or acquired, is the most common cause of bradydysrhythmias in childhood.

Sick Sinus Syndrome (Bradycardia Tachycardia Syndrome)

Sick sinus syndrome occurs by either decreased sinus impulse formation or sinus node exit block, caused by direct injury to the sinus node.[1,13] In children, this usually follows injury, especially Mustard's procedure for correction of transposition of the great vessels.[23] but may rarely be due to cardiomyopathies, myocarditis, or ischemia. The ECG manifestations include profound, unresponsive sinus bradycardia or periods of sinus arrest, with or without occurrence of a subsidiary pacemaker. This escape rhythm may be nodal or ventricular, and occasionally atrial fibrillation may occur, which is unresponsive to usual therapy. The symptoms are those of Stokes-Adams attacks, or hypoprofusion from profound bradycardia.

Recognition of sick sinus syndrome requires clinical suspicion in the setting of sinus bradycardia, sinus arrest, or the concurrence of bradycardia and tachycardia. Diagnosis requires intracardiac electrophysiologic determination of sino-atrial conduction and sino-atrial recovery time, following atrial pacing.[17] In symptomatic patients permanent pacing is almost always required.

THERAPY

The underlying principles of therapy of circulatory failure are as important in treating cardiac dysrhythmias as in other causes of circulatory failure. Patients should be oxygenated, perfusion should be optimized, and the underlying condition should be treated. The correction of any metabolic and electrolyte abnormalities is obviously required. However, in the face of a life-threatening dysrhythmia, such as ventricular tachycardia or supraventricular tachydysrhythmia, the only therapeutic maneuver which will be of permanent benefit is correcting the rhythm disturbance.

Therapy of abnormal cardiac rates and rhythms in children may vary from merely treating the underlying condition to more invasive pharmacologic or even electrocardioversion techniques. The choice of this therapy is dictated by the child's hemodynamic status and by the electrocardiographic diagnosis. Obviously, the therapy should entail the least risk. Table 8.1 summarizes the pharmacologic agents most commonly used to treat dysrhythmias in children.

Tachydysrhythmias

The correction of a sinus tachycardia is almost never indicated. Removal of the chronotropic drive, which may be the only factor in providing adequate cardiac output in the infant and small child, can be disastrous. The ability to compensate with increased stroke volumes may not be fully developed in this age group. Using a beta-blocker in order to treat a child with tachycardia secondary to volume contraction, fever, or cardiac failure from any cause in order to decrease the sinus rate is obviously extremely dangerous. However, differentiation and recognition of cardiac dysrhythmias other than sinus tachycardia are necessary, and therapy may be indicated. In the absence of syncope, alterations in the level of consciousness, or decreased myocardial perfusion, urgent therapy may not be required. It is essential to tailor the rapidity of therapy with the urgency of the situation. Mild congestive failure resulting from SVT can await slow conversion with digoxin, whereas an unconscious patient with shock from ventricular tachycardia obviously requires urgent cardioversion.

Supraventricular Tachydysrhythmias

For all presentations of supraventricular tachydysrhythmia, physiologic maneuvers to increase vagal tone and interrupt the irregular circus movement of electrical depolarization is indicated and may prove rapidly successful in converting SVT to sinus rhythm. However, before trying any of these maneuvers, it should be noted that profound bradydysrhythmias may result and, therefore, one should think ahead of therapy that is aimed at treating bradycardia. Frequently used physiologic maneuvers in older children include carotid sinus massage and inducing the Valsalva maneuver. This latter maneuver can be induced in younger children by merely applying abdominal pressure, which frequently leads to a voluntary "bearing down" response in children. Occular pressure can be efficacious; however, this technique does carry with it the risk of retinal detachment. Eliciting the diving reflex constitutes another therapeutic modality.[8] This is best accomplished by providing a cold (0°C, iced water) stimulus to the head or face of the child. This technique has been shown to rapidly convert supraventricular tachycardia in neonates and small infants. The same caveat holds true for the diving reflexes as for other physiologic means of aborting supraventricular dysrhythmia since profound bradycardias and even asystole have been reported.[3]

Further therapy of supraventricular tachycardia depends on the situation. If time and the patient's condition allow, pharmacologic therapy is certainly indicated. Digitalization remains the cornerstone for the therapy of supraventricular tachycardias and is indicated no matter how the rhythm is eventually terminated.

Table 8.1. Drug Therapy for Dysrhythmias

Drug	Indication	Route	Dose	Drug Level	Side Effects
Atropine	Bradycardias	IM, IV bolus	.01 mg/kg not <.1 mg	—	Flushing, tachycardia Fever, pupillary dilatation
Bretylium	VT, VF Recurrent	IV bolus	5 mg/kg IV over 8 min	—	Hypotension
Digoxin	SVT, AF	PO, IM, IV	See digitalizing schedule	1–3 ng/ml	Dysrhythmias Conduction delay Diarrhea, nausea, vomiting
Disopyramide	SVT, PVCs	PO	2–5 mg/kg	—	
Edrophonium	SVT	IV	.04 mg/kg × 3		Profound bradydysrhythmias
Isoproterenol	AV dissociation	IV infusion	0.1–1.0 μg/kg/min titrated	—	PVCs, tachycardia
Lidocaine	VT, PVCs	IV bolus Infusion	1–3 mg/kg repeat if necessary 30–50 μg/kg/hour	1–6 μg/ml	Convulsions

Methoxamine	SVT	IV infusion	5–15 μg/kg/min, titrate to BP	—	Hypertension
Phenylephrine	SVT	IV infusion	.5–5 μg/kg/min titrate to BP	—	Hypertension
Phenytoin	PVCs, VT	IV bolus, PO	1–2 mg/kg	10–20 μg/ml	Heart block
Procainamide	AF, PVCs	IV bolus, infusion, PO	3–10 mg/kg	3–12 μg/ml	Nausea, vomiting Sudden death
Propranolol	SVT, PVCs	IV bolus	.01–.1 mg/kg slowly	20–150 ng/mg	Hypotension, asystole Bronchospasm
Quinidine	SVT, PVCs, AF	PO	15–60 mg/kg/day ÷ 4	2–8 μg/ml	PVCs, AV block Hypotension
Verapamil	SVT	IV bolus, PO	.05–.15 mg/kg over 15 mins × 2	100–300 ng/ml	Hypotension

Rapid digitalization over 4 to 6 hours can be accomplished by using digitalizing schedules as reported elsewhere in this book. Clearly, intravenous digitalization is indicated if there is any circulatory compromise. Digitalization frequently converts the supraventricular tachydysrhythmia to sinus rhythm. Continuation of digitalis in children who have presented with supraventricular tachycardia is prudent. Although there is little evidence that it prevents further attacks, it certainly aids the rapidity of conversion of subsequent attacks.

The use of digoxin in treating supraventricular tachycardia, or for that matter, atrial fibrillation and flutter, in children with WPW is not recommended. Antergrade conduction through the accessory conducting pathway is facilitated by digoxin, and a rapid ventricular response and even ventricular fibrillation may occur. Although rare, sudden death in children with WPW has been reported during digoxin treatment.[7]

Propranolol, a beta-blocker, which also prolongs atrioventricular nodal conduction and enhances the refractoriness of conducting pathways, is useful in converting a supraventricular tachydysrhythmia to a sinus rhythm. Urgent therapy may be given intravenously, and this may be repeated after an hour if the hemodynamic status is not adversely affected by propranolol. Propranolol therapy for SVT seen in Wolff-Parkinson-White syndrome is particularly effective. In refractory SVT, the use of either quinidine or procainamide in relatively high doses can also block nodal conduction of the SVT and convert the rhythm to a sinus rhythm.

Another interesting pharmacologic approach to conversion of SVT includes using alpha-adrenergic stimulant drugs to elevate peripheral vascular resistance and thus, blood pressure, leading to a reflex vagal stimulation of the myocardium. Phenylephrine and methoxamine have been reported as useful for this purpose. Titrating the blood pressure to twice baseline may be required. Similarly, the cholinesterase inhibitor, edrophonium bromide, has been used to increase endogenous acetylcholine and thus increase vagal tone. Frequently, however, these maneuvers are only temporarily useful in terminating the supraventricular tachydysrhythmia. Therefore, some pharmacologic maneuver, such as digitalization, is also necessary to interrupt the conduction of the aberrant pathways in order to prevent recurrence of supraventricular tachydysrhythmia.

Recently, the slow calcium-channel blocker, verapamil, has become the treatment of choice for supraventricular tachydysrhythmia that is resistant to digoxin in adults.[20,24] European use of this drug has shown it to be particularly helpful intravenously for converting supraventricular tachycardia in children. It is an alternative to propranolol as first line treatment for supraventricular tachycardia due to WPW. It should be noted that all slow calcium channel blockers are both myocardial depressants and peripheral vasodilators. Hypotension is frequently seen with intravenous verapamil after conversion of the supraventricular dysrhythmia and may require treatment. Its use following beta-blockade is not recommended. The place of verapamil and the other slow calcium channel blockers in long-term therapy of supraventricular tachycardia in children is not yet defined.

In patients who are, or become acutely hypoperfused, hypotensive, and acidotic, more urgent therapy is obviously required. This is generally the case in neonates with congestive heart failure due to supraventricular tachycardia. In this case, direct current cardioversion with a dose of 0.5 to 2 joules/kg is usually effective. Synchronized cardioversion is, of course, indicated, and recurrent cardioversion may be required. If the first attempts at cardioversion are unsuccessful, the dose may be increased up to 5 joules/kg. Obviously, sedation and anesthesia should be considered before cardioversion and all precautions should be taken to secure and maintain the child's airway and ventilation. Previous digitalization, although best avoided, is not a contraindication to electrical cardioversion, and, in the face of a life-threatening supraventricular tachycardia with hemodynamic collapse, electro-cardioversion is the indicated therapy. Maintenance therapy with either digoxin or one of the other above-mentioned drugs should be instituted immediately after conversion to sinus rhythm.

Finally, mention should be made of overdrive electrical pacing, which is often successful if cardioversion fails. By directly pacing the atria at a rate greater than the SVT for 1 to 2 minutes, and then suddenly discontinuing the pacing, conversion to sinus rhythm may occur. This is practical if atrial pacing wires are already in place, such as following cardiac surgery, but is more difficult in the absence of previously placed leads. If the hemodynamic compromise is severe, cardioversion should be attempted before placement of a means of cardiac pacing.

Atrial Fibrillation and Atrial Flutter

The treatment of both atrial flutter and atrial fibrillation is similar to that for supraventricular tachydysrhythmias. An attempt at converting both atrial fibrillation and atrial flutter even in the presence of cardiac compromise is best made by initial intravenous digitalization. In the face of adequate hemodynamic stability, this may be achieved over 24 hours. If conversion has not been successful by this time, procainamide or quinidine have been found useful. With evidence of hemodynamic compromise, atrial fibrillation and flutter can be converted by more rapid intravenous digitalization or intravenous procainamide; however, use of either of these drugs is frequently to no avail in small children. The addition of propranolol may be useful to slow ventricular response. In the face of resistant atrial flutter and fibrillation or an urgent requirement for therapy, electrical cardioversion—again with direct current counter-shock—should be considered. The initial dose for converting atrial flutter or atrial fibrillation is similar to that for supraventricular tachycardia; however, lower doses, approximately 0.25 to 0.5 joules/kg, are frequently efficacious. The use of digoxin to treat atrial flutter or fibrillation is not recommended in WPW syndrome for reasons described above.

The therapy of nonparoxysmal atrial tachycardias or AV nodal tachydysrhythmias is often difficult. Thorough investigation for underlining metabolic and electrolyte abnormalities is indicated. Digitialization is frequently unhelpful and may aggravate the recurrence of these supraventricular tachydysrhythmias. Quinidine and procainamide are the cornerstone of medical therapy. However, as mentioned above, these supraventricular tachydysrhythmias are frequently refractory to therapy. Calcium antagonists or disopyramide[16] are sometimes effective therapy.

Ventricular Arrhythmias

The therapy for ventricular tachycardias is directed by the clinical condition of the child. However, even in the absence of hemodynamic compromise, ventricular tachydysrhythmias should be treated, especially if the child is, for any reason, critically ill. The lone PVC may indicate myocardial damage, but more importantly, may herald further decompensation of ventricular rhythm. It should be noted that if the ventricular ectopic beats are due to either conduction delay or an absence of higher pacemaker potentials, then therapy should be directed toward increasing either sinoatrial depolarization or AV conduction through the normal pathways to suppress ectopic ventricular foci.

The acute therapy of premature ventricular contractions is intravenous lidocaine. If premature ventricular contractions become greater than six per minute, appear to be occurring on the T wave, or are multifocal, then lidocaine therapy as an intravenous bolus is indicated. If this is unsuccessful in decreasing the frequency of premature ventricular contractions, it may be repeated, and it may be necessary to start a continuous intravenous lidocaine infusion. Serum lidocaine levels are useful to guide therapy. Intravenous procainamide is the next line of therapy and may be continued either orally or intravenously to prevent recurrence. Alternatively, oral quinidine is very effective in suppressing PVCs but is not recommended intravenously. Disopyramide, a new quinidine-like drug, is a successful oral agent to prevent or suppress PVCs, and although not yet available for intravenous use in the United States, it is also very effective for emergent intravenous treatment of PVCs.[16]

The treatment of ventricular tachycardia depends on the hemodynamic status of the patient. If blood pressure and perfusion are maintained then pharmacologic therapy may be indicated, and the drug of first choice is intravenous lidocaine. If VT persists after repeating lidocaine twice and instituting a continuous infusion, then further therapy is required. Intravenous procainamide or phenytoin is often successful in this setting. Recent use of the adrenergic nerve blocking drug, bretylium tosylate, intravenously, has proven very salutory in terminating VT and VF in adults, and should be considered in children with resistant VT.[10,15] Again, intravenous disopyramide has proven very useful in Europe in the management of VT. The long-term prophylactic therapy for VT includes oral quinidine, procainamide, propranolol, phenytoin, or disopyramide. Failure of conversion of ventricular tachycardia by pharmacologic means or the occurrence of hemodynamic compromise during VT requires urgent therapy. Electrocardioversion is the therapy of choice in the face of hemodynamic compromise. Again, the anesthetic and airway management aspects of the child should be taken into account before attempting ventricular countershock. Doses of 1 to 4 J/kg may be tried and increased until sinus rhythm is achieved. Finally, mention of electrical overdrive pacing should be made. Frequently, either rapid atrial or ventricular pacing may suppress the ectopic focus of VT and successfully lead to conversion to sinus rhythm when drug therapy has failed.

Ventricular Fibrillation

Ventricular fibrillation demands immediate treatment. It calls for full cardiopulmonary resuscitation with airway management and immediate conversion of the arrhythmia by direct countershock. Direct countershock is started with 2 J/kg and doubled until cardioversion occurs. Correction of underlying acidosis with bicarbonate, airway maintenance, intubation, and ventilation with 100 percent F_{IO_2} is essential. If an underlying electrolyte abnormality is suspected, it must be rapidly treated. Concurrent with electroconversion, intravenous lidocaine should be administered and repeated if there is any evidence of deterioration of the resulting rhythm. Intravenous bretylium tosylate may also be useful.

The discussion of fine versus coarse ventricular fibrillation has, in the past, been confusing. Coarse, obvious ventricular fibrillation with disorganized, irregular electrical activity on the ECG is frequently responsive to electrical cardioversion, whereas fine ventricular fibrillation, which may be manifest by mere diversions from an isoelectric ECG or indeed, by what appears to be an absolutely isoelectric ECG, is less successful. It is frequently useful to convert fine ventricular fibrillation (or what may appear to be asystole) to coarse ventricular fibrillation or ventricular tachycardia. This can be achieved with the administration of potent catecholamines such as epinephrine and isoproterenol, and occasionally by intravenous calcium, rendering the dysrhythmia more amenable to electrical cardioversion. The occurrence of ventricular fibrillation, no matter how rapidly converted, requires continuous, aggressive monitoring and therapy.

Bradydysrhythmias

Asystole

Sinus bradycardias require therapy only if there is hemodynamic compromise manifest by hypoperfusion and low blood pressures. The first therapy of choice is intravenous atropine. In the absence of a severely compromised sinus node such as in sick sinus syndrome, this frequently increases heart rate by blocking vagal action and alleviates the problem. This therapy is also useful for treatment of lower escape rhythms from either a junctional or ventricular site. If atropine is unsuccessful, intravenous isoproterenol frequently, is efficacious. If either of these therapies is unsuccessful, electrical pacing of the heart may be mandated.[6]

Bradycardias due to conduction delay are treated either by therapy aimed at improving conduction or by providing electrical cardiac pacing at the ventricular level. Atropine is always used initially; however, this frequently is unsuccessful. Intravenous isoproterenol or even epinephrine may be required for either congenital or surgically acquired conduction interference, and this may provide time for further transthoracic or transvenous pacemaking to be instituted as required. In the face of hemodynamic compromise with conduction delay, consideration should always be given to providing at least temporary, if not permanent, electrical pacemaking support for the myocardium.

Asystole is obviously life-threatening and requires emergent therapy for cardiac arrest. Before success can be achieved, some form of electrical activity must be obtained, and this is outlined in the section *Therapy for Cardiac Arrest*.

SUMMARY

Understanding the underlying physiology of the infant and child's heart indicates the necessity for maintenance of sinus rhythm and guides the therapy of the dysarrhythmias. Rapid recognition of abnormal ECG patterns and analysis of the underlying hemodynamic status indicates which therapy is required for the particular arrhythmia. Care to provide routine critical care for the child, as well as specific antidysrhythmic therapy, generally leads to successful therapy of cardiac dysrhythmias.

REFERENCES

1. Alpert MA, Flaker GC 1983 Arrhythmias associated with sinus node dysfunction. Journal of the American Medical Association 250: 2160
2. Anderson PAW, Rogers MC, Canent RB, Spach MS 1972 Reversible complete heart block following surgery: analysis with his bundle electrograms. Circulation 46: 514
3. Bisset GS, Gaum W, Kaplan S 1980 The ice bag: a new technique for interruption of supraventricular tachycardia. Journal of Pediatrics 97: 593
4. Downing SE, Talner NS, Gardner TH 1965 Ventricular function in the newborn lamb. American Journal of Physiology 208: 931
5. Friedman WF 1972 Intrinsic properties of the developing heart. Progressive Cardiovasular Disease 15: 87
6. Gamble WJ, Ownes JP 1977 Pacemaker therapy for conduction defects in the pediatric population. IN: Roberts NK, Gelband H (eds) Cardiac arrhythmias in the neonate, infant and child, Appleton-Century-Crofts, New York
7. Gillette PC, Garson A, Porter CJ, McNamara DG 1983 In: Adams FH, Emmanouilides GC (eds) Heart disease in infants and adolescents. 3rd edn, Williams & Wilkins, Baltimore
8. Grahame IFM, Hann IM 1978 Use of the driving reflex to treat supraventricular tachycardia in an infant. Archives of Diseases in Childhood 53: 515
9. Guntheroth WG 1965 Pediatric Electrocardiograms. W B Saunders, Philadelphia
10. Heissenbuttel RH, Bigger JT 1979 Bretylium tosylate: A newly available anti-arrhythmic drug for ventricular arrhythmias. Annals of Internal Medicine 91: 229
11. Heymann MA, Rudolph AM 1973 Effect of increasing preload on right ventricular output in fetal lambs in utero. Circulation 48: 37
12. Husson GS, Blackman MS, Rogers MC, Bhavati S, Lev M 1973 Familial congenital bundle branch system disease. American Journal of Cardiology 32: 365
13. Kaplan BM, Langendorf R, Lev M, Pick A 1973 Tachycardia-bradycardia syndrome (so-called "sick sinus syndrome"). American Journal of Cardiology 31: 497
14. Karhunen P, Luomäki K, Heikkilä J, Eisalo A 1970 Syncope and Q-T prolongation without deafness: the Romano-Ward syndrome. American Heart Journal 80: 820
15. Koch-Wester J 1979 Bretylium. New England Journal of Medicine 300: 473
16. Koch-Wester J 1979 Disopyramide. New England Journal of Medicine 300: 957
17. Kugler JD, Gillette PC, Mullins CE, McNamara DG 1979 Sinoatrial conduction in children: an index of sinoatrial node function. Circulation 59: 1266
18. Macartney FA 1980 Heart and circulation. In: Godfrey S, Bower JD (eds) Clinical pediatric physiology. Blackwell Scientific Publications, Oxford
19. Moe GK, Mendez C 1973 Physiologic basis of premature beats and sustained tachycardias. New England Journal of Medicine 288: 250
20. Porter CJ, Gillette PC, Garson A, Hesslein PS, Karpawich PP, McNamara DG 1981 The effects of verapamil on supraventricular tachycardia in children. American Journal of Cardiology 48: 487
21. Rogers MC, Zahka KG, Nugent SK, Gioia FR, Epple L 1980 Electrocardiographic abnormalities in infants and children with neurological injury. Critical Care Medicine 8: 213
22. Rudolph AM, Heymann MA 1976 Cardiac output in the fetal lamb: The effects of spontaneous and induced changes in heart rate and left ventricular output. American Journal of Obstetric Gynecology 124: 183
23. Schiller MS, Levin AR, Haft JI, Engle MA, Ehlers KH, Klein AA 1977 Electrophysiologic studies in sick sinus syndrome following surgery for d-transposition of the great arteries. Journal of Pediatrics 91: 891
24. Soler-Soler J, Sagristá-Sauleda J, Cabrera A, Sauleda-Parés J, Iglesias-Berengué J, Permanyer-Miralda G, Roca-Llop J 1979 Effect of verapamil in infants with paroxysmal supraventricular tachycardia. Circulation 59: 876
25. Vetter VL, Rashkind WJ 1983 Congenital complete heart block and connective-tissue disease. New England Journal of Medicine 309: 236

9
Cardiopulmonary Resuscitation

Mark S. Schreiner, Robert G. Kettrick, and Stephen Ludwig

Cardiopulmonary resuscitation (CPR) is a sequence of interventions whose aim is to restore vital functions and prevent a threatened death from occurring. The immediate goal is to restore ventilation and circulation so that oxygen and other substrates are delivered to the myocardium and brain to prevent death. The long-term goal is the prevention of the morbidity secondary to the cardiopulmonary arrest and resuscitation so that the victim can return to prearrest function.

Recommendations for adult CPR are primarily designed to prevent death following ventricular dysrhythmias and myocardial infarction. Pediatric recommendations[19,29,52,53] are largely based on the adult experience, although dysrrhythmias are rarely the cause of cardiac arrest in children. The same orderly progression through the assessment and management of the ABCs—airway, breathing, and circulation— is utilized. Ideally, resuscitation should be performed by a trained team of physicians, nurses, respiratory therapists, and other support personnel. Often, however, physicians who have little contact with pediatric patients may be called upon to resuscitate children. Lack of familiarity with drug dosages, and difficulty in the technical procedures of establishing intravenous access and tracheal intubation are but a few of the problems that help create an atmosphere of anxiety and confusion. This chapter emphasizes the knowledge and performance skills needed for supporting the pediatric patient and some of the newer areas of research that may modify the future practice of CPR.

OVERVIEW

There are no data for the annual incidence of pediatric resuscitations in the United States. Two reviews of resuscitations performed at The Children's Hospital of Philadelphia lend some perspective to the epidemiology of the cardiac arrest in childhood. Ludwig et al retrospectively examined all resuscitations between 1976 and 1980 which were attended by a resuscitation team.[24] Resuscitations in the operating rooms, intensive care units and cardiac catheterization laboratories were excluded from evaluation. A total of 130 resuscitations were reviewed (Fig. 9.1). During that same period, there were approximately 6,000 admissions and 140,000 outpatient visits per year.

The most striking feature of the data was the young age of the patients. The

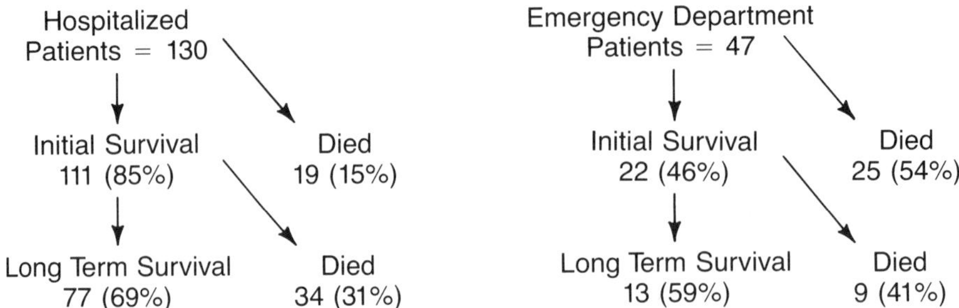

Fig. 9.1. Outcome of pediatric cardiopulmonary resuscitation. The percentages indicate the percent of each subgroup and not the entire patient population.

mean age was nearly 2 years with a range of 2 weeks to 16 years, but the median age was only 5 months. O'Rourke,[30] Nichols et al,[26] and others[23] have confirmed the tendency for arrest to occur in young children.

The second striking feature was the wide range of diagnoses in the patients requiring life support as shown in Table 9.1. Cardiac arrest in adults is dominated by patients with coronary artery disease. In this series, the most common etiologies were conditions that involved the respiratory system and not cardiac disease. Cardiovascular dysfunction secondary to congenital disorders, sepsis, and dehydration were approximately half as common as the respiratory disorders.

Patients who were outside of the hospital were more likely to have arrested from sudden infant death syndrome (SIDS) and trauma. Near drowning, SIDS, upper airway obstruction, infection, and trauma (motor vehicle accidents, child abuse, and miscellaneous causes) were the dominant diagnoses leading to cardiac arrest in O'Rourke's survey of out-of-hospital arrests.

The etiology of arrest has important implications for the mechanism of arrest, the therapy required, and the ultimate survival and morbidity. In childhood, arrest is usually due to a primary respiratory event with subsequent hypoxia and acidosis. Cardiac arrest is secondary to severe hypoxia and usually starts with bradyarrhythmias. If no intervention occurs, the rhythm proceeds to asystole. Resuscitation from bradyarrhythmias has been shown to have a much poorer outcome in adults then does resuscitation from ventricular tachyarrhythmias.[17,25,46] In many cases, by the time resuscitative efforts have been initiated, significant irreversible organ damage has occurred. This is especially true in the out-of-hospital arrest where recognition and bystander management of arrest may be delayed.

In a second study at The Children's Hospital of Philadelphia, Nichols et al prospectively reviewed 47 consecutive inpatient and outpatient cardiac arrests.[26] This study attempted to delineate those features which were likely to predict a successful resuscitation and long-term post-resuscitation survival. Of the 47 patients, 27 of them (54 percent) were short-term survivors (greater than 24 hours), but only 18 of the 47 children (38 percent) survived long term (discharge from the hospital). Inpatients fared much better than out-patients (44 percent long-term survival versus 23 percent).

The two best predictors of survival were the magnitude of the intervention

Table 9.1. Diagnoses of 130 Patients Requiring Life Support by System*: The Children's Hospital of Philadelphia, 1976–1980

Diagnoses	Number of Patients	(total)
Respiratory		**(71)**
Bronchiolitis	3	
Pneumonia	16	
Aspiration	6	
Bronchopulmonary dysplasia	26	
Respiratory failure/chronic lung disease	5	
Primary apnea	4	
Asthma	2	
Epiglottitis	2	
Tracheostomy obstruction	3	
Other	4	
Cardiovascular		**(36)**
Congenital heart disease	15	
Septic shock	9	
Dehydration	4	
Congestive heart failure	6	
Other	2	
Central Nervous System		**(34)**
Acute hydrocephalus	11	
Head trauma	6	
Status epilepticus	4	
Tumor	5	
Meningitis	4	
Other	4	
Gastrointestinal		**(8)**
Trauma	1	
Necrotizing enterocolitis	3	
Bowel perforation	1	
Bowel obstruction	2	
Tracheoesophageal fistula	1	
Miscellaneous		**(26)**
SIDS	6	
Noncardiac anomalies	6	
Other	14	

* 130 patients with 175 diagnoses.
(Modified from Ludwig S, Kettrick RG, Parker M 1984 Pediatric cardiopulmonary resuscitation: a review of 130 cases. Clinical Pediatrics 23:71.)

required and the rapidity of response; two obviously interrelated variables. Long-term survival occurred in 11 of 12 patients (92 percent) who required ventilation and oxygen alone to achieve hemodynamic stability. Long-term survival was achieved in 4 of 8 children who required only 1 dose of bicarbonate and epinephrine, and in 2 of 5 children (40 percent) who required 2 doses in addition to oxygen and ventilation. Of the 20 patients who required more than 2 doses of bicarbonate and epinephrine, there were no long-term survivors.

When the time required to achieve hemodynamic stability was examined, similar results were obtained. If CPR lasted less than 15 minutes, 12 of 20 patients survived long term. Only 4 of 25 patients who required more than 15 minutes of resuscitation were long-term survivors. The longest resuscitation that produced a long-term survivor lasted 45 minutes.

The presence or absence of pupillary and motor reflexes at the time CPR was initiated was not predictive of survival, and should not be used in decision making. If adequate perfusion was achieved, pupillary reflexes returned to normal and flaccidity proved reversible.

This experience has shown that CPR can be successful in resuscitating a substantial proportion of children. Combining the populations of the study by Ludwig et al[24] and the study by Nichols et al.[26] 85 percent of the 130 inpatients were resuscitated, while 59 percent survived to be discharged. The result from the emergency room was less encouraging with 46 percent initial survivors and 28 percent long-term survivors (Fig. 9.1).

The poor prognosis for patients with out-of-hospital arrest is understandable but frustrating and difficult to remedy. In order to reverse the primary respiratory problem precipitating cardiac arrest, immediate airway intervention and ventilation is required. Because of technical and emotional barriers, paramedics are more likely to provide better basic and advanced life support for adult arrest victims than they do for children. Thus, pediatric patients are more likely than adults to reach the emergency room without the benefit of optimal prehospital care. Absent or inadequate prehospital ventilatory care lengthens the period of hypoxia and hypoperfusion and contributes to the high mortality and high central nervous system morbidity in those who do survive.[11,30] The improved prognosis for survival with in-hospital arrests compared to the emergency department arrest is also probably related to successful intervention prior to the development of severe bradycardia or asystole.

Other obstacles in providing successful resuscitation involve the difficulty in obtaining intravenous access and the inability to adjust dosages and equipment size to the needs of a wide variety of patients and the inability to overcome the psychological barriers involved when a child arrests. The ability to remain flexible to the variety of demands placed by small patients comes only with preparation and experience.

MANAGEMENT OVERVIEW

Initiation of CPR in children involves the same sequence of assessments and interventions as in adults. Consciousness is assessed by the shake and shout maneuver. In the absence of response, it is assumed that the brain is no longer receiving adequate oxygen, and the basic life support sequence of evaluation and management is initiated.

First, the airway is opened by maneuvering the mandible and its associated block of soft tissue forward and off the posterior pharyngeal wall. If air movement can be detected by listening and feeling, and if chest wall movement is observed, then continued airway support with supplemental oxygen should be provided. If the patient is not breathing spontaneously, then ventilation must be provided, the exact route dependent on the equipment available. Once adequate ventilation is established, the adequacy of circulation is assessed by palpation of brachial, carotid, or femoral arterial pulsations. In the absence of peripheral pulses, closed chest massage is initiated. Restoration of peripheral pulsations and spontaneous ventilation and improvement in the level of consciousness are signs that adequate oxygen and substrate is being delivered to the central nervous system and myocardium.

AIRWAY

Evaluation

The evaluation and establishment of an adequate airway should have the highest priority. Since most children suffer respiratory arrest with subsequent secondary cardiac arrest,[23] early reestablishment of an adequate airway is crucial to successful management. Visual inspection of chest and abdominal wall movement, coupled with auscultation for breath sounds over the mouth and nose should be done immediately. The rescuer's cheek or hand should be used to feel for air movement to confirm that gas exchange is taking place. If there is spontaneous respiratory effort but no evidence of air movement, then a presumptive diagnosis of airway obstruction is made.

Management

Relief of airway obstruction is accomplished by placing the patient's head in the "sniffing" position. The cervical spine is gently flexed on the thoracic spine, and the occiput is gently extended on the cervical spine. Excessive extension may cause obstruction in a small child and should be avoided. Pulling or lifting the chin will move the mandibular block of tissue forward and off of the posterior pharyngeal wall. The fingers should be placed behind the angle of the jaw to push or pull the jaw forward. This will move the lower central incisors anterior to the upper central incisors. If these noninvasive maneuvers fail, then more invasive airway adjuncts should be utilized. Table 9.2 lists the airway equipment which should be available for pediatric patients.

Artificial Airways

Oropharyngeal airways

Oropharyngeal airways are used for re-establishing airway patency. The airway serves several purposes: it supports the mandibular block of tissue and serves as an airway stent; the bite block portion of the airway prevents the central incisors from forcefully obstructing an orotracheal tube; and lastly, the airway provides an air channel and conduit for a suction catheter.

To determine the proper size, the airway should be placed along the side of the face. With the flange at the level of the central incisors, the tip should just reach the angle of the mandible. An airway that is too long may prove hazardous by provoking vomiting or laryngospasm. An airway that is too short may be ineffective. The airway should be placed while holding the tongue forward in the floor of the mouth. A tongue blade (wooden tongue depressor) or laryngoscope blade can be used. Placement of an oropharyngeal airway without these aids is likely to traumatize the upper airway or cause obstruction by forcing the tongue backwards.

Table 9.2. Airway Equipment Kit for Pediatric Resuscitation

1. Laryngoscope handle with knurled finish
2. Laryngoscope blades:
   Miller 0, 1, 2, 3
   MacIntosh 2, 3, 4
   Wis-Hipple 2.5
3. Oropharyngeal airways: Guedel sizes 00, 0, 1, 2, 3, 4
4. Nasopharyngeal airways: French sizes 12, 16, 20, 24, 28
5. Endotracheal tubes: inside diameter sizes
   Uncuffed—2.5, 3.0, 3.5, 4.0, 4.5, 5.0, 5.5, 6.0
   Cuffed—6.0, 7.0, 8.0
6. Stylet: infant, adult
7. Magill forceps: child, adult
8. Extra batteries and laryngoscope lamps
9. Suction catheters: French sizes 6, 8, 10, 12, 14
10. Masks: neonatal, infant, child, adult

Nasopharyngeal airways

Nasopharyngeal airways are an alternative device to oropharyngeal airways in stenting the tongue off of the posterior pharyngeal wall. The proper length is equal to the distance from the nares to the tragus of the ear. Commercially available airways or an endotracheal tube cut to the proper length may be used. The main limitation in using this device is the tendency during insertion to traumatize the vascular nasopharyngeal adenoidal tissue that is often hypertrophied in childhood.

Esophageal obturator airways

Esophageal obturator airways are not designed for use in children and use is therefore not recommended.

Tracheal tubes

The purpose of the tracheal tube is to provide a stable, reliable airway. They are used to overcome airway obstruction, to facilitate adequate ventilation and oxygenation, and to protect the lower respiratory tract from contamination from aspiration. The appropriate size can be estimated from the formula:

$$\text{ID (mm)} = \frac{\text{age (yrs)} + 16}{4}$$

where ID is the inside diameter. It is prudent to have a tube one half size larger and one half size smaller available. Uncuffed tubes are used in children below 10 years of age because the cricoid ring forms a natural narrowing which provides a seal.[13] Beginning at 10 years of age, cuffed tubes should be substituted for uncuffed tubes. The cuff effectively adds one half size to the tube so that for the 10-year-old, a 6.0 mm ID cuffed tube is usually appropriate.

Endotracheal tubes should be translucent to facilitate visual inspection for occlusion. They should have a radiodense marker so that their position can be confirmed by x-ray, and optimally, they should have a ring marker that signifies the proper placement at the vocal cords. Although the ring marker may be helpful in reducing the incidence of endobronchial intubation, it does not guarantee correct tube placement. All tracheal tubes should have depth markings on the tube wall to serve as reference points for proper tube positioning, and have the internal diameter clearly labeled in a visible location. All tracheal tubes should meet the American National Standards Institute (ANSI), Committee Z-79 standards.

Laryngoscopy and Intubation

In the setting of CPR, directly visualized orotracheal intubation should be performed. Nasal intubation and fiberoptic facilitated intubation take far more time and require a greater degree of expertise. Blind nasal intubation in small children and in patients who are not spontaneously ventilating can be a very difficult maneuver.

The purpose of laryngoscopy is to allow direct visualization of the larynx by aligning the mouth, pharynx, and trachea. This is best accomplished by placing the patient's head in the sniffing position prior to laryngoscopy. Infants have a large head relative to the rest of their body so that minimal additional support under the occiput is needed. Older children may benefit from padding under the occiput to flex the cervical spine on the thoracic spine.

Children have anatomic differences which need to be recognized to facilitate intubation.[13] The larynx in the infant is more anterior and more cephalad in proportion to the rest of the body than in the adult. Overextension may move it even further anterior making visualization difficult. The epiglottis is shaped like an inverted U or V in contrast to the relatively more flat epiglottis of the adult. It is longer and less flexible than in the adult and it assumes a 45 degree angle to the anterior pharyngeal wall. These anatomic differences make the epiglottis difficult to lift with a curved laryngoscope blade in infants and small children. Therefore, a straight blade is preferable to allow direct elevation of the epiglottis and visualization of the larynx.[29]

The laryngoscope should be inserted into the right side of the mouth and advanced along the right side of the tongue. As the tip of the blade is advanced, the tonsillar pillars are identified, and as the blade is advanced further, the epiglottis should be visualized. The tip of the blade is then positioned under the epiglottis. Once the tip is in position, the blade is moved to the midline, pushing the tongue to the left side of the mouth, and leaving the right one-third of the mouth to serve as a channel for passage of the tracheal tube. The tracheal tube should be styletted, with the curvature resembling a hockey stick, and caution should be taken to ensure that the stylet does not protrude beyond the end of the tube or through the side hole if a Murphy-style tube is used. The tracheal tube is passed down the right side of the mouth and through the glottis until the ring marker on the tube is positioned at the vocal cords. With the ring marker in this position, the tip of the tube should be in mid-tracheal position. Tubes with triple ring markers should be advanced until the second marker is at the vocal cords. The depth marking on the side of the tube corresponding to the gum or teeth line should be noted.

In infants, the thin chest wall will readily transmit sounds. Listening for equality of breath sounds over the anterior chest wall may be deceiving, and esophageal intubation may be missed if one neglects to listen over the stomach. To confirm that the tracheal tube is in the proper location, breath sounds should be auscultated in both axillas, condensation within the lumen of the tube should be evident on exhalation, and the absence of breath sounds over the stomach noted. The chest should rise symmetrically with ventilation. If chest movements or breath sounds are not present and equal, then the tube should be repositioned. The carina can be identified by advancing the tube until breath sounds disappear entirely on one side, and then pulling back 2 cm in infants, and 3 cm in the older child. When time permits, radiographic confirmation of proper placement may be obtained. The tube should lie with the tip at the second or third thoracic vertebral body on an anteroposterior (AP) chest film; this usually corresponds to a position beyond a line drawn between the medial heads of the clavicles.

Once an airway has been established with a tracheal tube, it should be firmly secured to prevent accidental extubation. Nothing is more frustrating and dangerous than losing what should be a secure airway. The skin should be dried and cleansed, and tincture of benzoin applied. The adhesive tape should be tightly applied to prevent any movement of the tube. The movement of the mandible may cause movement of the tub, and therefore, the tape should be concentrated on the fixed maxillary portion of the face.

BREATHING

Evaluation

Once an airway has been established, the sequence of looking, listening, and feeling for gas exchange should be repeated. In infants, ventilation is assessed by observing movement of the lower chest and abdomen, whereas in older children and adolescents there should be expansion of the upper chest as in adults. Chest movement is not a guarantee of adequate ventilation. Auscultation over the trachea to confirm gas movement in the central airway followed by auscultation for breath sounds is helpful.

Management

If, after establishment of an airway, the patient is breathing spontaneously, supplemental oxygen should be administered and the patient closely monitored. Initially, 100 percent oxygen should be given. Children are quite resistant to the effects of respiratory acidosis, but are not tolerant of even short periods of hypoxia. A wide variety of devices are available for delivery of supplemental oxygen. Nasal cannulas, oxygen hoods or tents, and oxygen masks can provide between 24 and 100 percent oxygen. The adequacy of oxygenation should be assessed by arterial blood gas analyses or reliable noninvasive means, such as oximetry.

If, after establishment of an adequate airway, gas exchange is not adequate, artificial ventilation should be started. The recommended rates for rescue breathing in infants and children are shown in Table 9.3. If adjuncts for mechanical ven-

Table 9.3. Ventilation/Compression Schedule for Pediatric Resuscitation

	Infant	Child	Adolescent*
Compression (rate/min)	100	80	60
Depth of compression (cm)	1–2.5	2.5–4	4–5
Ventilation (rate/min)	20	16	12

* Two-person rescue.

tilation are not immediately available, then an expired air technique should be used. Mouth to nose, mouth to mouth and nose, mouth to mouth, and mouth to tube are all acceptable techniques. Trial and error will determine which will work best for any individual patient. Care must be taken not to apply excessive force when ventilating infants and small children. During rescue breathing for an infant, puffs of air should be used which are sufficient to make the chest rise. Larger volumes delivered to the pharynx may distend the stomach and compromise the diaphragm, while excessive volumes delivered to the trachea may produce barotrauma.

Oxygen Delivery Devices

Face masks

Face masks are made of rubber or a variety of plastics. Clear masks are preferable for CPR in order to see the mouth to assess color and see the presence of vomitus or secretions. The mask should rest securely on the nasal bridge and maxillary bones and should fit between the lower lip and the chin. The Rendell-Baker-Soucek type mask has been used extensively for infants and small children but has several disadvantages. It does not have a soft cuff, it is usually not clear, and it is often difficult to get a good mask fit. Palme et al[32] recently reported their evaluation of five different neonatal masks. They examined the amount of "leakage" around each mask during positive pressure ventilation, and found the Rendell-Baker-Soucek mask was the most difficult to use. Inexperienced personnel are more likely to have difficulty with this type of mask, compared to one with a soft pneumatic cuff. The pneumatic cuff design allows a secure fit with a variety of facial contours. Consideration should be given to using the Laerdal mask (Laerdal, Stavanger, Norway), which was the preference of Palme, or a new clear plastic mask with a pneumatic cuff manufactured by Vital Signs, Inc. (Totowa, NJ).

Hand squeezed, self inflating resuscitators

Hand squeezed, self-inflating resuscitators are the most commonly used resuscitators for infants and children and may be used with either mask or tracheal tubes. They refill independently of gas flow. In order to provide close to 100 percent oxygen, an oxygen reservoir or demand valve is attached. Without the reservoir or demand valve, these units may deliver low concentrations of oxygen. A pop-off valve prevents delivery of high pressures. The major advantage of these devices is that even if proper mask fit cannot be maintained continuously, the bag will reinflate and ventilation will not be interrupted.

Anesthesia bag

These resuscitators are usually either Mapleson A or Mapleson D systems and depend on continuous gas flow to refill the bag. An exit port must be present to prevent CO_2 from accumulating in the reservoir. These devices will deliver 100 percent oxygen, and if connected to a blender can deliver any concentration desired. Their main disadvantage is that they require skill and experience to use. If an inadequate mask fit is present, the bag will deflate and it will be impossible to continue ventilation. To detect high pressures being delivered to the patient, a manometer may be placed in line.

CIRCULATION

Reestablishment of adequate circulation may often be accomplished by airway manipulation and ventilation alone. The frequency with which this can be expected to occur depends on the location of the arrest. In hospitalized patients, approximately 30 percent will need airway and ventilatory support alone, but emergency room patients will only rarely be resuscitated without cardiac massage and pharmacologic intervention.[23,24]

While airway and ventilatory management are well established, recent research has called into question the mechanism and optimal management of external cardiac massage. In 1960 Kouwenhoven et al[21] reported effective cardiac massage without thoracotomy by using what is now known as conventional CPR (CCPR). The advantage of CCPR over open chest CPR (OCCPR) was its widespread applicability. Because of the success of CCPR it appeared that OCCPR had been relegated to a position of historical interest. Recent reports[2,40], however, document the superiority of OCCPR in maintaining coronary and cerebral perfusion over CCPR in dogs. Diastolic blood pressures were higher and venous pressures lower during OCCPR, maintaining higher perfusion pressures. OCCPR not only provided higher perfusion pressure, but also a significantly higher survival rate and a better neurologic outcome compared to CCPR. These two studies are consistent with previous reports of successful resuscitation in adults with OCCPR after failed CCPR.[12]

Jackson and colleagues measured central blood flow (CBF) prearrest and during three types of resuscitation: CCPR, CCPR plus epinephrine infusion, and OCCPR.[18] CCPR maintained CBF at only 10 percent of prearrest levels, while the addition of epinephrine infusion increased CBF to 36 percent of the prearrest baseline. However, OCCPR resulted in CBF that was 156 percent of the prearrest level. OCCPR produced excellent systolic and diastolic pressures in addition to the elevated CBF.

The exact role of OCCPR is unclear at present and further research is required. The role in children is even more poorly defined than in adult patients because the mechanism for blood flow may not be the same. Kouwenhoven et al.[21] proposed that the mechanism for CCPR was compression of the heart between the sternum and the vertebral column. This mechanism was largely accepted with few dissenting opinions.[47] More recently, it has been demonstrated that this mechanism is inadequate to explain forward flow of blood in the majority of adults. The accepted mechanism at this time is the concept of a thoracic pump, and the history behind its development is well reviewed.[22,41,51] The theory behind the thoracic pump is that the heart is a passive conduit for blood, and forward flow is generated by an increase in the intrathoracic pressure. The generalized increase in pressure is transmitted equally to all chambers of the heart and to the great vessels. Forward flow is not generated because of an intrathoracic pressure gradient between the various chambers, but rather because of the extrathoracic pressure gradient between the carotid arterial system and the jugular veins. Jugular venous pressure is lower than that on the arterial side first because of the increased tendency of the thinner walled vessels to be compressed at the thoracic inlet, and second because of the presence of venous valves preventing backward flow of blood. The third factor responsible for forward flow is the decreased capacitance of the arterial system as compared to the venous system. An equal volume of blood translocated to the arterial and venous systems will generate a higher pressure on the arterial side.

Supporting evidence for the thoracic pump mechanism comes from several sources. One of the more important is the successful maintenance of cardiac output and consciousness during cough-induced CPR.[10] Cary and his co-workers demonstrated that increasing the pleural pressure by increasing the strength of the cough provided a greater flow.[5] In studies performed in dogs, Rudikoff and co-workers[36] demonstrated that the pressure in the right atrium, left ventricle, aorta, pulmonary artery, and esophagus (assumed to be equal to intrathoracic pressure) were all identical. The equality of pressures is consistent with forward flow being secondary to the generalized increase in intrathoracic flow. These observations have opened up new areas of research in CPR whose aim is to find ways of modifying CCPR in order to increase cardiac output.

Rudikoff et al, in addition to demonstrating that the thoracic pump was the probable mechanism for forward flow, also postulated that maneuvers that increase intrathoracic pressure at the time of compression would increase flow.[36] They showed that maintaining inflation of the lungs during compression could increase aortic pressure and carotid flow. This is now referred to as simultaneous-ventilation-compression CPR (SVC-CPR). Abdominal binding to prevent diaphragmatic paradoxical motion and thereby increase intrathoracic pressure also increases aortic systolic pressure and carotid blood flow.[6]

The role for SVC-CPR and abdominal binding in the clinical setting is as yet uncertain. What has become clear is that increased pressure in the aorta and increased common carotid blood flow does not mean that cerebral or coronary blood flow has increased or that neurologic recovery will improve. The reasons for this observation are many. The common carotid artery supplies the face and other extracranial vessels in addition to the intracranial contents. The vertebral arterial flow is not accounted for by the measurement of common carotid flow, and these vessels are capable of supplying adequate CBF by themselves in the dog. A third source of CBF, the anterior spinal arteries, is also ignored. In order to demonstrate that CBF has indeed been increased by a modification of CCPR, direct measurement of CBF needs to be made.[35] Increased common carotid blood flow may not result in increased cerebral blood flow for another reason. Rogers et al demonstrated that the increase in intrathoracic pressure in SVC-CPR was attended by dramatic increases in intracranial pressure (ICP).[34] Increases in ICP diminish the cerebral perfusion pressure and may offset the advantage of increased systolic pressure.

A further limitation of CCPR and its modifications is the limited coronary blood flow. Coronary blood flow during CCPR appears to be secondary to the aortic right atrial pressure gradient during relaxation. Maintaining a high diastolic pressure with alpha agonists would be expected to improve coronary perfusion.[33,37,47] Factors which increase intrathoracic pressure prior to compression of the chest might be expected to decrease the pressure gradient between right atrium and aorta, and thereby decrease coronary flow.[51]

The advantage of OCCPR is that an increase of intrathoracic pressure is not required for forward flow. Coronary flow is therefore preserved, and there is no increase in ICP which enhances the cerebral blood flow as well.

While it is clear that the thoracic pump mechanism is responsible for flow in most adult patients, it is less clear what the primary mechanism of flow is in infants and children. Their thinner walled, more compliant chests may allow direct compression of the heart, and might be more analogous to OCCPR than CCPR in the adult. The mechanism of blood flow in CCPR in older children and adolescents is probably similar to CCPR in adults.

The role of abdominal binding, SVC-CPR, and OCCPR is still experimental and needs to be investigated further. Although the following sections follow current recommendations, it can be expected that modifications will be made in the future as some of the exciting research in this area comes to fruition.

Evaluation

When adequate ventilation has been established, the effectiveness of circulation needs to be rapidly evaluated by (1) observing the color of the patient's skin and mucous membranes and (2) palpating for a peripheral pulse. If the patient is cyanotic or ashen in color then the circulation needs to be augmented.

In children, the palpation of an apical pulse is not an adequate assessment of cardiac output and is not recommended. Palpation of a peripheral pulse is considered mandatory. A strong femoral or brachial pulse is evidence that cardiac output is adequate.

Measurement of blood pressure by manual palpation or auscultation is difficult in the arrest situation in infants and children. An automated Doppler or ultrasound device, or a Doppler device coupled with a manually inflated blood pressure cuff may be necessary in order to successfully measure low blood pressure. Although arrhythmias may not be the primary cause of arrest in most children, continuous ECG monitoring is helpful in assessing the development of dysrhythmias.

Management

The absence of peripheral pulses or the continuation of cyanosis despite adequate ventilation signals the need for further management. This can be divided into five phases: (1) initiation of external cardiac compression, (2) establishment of intravenous access, (3) administration of essential life support medications, (4) use of secondary resuscitative drugs, and (5) use of defibrillation.

External cardiac compression

Once the absence of peripheral pulses has been established, external cardiac compression should be initiated to reestablish at least a minimal circulation to the brain and the coronary arteries. Whatever mechanism of external cardiac compression in the pediatric patient is used, the data presented previously indicate that by using the current recommendations many children are salvageable.

Ludwig and Fleisher[23] have summarized six studies published between 1970 and 1985 on outcome from pediatric CPR. They found a wide variety of survival rates in these studies, but the differences probably represent differences in the patient populations (higher survival rates in the two studies with a large number of hospitalized patients), differences in the definitions of arrest employed by the various investigators, and possible differences in postresuscitative care. They propose a standardized format for record-keeping, and standard definitions of outcome that will allow comparison of results between institutions.

The updated standards for pediatric CPR recommend that chest compression in children be over the lower one third of the sternum.[42a] This is a change from the midsternal location. Preliminary data reported by Orlowski[28] favored this approach. This technique resulted in higher mean arterial pressures and stroke volumes. While there is a concern that compression over the lower third of the sternum may be hazardous, in Orlowski's study there were no liver lacerations, but only six patients were autopsied.

In the infant the midsternal location is found by spanning the sternum between the thumb and fifth finger and then judging the midpoint. This should coincide with the point at which the transnipple line intersects the sternum. Two or three fingers should be placed on the sternum, one finger width below the midsternal line.

The depth and rate of compression is based on the age of the child as shown in Table 9.3. Compression should be smooth, continuous, and uninterrupted. Irregular compressions may appear to produce adequate amplitude pressure pulses on a monitor, but the blood flow is unlikely to be optimal. Taylor et al[44] have demonstrated that blood flow is related to the duration of compression. The optimal duration was 60 percent of the compression-release cycle. In fact, changing the compression rate at a constant compression-release ratio does not appear to effect cardiac output.

Because the child has a relatively large occiput, neck extension may elevate the shoulders and upper thorax off of the firm resuscitation surface. This may result in a dead space which will absorb the force of compression unless a firm wedge is used to fill this gap. Placing a towel or the rescuer's hand beneath the upper thorax will prevent the effort of the compression from being dissipated. Compressions may then be applied with two fingers or with one hand in the older child. The technique developed by Thaler and Stobie[45] avoids this problem. When using this technique, the rescuer links his fingers beneath the thoracic spine and compresses with his thumbs. This method is quite comfortable for the rescuer when used on a newborn patient. When used on infants larger than the newborn, care must be taken to avoid encircling the chest and limiting the respiratory expansion of the thorax.

Mechanical chest compressors should not be used in children. Their safety and efficacy in pediatric patients has yet to be established.

Intravenous access

The placement of an intravenous line may be the most frustrating and time consuming aspect of pediatric life support. A central route is preferable whenever possible, but even a small "butterfly" is better than no access at all. However, peripheral sites may be inadequate for rapid delivery of drugs to the central circulation. Intracardiac instillation of medications is dangerous and should be avoided except under extreme circumstances. If an intravenous route can not be rapidly secured, resuscitation medications can be given by routes other than intravascular ones.[27] Atropine, epinephrine, and lidocaine can be given by the intratracheal route.[14] Absorption of intratracheal drugs is excellent, with a rapid onset of action, and a prolonged duration. The drug doses are the same as those recommended for intravenous administration. They should be delivered deep into the lungs followed by a period of hyperinflation. Berg[1] has reviewed the use of the intraosseous route by which most resuscitation drugs can be given by bolus or continuous infusion.

During CPR in the pediatric patient, access to the subclavian vein is both difficult and hazardous. Pneumothorax and hemothorax are frequently associated complications. The two vessels that we have used with the most success are the femoral vein, and the external jugular vein. The femoral vein can be located by palpating the femoral artery and moving just medially to it. In the event that there is no palpable pulsation, then the vein may be located by finding the midpoint between the symphysis pubis and the anterior superior iliac spine. The vein should be approached at a 30 to 45 degree angle to the skin, at a point 2 to 3 cm below the inguinal ligament to avoid entering the peritoneal cavity.

The external jugular vein has the disadvantage that it cannot be used until the airway is secured. It may be located by placing the child in a 20 degree head-down position. With the patient at this angle, the vein will usually fill and be visible as it courses over the sternocleidomastoid muscle. If there is an unsuccessful attempt at cannulating this vessel, a hematoma usually forms, and further attempts are likely to result in failure.

In cannulating either of these vessels we recommend using the Seldinger technique. We use a 22 gauge, thin walled, short bevel needle to introduce a 0.018 inch wire, and then a flexible Teflon or polyurethane catheter. If the Seldinger technique is not successful, then a surgical cutdown should be attempted. The lesser saphenous vein located superior and anterior to the medial malleolus is commonly used. The femoral and brachial vein are also excellent sites for cutdowns. This method is more time consuming and requires more expertise than percutaneous cannulation.

Essential drugs

Essential drugs for advanced life support are oxygen, sodium bicarbonate, epinephrine, atropine, calcium, and glucose. Table 9.4 shows the drug dosages for pediatric patients. Dosage should be based on the patient's weight. As this is usually not known for arrest victims in the emergency department, the weight should be estimated either by experience or by using a growth chart and finding the weight at the 50th percentile for the child's age.

Oxygen The effectiveness of oxygen therapy and ventilation alone at resuscitating a large percentage of pediatric patients emphasizes that in the context of cardiopulmonary arrest, it is an essential drug. Low cardiac output during external cardiac massage will result in high tissue extraction of delivered oxygen and a resultant low venous saturation in blood returning to the heart. Shunting may

Table 9.4. Essential Life Support Drugs

Sodium bicarbonate	1 mEq/kg IV
Epinephrine	10 μg/kg IV or IT*
Atropine	0.01 mg/kg IV or IT (min 0.2 mg)
Calcium chloride	10 mg/kg IV
Calcium gluconate	30 mg/kg IV
Glucose	1.0 g/kg IV

* IT = intratracheal

occur from right to left at the pulmonary or cardiac level. Ventilation perfusion matching may be far from optimal. The result of these factors is hypoxemia.

Any patient who is suspected of having decreased oxygen delivery to the tissues should receive supplemental oxygen. This should be in the form of 100 percent oxygen until the patient has been stabilized, and arterial blood gas analysis demonstrates that lower concentrations will be safe. The issue of oxygen toxicity is inconsequential in the resuscitation setting and should not be of concern.

The physician should be familiar with the capabilities of a variety of delivery systems, and understand their limitations in providing supplemental oxygen. Expired air ventilation can be expected to provide between 17 and 21 percent oxygen. Self-inflating resuscitation bags will provide 21 percent oxygen without a supplemental oxygen source, and when connected to an oxygen source they can deliver between 30 and 60 percent. In order to approach 100 percent oxygen delivery, a reservoir bag or demand valve is necessary. An anesthesia bag will deliver 100 percent oxygen. No matter what system is used, blood gas analysis is needed to document the adequacy of ventilation, acid-base balance, and oxygenation.

Epinephrine Epinephrine is the essential catecholamine for CPR. Its main effect is to ensure an adequate coronary perfusion pressure. The importance of maintaining a coronary perfusion pressure of at least 30 to 40 mmHg was recognized nearly 80 years ago by Crile and Dolley.[9] Redding examined the effectiveness of CPR, CPR with abdominal binding, and CPR with methoxamine in dogs.[33] He found that "there was complete correlation between return of spontaneous circulation and the development of aortic diastolic pressures above 40 mmHg, as well as complete correlation between failure of resuscitation and aortic diastolic pressures below 40 mmHg in all 100 dogs. . . ." Both methoxamine and abdominal compression were effective in elevating the aortic diastolic pressure. Recently, Sanders et al[39] have shown that if the coronary perfusion pressure can be kept above 30 mmHg with large doses of epinephrine, then resuscitation was possible even after 30 minutes of fibrillation. If the coronary perfusion pressure could not be kept above 30 mmHg, then the dogs were not resuscitatable by external massage. In a related study, four of five dogs whose perfusion pressure were less than 30 mmHg after 15 minutes of external massage could be resuscitated with 4 minutes of open massage and defibrillation.[40] None of the dogs who received an additional 4 minutes of closed chest massage could be successfully resuscitated after difibrillation. During open chest massage the aortic diastolic pressures consistently remained above 40 mmHg

Epinephrine has both alpha- and beta-adrenergic effects, but the primary effect is that of vasoconstriction to maintain the coronary perfusion pressure. Otto et al[31] demonstrated that the beta effect of epinephrine was not essential for successful resuscitation in dogs. The animals were randomized to receive phenoxybenzamine, propranolol, both drugs, or no drug prior to a 5 minute asphyxial arrest. All of the animals who received phenoxybenzamine died despite external cardiac massage, ventilation, and epinephrine. Six of eight animals who received propranolol and seven of eight in the control group were successfully resuscitated. Brillman et al[4] have recently confirmed these findings by demonstrating that phenylephrine was as effective as epinephrine in a canine cardiac arrest model. The beta effects of epinephrine may provide vasodilatation of the coronary and the cerebral vasculature and an inotropic and chronotropic effect, but there is no proof that these effects are essential.

The indications for epinephrine include asystole, electromechanical dissociation, and hypotension. It is also used to change a fine fibrillatory pattern to a coarse one prior to defibrillation. Coarse fibrillation is felt to be more easily converted to a sinus rhythm.

The initial dose of epinephrine for asystole or electro-mechanical dissociation is 10 μg/kg IV, or 0.1 ml/kg of a 1:10,000 dilution. Subsequent doses should be determined by the initial response. If there is an inadequate response, the second dose should be doubled to 20 μg/kg. If this is unsuccessful, the dose should be again doubled. This is a safe approach provided that there is no underlying cardiovascular disease. The epinephrine should be administered as a 1:10,000 concentration. The same dose and concentration may be used for intratracheal administration.

There is still a substantial amount that is not known about the use of epinephrine in humans. Even the optimal dosage of epinephrine is uncertain. Kosnik et al[20] have recently investigated the dose response of epinephrine on aortic diastolic pressure in dogs. In their model, increasing the dose of epinephrine did not increase the coronary perfusion pressure compared to a control group, although aortic diastolic pressure was augmented. The use of high dose epinephrine infusion by Jackson et al[18] resulted in higher cerebral blood flow in dogs as compared to CCPR alone. The role of high dose infusion, optimal dosage and interval between doses of epinephrine, and pure alpha agents are all areas of active current research.

For the treatment of hypotension, epinephrine may be given as a bolus starting at a dose of 1.0 μg/kg or as an infusion starting at a dose of 0.02 to 0.05 μg/kg/min and increased to a maximum of 0.5 μg/kg/min. It is preferable to give epinephrine by a central route, but it can be given through a peripheral intravenous route as well.

Epinephrine is a relatively safe drug with few untoward effects seen in the pediatric patient. The main hazard is the production of arrhythmias. Supraventricular or ventricular tachycardias or ventricular fibrillation may be seen. Whenever possible the intracardiac route should be avoided.

Sodium bicarbonate The metabolic consequences of cardiopulmonary arrest are progressive respiratory and metabolic acidosis. Historically, the treatment of the metabolic component of acidosis has been sodium bicarbonate. Bicarbonate works by combining with hydrogen ions to make carbonic acid, and this rapidly leads to the production of carbon dioxide and water.

Acidosis may impair cardiac and circulatory function. It impairs myocardial contractility and may predispose to ventricular arrhythmias. Children are more resistant to the effects of acidosis than adults, and it is unclear at exactly what level of acidosis these dangers occur.

Bicarbonate is indicated for any patient with suspected metabolic acidosis including the patient with several minutes of cardiac arrest. The initial dose of sodium bicarbonate is 1 mEq/kg IV. For children less than 6 months of age this may be given as half strength bicarbonate to avoid acute hyperosmolarity. In children over 6 months of age it is administered as a full strength solution. Subsequent doses may be based on arterial blood gas analysis in order to avoid overcorrection and the consequences of excess administration.

Subsequent dosages can be calculated using the patient's weight in kilograms, and the base deficit calculated from the blood gas.

$$\text{mEq bicarbonate} = \frac{(\text{base deficit} \times \text{weight} \times 0.4)}{2}$$

The bicarbonate distribution space is 40 percent of total body weight and hence the correction factor of 0.4. It is customary to correct by half the calculated deficit to avoid overcorrection.

Bicarbonate therapy is not without hazard.[3] In the context of inadequate ventilation, the administration of bicarbonate may rapidly lead to elevated PCO_2 levels. Since carbon dioxide is readily permeable across cell membranes and bicarbonate is not, the rapid elevation in carbon dioxide level can lead to exacerbation of intracellular acidosis. Clancy et al[7] noted a transient myocardial depression in the intact dog heart following bicarbonate administration, which they attributed to an elevation of intramyocardial PCO_2 and hence, the development of intracellular acidosis. Administration of bicarbonate has also been shown to lead to cerebrospinal fluid acidosis.

Another untoward effect of bicarbonate therapy is the development of the hyperosmolar state. During cardiac arrest, there is a gradual increase in serum osmolarity, and the administration of bicarbonate will add to this trend.[38] Over zealous administration of bicarbonate will lead to a subsequent metabolic alkalosis and hypernatremia. Bicarbonate will also inactivate catecholamines and precipitate calcium salts from solutions. The administration of bicarbonate must be followed by saline flush to prevent these complications. Intratracheal administration causes atelectasis, is irritating to the airways, and destroys surfactant. Its administration should therefore be limited to the intravenous route.

Bishop and Weisfeldt[3] showed that if preexisting acidosis is not present, then ventilation alone can prevent the development of acidosis. The administration of bicarbonate did not substantially alter the outcome of CPR, or elevate the pH. These results were recently confirmed in a canine model by Sanders et al.[38] In dogs that were arrested for 3 minutes prior to the initiation of CPR, ventilation and chest compression alone resulted in normalization of pH for about 18 minutes. The pattern seen was an initial respiratory alkalosis which peaked at 8 minutes and then a gradual decline in pH as the metabolic acidosis became more pronounced.

In summary, because of the potential complications of bicarbonate, its administration should be based on a rational plan. It should not be used without first establishing adequate ventilation. In the experimental model, there is evidence that ventilation alone will correct metabolic acidosis of brief duration. If metabolic acidosis is suspected to be of other than brief duration, bicarbonate should be given without waiting for blood gas analysis, but all susbsequent doses should be based on the laboratory findings.

Atropine Atropine is a parasympatholytic drug that is a competitive antagonist to acetylcholine. It has a peripheral vagolytic effect that results in an increased heart rate. It increases the rate of discharge at the sinoatrial (SA) node and increases the rate of conduction through the artrioventricular (AV) node. It is used to increase the heart rate during bradycardia associated with hypotension or during symptoms of central nervous system or myocardial dysfunction. It is also useful to improve conduction during second- or third-degree heart block. Atrial and ventricular tachyarrhythmias may be seen, and in adults tachycardia can cause myocardial ischemia.

In addition to its vagolytic effects, atropine can stimulate the medullary vagal nucleus. At higher doses, this can lead to restlessness, irritability, and hallucinations. At low doses mild cardiac slowing may be seen. This is not usually observed with rapid intravenous infusion, provided the minimum recommended dosage is administered.

The dose of atropine is 0.01 mg/kg IV. The minimum dose for resuscitation is 0.20 mg, and can be repeated every 5 to 10 minutes to a maximum total dose of 2.0 mg. Atropine may be safely given by the intratracheal route.

Calcium Calcium increases myocardial contractility, ventricular excitability, and conduction velocity within the ventricle. Calcium has previously been recommended for resuscitation when there is asystole or electromechanical dissociation. It is also useful as an inotropic agent.

The dose of calcium and the route of administration depends on the calcium salt used. Calcium chloride must be given into a central vein at an initial dose of 10 mg/kg. Calcium gluconate can be administered into a peripheral vein, but the dosage is three times the chloride dose on a weight basis, or 30 mg/kg. Cote et al[8] have demonstrated that equimolar dosages of calcium gluconate and calcium chloride resulted in equivalent changes in serum-ionized calcium values. The hemodynamic changes were the same regardless of which salt was administered, and there was no advantage of one preparation over the other. Regardless of which form is used, the drug should be given as a slow infusion with continuous heart rate monitoring for the appearance of bradycardia. Rapid infusion can cause arrest in asystole. This may be an untreatable situation. Extra caution should be taken for digitalized patients who are more prone to calcium-induced dysrhythmias. Calcium administration may be repeated, but therapy should be guided by the results of serum-ionized calcium measurements.

Currently, there is a substantial amount of investigation into the role of intracellular calcium and post-ischemic cellular death, and the role of calcium antagonists at preventing this phenomena.[42,43] The new recommendations are therefore to give calcium only when there is documented hypocalcemia, hyperkalemia, hypermagnesemia, or calcium-channel blocker overdosage.[42b]

Glucose Hypoglycemia is a frequent occurrence in the arrested infant and child.

Table 9.5. Useful Life Support Drugs

	Initial Dose	Subsequent Dose
Lidocaine	1 mg/kg IV or IT	10–20 μg/kg/min IV
Bretylium	5 mg/kg IV	10 mg/kg IV
Dopamine	10μg/kg/min IV	
Isoproterenol	0.1 μg/kg/min IV	
Furosemide	1 mg/kg IV	2 mg/kg IV
Naloxone	0.01 mg/kg IV	Repeat
Methylprednisolone	30 mg/kg IV	
Dexamethasone	1 mg/kg IV	
Defibrillation current	2 joules/kg	4 joules/kg

They have limited glycogen stores to convert rapidly to glucose, and these may have been depleted prior to arrest by the underlying precipitating illness. For these reasons, glucose should be considered an essential drug in the pediatric patient. The initial dose of glucose is 1.0 g/kg IV, or 0.25 ml/kg of a 25 percent solution. Hyperglycemia and hyperosmolarity are potential complications, but these should not be of concern with a single dose.

Secondary resuscitation drugs
There are a number of other drugs that are useful and should be available for resuscitations, but these medications are not used commonly during pediatric resuscitation. Ludwig et al[24] examined drug utilization during pediatric CPR. Lidocaine was used in only 3 of 130 resuscitations, and direct current was used in only 4 of the 130. Table 9.5 lists some of the more useful secondary medications, the more important of which will be discussed.

Lidocaine Lidocaine is an amide local anesthetic which has several beneficial effects on the heart. Lidocaine decreases the automaticity of ventricular pacemakers, increases the threshold for fibrillation, and is useful in terminating reentrant ventricular arrhythmias. Ventricular fibrillation is uncommon in pediatric resuscitations, but when it occurs, lidocaine is the drug of choice. The initial dose is 1 mg/kg IV. This dose can be repeated at 5 minute intervals to a total of 3 mg/kg. Lidocaine can be given by the intratracheal route. It necessary, lidocaine can be given as an infusion, with an initial infusion rate of 10 to 20 μg/kg/min.

Lidocaine's adverse reactions are those common to local anesthetics. Usually, central nervous system symptoms appear first, and then in higher doses cardiac toxicity may appear. The initial symptoms are tinnitus, perioral numbness, nausea, vomiting, lethargy, and disorientation. Although at low doses lidocaine is an anticonvulsant, at higher levels seizures and coma can occur. The cardiac symptoms include depression of myocardial contractility and ventricular irritability. At high serum levels there is slowing of atrioventricular and ventricular conductivity with resultant heart block and even asystole.

Lidocaine is metabolized in the liver. Children with hepatic dysfunction because of congestive heart failure or other chronic disease need lidocaine levels monitored to prevent toxicity. The volume of distribution is decreased in patients with congestive heart failure. Because of this, the initial dosage employed for these patients needs to be reduced.

Bretylium In the event that lidocaine and countershock are not successful in terminating ventricular arrhythmias, bretylium tosylate may be employed. Bretylium significantly increases the threshold for ventricular fibrillation by a mechanism that is incompletely understood. Bretylium may be given by the intravenous or intramuscular route in a dose of 5 mg/kg. If fibrillation is not successfully terminated with countershock, then a dose of 10 mg/kg should be administered and defibrillation again attempted. The total dose should not exceed 30 mg/kg.

The most important side effect seen with bretylium administration is hypotension, an effect that is magnified by standing. Hypotension is secondary to bretylium's inhibition of norepinephrine release. Nausea and vomiting are also common untoward effects of bretylium administration and should be anticipated by the resuscitative team.

Dopamine Dopamine is a catecholamine which has alpha- and beta-adrenergic effects. It is unique among currently available catecholamines because of its action on dopaminergic receptors, effects which increase renal and mesenteric blood flow. These effects occur at low dosages between 2 and 10 μg/kg/min. At higher dosages the alpha effects may begin to offset the increase in renal blood flow. The cardiac effects of dopamine include a positive inotropic and chronotropic effect. This is due to dopamine's action at beta-1 receptors and release of norepinephrine from nerve terminals. At low dosages dopamine will have minimal effect on peripheral vasculature. At intermediate dosages between 5 and 20 μg/kg/min, there is progressively more beta-adrenergic effect, with an increase in contractility, stroke volume, and cardiac output. As the dosage is increased, peripheral alpha effects cause vasoconstriction. The increase in cardiac output coupled with the increase in peripheral resistance results in an increase in blood pressure. At doses above 20 μg/kg/min the alpha effects predominate, and there is marked vasoconstriction, not only peripherally, but in the renal and mesenteric beds as well.

Dopamine is not useful during initial resuscitative efforts in the arrested patient. It is indicated for the patient with hypotension unresponsive to adequate volume replacement or in situations where blood pressure support is needed while volume replacement is being infused.

Dopamine has a very short half-life which allows its effects to be closely titrated. It may cause hypertension, arrhythmias, nausea, vomiting, and vasoconstriction. Blood pressure should be closely monitored during administration as should urine output. In the shock state, excessive renal vasoconstriction can readily lead to impairment in renal function.

Defibrillation

As mentioned previously, ventricular fibrillation is not common in pediatric patients. Because fibrillation is uncommon, ECG confirmation should be obtained prior to attempted coutershock. The precordial thump is not recommended in the pediatric age range.

Defibrillation works by producing a mass depolarization of myocardial cells with the hope that spontaneous sinus rhythm will resume. Termination of ventricular fibrillation will be more successful if hypoxia and acidosis are corrected before defibrillation is attempted. If the arrest was unobserved, or if a prolonged interval of diminished perfusion has elapsed, then sodium bicarbonate should be administered, and the patient ventilated with 100 percent oxygen. Fine fibrillation is more difficult to convert to sinus rhythm, and epinephrine should be administered in an attempt to convert to a coarse fibrillation pattern.

Standard adult defibrillator paddles are 8 cm in diameter. These may not be appropriate for all pediatric patients, and pediatric paddles, which are 4.5 cm in diameter, should also be available. The paddles should make complete and uniform contact with the chest wall. The electrodes need to be carefully placed on the small chest to prevent electrical bridging and possible skin burns.

There are two acceptable placements for the electrodes. An AP placement is considered acceptable, but is awkward and often impractical. The more common method is to place one electrode to the right of the sternum below the clavicle, and to place the second electrode in the left midclavicular line at the level of the xyphoid. Firm pressure should be applied to ensure uniform contact with the skin, and no personnel should have contact with either the bed or the patient.

The recommended dose of current for defibrillation is 2 joules/kg.[15] If the first defibrillation attempt is not successful, the dose of current should be doubled to 4 joules/kg. If a third attempted at defibrillation is needed, the dose is again doubled to 8 joules/kg.

Myocardial injury may occur from excessive current or the use of multiple defibrillation attempts delivered within a brief time span. To prevent this, careful attention should be paid to the power output setting of the defibrillator unit. Proper paddle placement and the use of saline-soaked gauze sponges or electrode paste will minimize the incidence of skin burns.

Calcium antagonists

There is currently controversy about the role calcium antagonists have following cardiac arrest.[48] Ongoing research indicates that the intracellular calcium accumulation in vascular smooth muscle and neurons may be partly responsible for neuronal death following an ischemic anoxic insult. The role of calcium blockers in cerebral resuscitation has recently been reviewed by White et al,[49] and Shapiro.[42] Calcium-mediated vasospasm may cause diminished regional cerebral blood flow and cause a postarrest progressive hypoperfusion state (no reflow phenomenon).[48,49] In cat and monkey anoxic brain preparations, Hossman and Kleihues[16] found that neuronal function could be restored after up to 60 minutes of ischemic anoxia. This led to the conclusion that neuronal death may not occur during a 4 or 5 minute ischemic event or even shortly thereafter, but by events that occur after the arrest. These observations have lead to the use of calcium antagonists to try and prevent the no reflow phenomenon, and the additional cellular injury that occurs after resuscitation.

Experimentally, flunarazine, lidoflazine, verapamil, and $MgSO_4$ have been shown to maintain cerebral blood flow and cerebral oxygen consumption after a 20 minute arrest in dogs.[48,50] All of these drugs have calcium antagonist properties. A recent study by Steen et al[43] demonstrated that nimodipine, when given 5 minutes following a 17 minute complete cerebral ischemic arrest, dramatically improved neurologic outcome 96 hours postresuscitation in a primate model. While all of these reports are encouraging, problems remain. First, each of the calcium antagonists has slightly different properties and it is not clear which agent is likely to be the most beneficial. Second, the experience with barbiturates and cerebral resuscitation dictates that clinical studies in humans should be approached cautiously, and only after adequate experience with animals. Third, the calcium antagonists have negative inotropic effects, and whether their use will negatively affect the ability to resuscitate the heart during a cardiac arrest remains to be seen. At the current time, it is too early to recommend the use of these drugs following cardiac arrest. Shapiro's admonition that "one should not forget that rapid restoration and maintenance of normal cerebral perfusion pressure and tissue oxygenation remains the mainstay of post-cardiac-arrest neuroresuscitative therapy" best sums up the state of the art.[42]

DISCONTINUATION OF CPR

Discontinuation of life support is largely determined by whether or not the cardiovascular system can be supported without external or internal cardiac massage. If cardiac function cannot be maintained without cardiac massage despite technologic and pharmacologic support, then CPR should be discontinued. Ventilatory support is technically more readily accomplished, and the need for controlled ventilation should not be a determining factor in terminating life support, while it is difficult to establish fixed criteria for cessation of chest massage. Pre-existent illness, arrest time prior to initiation of CPR, and length of the resuscitative effort are some of the contributing factors.

Brain death is becoming a widely accepted criterion for terminating mechanical life support. Brain death remains a clinical diagnosis that requires a series of observations with an interval of time between examinations. These observations are best made in the intensive care unit, and with supportive laboratory studies such as the electroencephalogram, cerebral angiography, and brain scans to confirm the absence of cerebral metabolic activity or blood flow. We have seen drug overdose, infant botulism, and postictal depression misdiagnosed as brain death in the emergency department, and we are therefore reluctant to make this diagnosis in that setting.

In the final analysis, the decision to terminate CPR should be the responsibility and judgment of the senior physician attending to the child.

REFERENCES

1. Berg RA 1984 Emergency infusion of catecholamines into bone marrow in children. American Journal of Diseases of Children 138: 810
2. Bircher N, Safar P 1985 Cerebral preservation during cardipulmonary resuscitation. Critical Care Medicine 13: 185
3. Bishop RL, Weisfeldt ML 1976 Sodium bicarbonate administration during cardiac arrest. Effect on arterial pH, PCO_2, and osmolality. Journal of the American Medical Association 235: 506
4. Brillman JC, Sanders AB, Otto CW, Rahmy H, Bragg S, Ewy GA 1985 Comparison of epinephrine and phenylephrine for resuscitation and neurologic outcome of cardiac arrest in animals. Annals of Emergency Medicine 14: 495
5. Cary JM, Ross BK, Krugmire R, Newman BH, Butler J 1978 Coughing causes systemic blood flow. Chest 74: 332
6. Chandra Nisha, Snyder LD, Weisfeldt ML 1981 Abdominal binding during cardiopulmonary resuscitation in man. Journal of the American Medical Association 246: 351

7. Clancy RL, Cingolani HE, Taylor RR, Graham TP, Gilmore JP 1967 Influence of sodium bicarbonate on myocardial performance. American Journal of Physiology 212: 917
8. Cote CJ, Daniels AL, Drop LJ 1984 Comparative hemodynamic and ionized calcium effects of calcium gluconate and calcium chloride. Anesthesiology 61: A422
9. Crile G, Dolley DT 1906 Experimental research into resuscitation of dogs killed by anesthetics and asphyxia. The Journal of Experimental Medicine 8: 713
10. Criley JM, Blaufuss AH, Kissel GL 1976 Cough-induced cardiac compression. Self-administered form of cardiopulmonary resuscitation. Journal of the American Medical Association 236: 1246
11. Cummins RO, Eisenberg MS 1985 Prehospital cardiopulmonary resuscitation. Is it effective? Journal of the American Medical Association 253: 2408
12. Del Guercio LRM, Eins NR, Cohn JD, Coomaraswamy RP, Wollman SB, State D 1965 Comparison of blood flow during external and internal cardiac massage in man. Circulation 31(suppl. I): 171
13. Eckenhoff JE 1951 Some anatomic considerations of the infant larynx influencing endotracheal anesthesia. Anesthesiology 12: 401
14. Greenberg MI, Roberts J, Baskin SI, Wagnenr DK 1980 The use of endotracheal medication for cardiac arrest. In: Budassi SA, Bander JJ, Kimmerle L, Eie KR (eds) Cardiac Arrest and CPR Aspen Systems Corporation, Rockville, MD
15. Gutgesell HP, Tacker WA, Geddes LA, Davis JS, Lie JT, McNamara DG 1976 Energy dose for ventricular defibrillation in children. Pediatrics 58: 898
16. Hossmann KA, Kleihues P 1973 Reversibility of ischemic brain damage. Archives of Neurology 29: 375
17. Iseri LT, Humphrey SB, Siner EF 1978 Prehospital brady-asystolic cardiac arrest. Annals of Internal Medicine 88: 741
18. Jackson RE, Joyce K, Danosi SF, White BC, Vigor D, Hoehner TJ 1984 Blood flow in the cerebral cortex during cardiac resuscitation in dogs. Annals of Emergency Medicine 13: 657
19. Kettrick RG, Ludwig S 1983 Resuscitation—pediatric basic and advanced life support. In: Fleisher GR, Ludwig S, Henretig FH, Ruddy R, Silverman BK, Templeton JM (eds) Textbook of Pediatric Emergency Medicine, Williams & Wilkins, Baltimore
20. Kosnik JW, Jackson RE, Keats S, Tworek RM, Freeman SB 1985 Dose-related response of centrally administered epinephrine on the change in aortic diastolic pressure during closed-chest massage in dogs. Annals of Emergency Medicine 14: 204
21. Kouwenhoven WB, Ing D, Jude JR 1960 Closed-chest cardiac massage. Journal of the American Medical Association 173: 1064
22. Luce JM, Cary JM, Ross BK, Culver BH, Butler J 1980 New developments in cardiopulmonary resuscitation. Journal of the American Medical Association 244: 1366
23. Ludwig S, Fleisher G 1985 Pediatric cardiopulmonary resuscitation: a review and a proposal. Pediatric Emergency Care 1: 40
24. Ludwig S, Kettrick RG, Parker M 1984 Pediatric cardiopulmonary resuscitation: a review of 130 cases. Clinical Pediatrics 23:71
25. Myerberg RJ, Conde CA, Sung RJ, Mayorga-Cortes A, Mallon SM, Sheps DS, Appel RA, Castellanos A 1980 Clinical electrophysiologic and hemodynamic profile of patients resuscitated from prehospital cardiac arrest. American Journal of Medicine 68: 568
26. Nichols DG, Kettrick RG, Swedlow DB, Lee S, Passman R, Ludwig S 1986 Factors influencing outcome of cardiopulmonary arrest in children. Pediatric Emergency Care 2: 1
27. Orlowski JP 1984 My kingdom for an intravenous line. American Journal of Diseases of Children 138: 803
28. Orlowski JP 1984 Optimal position for external cardiac massage in infants and children. Critical Care Medicine 12: 224
29. Orlowski JP 1983 Pediatric cardiopulmonary resuscitation. Emergency Medicine Clinic of North America 1: 3
30. O'Rourke PP 1986 Outcome of children who are apneic and pulseless in the emergency room. Critical Care Medicine 14: 466
31. Otto CW, Yakaitis RW, Blitt CD 1981 Mechanism of action of epinephrine in resuscitation from asphyxial arrest. Critical Care Medicine 9: 321
32. Palme C, Nystrom B. Tunell R 1985 An evaluation of the efficiency of face masks in the resuscitation of newborn infants. Lancet 1: 207
33. Redding JS 1971 Abdominal compression in cardiopulmonary resuscitation. Anesthesia and Analgesia 50: 668
34. Rogers MC, Nugent SK, Stidham GL 1979 Effects of closed-chest cardiac massage on intracranial pressure. Critical Care Medicine 7: 454

35. Rogers MC, Weisfeldt ML, Traystan RJ 1981 Cerebral blood flow during cardiopulmonary resuscitation. Anesthesia and Analgesia 60: 73
36. Rudikoff MT, Maughan WL, Effron M, Freund P, Weisfeldt ML 1980 Mechanisms of blood flow during cardiopulmonary resuscitation. Circulation 61: 345
37. Sanders AB, Ewy GA, Taft TV 1984 Prognostic and therapeutic importance of the aortic diastolic pressure in resuscitation from cardiac arrest. Critical Care Medicine 12: 871
38. Sanders AB, Ewy GA, Taft TV 1984 Resuscitation and arterial blood gas abnormalities during prolonged cardiopulmonary resuscitation. Annals of Emergency Medicine 13: 676
39. Sanders AB, Ewy GA, Taft TV 1983 The importance of aortic diastolic pressure during cardiopulmonary resuscitation. Journal of the American College of Cardiology 1: 609
40. Sanders AB, Kern KB, Ewy GA, Bailey L 1984 Improved resuscitation from cardiac arrest with open-chest massage. Annals of Emergency Medicine 13: 672
41. Sanders AB, Meislin HW, Ewy GA 1984 The physiology of cardiopulmonary resuscitation. An update. Journal of the American Medical Association 252: 3283
42. Shapiro H 1985 Post-cardiac arrest therapy: calcium entry blockade and brain resuscitation. Anesthesiology 62: 384
42a. Standards and Guidelines for Cardiopulmonary Resuscitation (CPR) and Emergency Cardiac Care (ECC). Part IV: Pediatric Basic Life Support. Journal of the American Medical Association 255: 2954, 1986
42b. Standards and Guidelines for Cardiopulmonary Resuscitation (CPR) and Emergency Cardiac Care (ECC). Part V: Pediatric Advanced Life Support. Journal of the American Medical Association 255: 2961
43. Steen PA, Gisvold SE, Milde JH, Newberg LA, Scheithauer BW, Lanier WL, Michenfelder JD 1985 Nimodipine improves outcome when given after complete cerebral ischemia in primates. Anesthesiology 62: 406
44. Taylor GJ, Tucker WM, Greene HL, Rudikoff MT, Weisfeldt ML 1977 Importance of prolonged compression during cardiopulmonary resuscitation in man. New England Journal of Medicine 296: 1515
45. Thaler MM, Stobie GHC 1963 An improved technique of external cardiac compression in infants and young children. New England Journal of Medicine 269: 606
46. Walsh CK, Krongrad E 1983 Terminal cardiac electrical activity in pediatric patients. American Journal of Cardiology 51: 557
47. Weale FE, Rothwell-Jackson RL 1962 The efficiency of cardiac massage. Lancet 1: 990
48. White BC, Winegar CD, Wilson RF, Hoehner PJ, Trombley JH 1983 Possible role of calcium blockers in cerebral resuscitation: a review of the literature and synthesis for future studies. Critical Care Medicine 11: 202
49. White BC, Winegar CD, Wilson RF, Krause GS 1983 Calcium blockers in cerebral resuscitation. Journal of Trauma 23: 788
50. Winegar CP, Henderson O, White BC, Jackson RE, O'Hara T, Krause GS, Vigor DN, Kontry R, Wilson W, Shelby-Lane C 1983 Early amelioration of neurologic deficit by lidoflazine after fifteen minutes of cardiopulmonary arrest in dogs. Annals of Emergency Medicine 14: 471
51. Wise RA, Summer WR 1983 Pulmonary mechanics and artificial support of the arrested circulation. Clinics in Chest Medicine 4: 189

Index

Page numbers followed by *f* indicate figures; numbers followed by *t* indicate tables